THE CHILD AND DEATH

It was a brisk, sharp January, just nine years ago.
I was six years old, but not too young to know
what piece of my life had been torn from the whole
by this tragedy which would torment my soul.
Still, I giggled when first told the news;
It had to be a trick, a thoughtless ruse!
But in a few lonely days I learned to lose.
It had happened—and that was how life had to be,
Yet I cried for days, for I believed that he
had died not of illness, but of me.

JORDAN WASSERTHEIL SMOLLER

THE CHILD AND DEATH

Edited by

OLLE JANE Z. SAHLER, M.D.

Assistant Professor, Pediatrics and Psychiatry,
University of Rochester,
School of Medicine and Dentistry,
Rochester, New York

THE C. V. MOSBY COMPANY

Saint Louis   1978

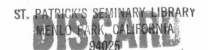

Copyright © 1978 by The C. V. Mosby Company

All rights reserved. No part of this book may be reproduced
in any manner without written permission of the publisher.

Printed in the United States of America

The C. V. Mosby Company
11830 Westline Industrial Drive, St. Louis, Missouri 63141

Library of Congress Cataloging in Publication Data

Main entry under title:

The Child and death.

Bibliography: p.
Includes index.
1. Terminally ill children—Psychology—Congresses.
2. Terminally ill children—Family relationships—
Congresses. 3. Children and death—Congresses.
I. Sahler, Olle Jane Z., 1944-
RJ47.5.C44   362.7'8'19607   78-18239
ISBN 0-8016-4288-4

C/M/M   9 8 7 6 5 4 3 2 1

CONTRIBUTORS

BRUCE H. AXELROD, M.D.

Assistant Professor of Psychiatry and Mental Health Sciences and Assistant Professor of Pediatrics, Medical College of Wisconsin, Milwaukee, Wisconsin

PATRICIA A. BALON, R.N.

Pediatric Nurse, Strong Memorial Hospital, University of Rochester, Rochester, New York

MARION J. BARNES, M.S.S.

Assistant Professor of Child Therapy, Division of Child Psychiatry, Case Western Reserve School of Medicine; Child Therapist, Hanna Perkins Therapeutic Nursery School and Kindergarten, Cleveland, Ohio

JoANN BELLE-ISLE, R.N., M.S.N.

Assistant Professor of Nursing and Clinician II, University of Rochester School of Nursing, Rochester, New York

SISTER MARY FRANCES LORETTA BERGER, B.V.M.

Librarian, Mundelein College, Chicago, Illinois

ALBERT C. CAIN, Ph.D.

Professor, Department of Psychology, University of Michigan, Ann Arbor, Michigan

BARBARA CONRADT, M.S.W.

Social Worker in Pediatrics and Hematology/Oncology, University of Rochester Medical Center, Rochester, New York

STANFORD B. FRIEDMAN, M.D.

Professor of Psychiatry and Human Behavior, Professor of Pediatrics, Director, Division of Child and Adolescent Psychiatry, and Head, Behavioral Pediatrics, Department of Psychiatry, University of Maryland School of Medicine, Baltimore, Maryland; President, National Sudden Infant Death Syndrome Foundation, Chicago, Illinois

PATRICIA E. GREENE, R.N., M.S.N.

Clinical Nurse Specialist, Pediatric Oncology, North Carolina Memorial Hospital, Chapel Hill, North Carolina

ROSE GROBSTEIN, R.S.W.

Chief Pediatric Social Worker and Lecturer, Department of Family, Community, and Preventive Medicine, Stanford University Medical Center, Stanford, California

JULIA HAMILTON, M.S.W.

Clinical Instructor (Social Work), Department of Pediatrics, Yale–New Haven Hospital, New Haven, Connecticut

JOAN E. HEMENWAY, M. Div.

Chaplain Supervisor, Presbyterian–University of Pennsylvania Medical Center; Associate Minister, First United Methodist Church of Germantown, Philadelphia, Pennsylvania

SHARON L. HOSTLER, M.D.

Associate Professor, Department of Pediatrics, University of Virginia School of Medicine; Pediatric Director, Children's Rehabilitation Center, University of Virginia Hospital, Charlottesville, Virginia

J. ALBIN JACKMAN, B.S., C.M.S.

Director of Family Services, Harry J. Will Funeral Homes, Inc., Detroit, Michigan

LORETTA KOPELMAN, Ph.D.

Associate Professor of Philosophy and Medicine, Department of Pediatrics, East Carolina School of Medicine, Greenville, North Carolina

HAL LIPTON, M.S.W.

Director, Department of Social Work, Children's Hospital National Medical Center, Washington, D.C.

IDA M. MARTINSON, R.N., Ph.D.

Professor of Nursing and Director of Research, School of Nursing, University of Minnesota, Minneapolis, Minnesota

STEPHEN W. MUNSON, M.D.

Assistant Professor, Departments of Psychiatry and Pediatrics, University of Rochester School of Medicine and Dentistry, Rochester, New York

JEFFREY D. REYNOLDS, M.S.Ed.

Special Education Teacher, Jefferson High School, Rochester City School District, Rochester, New York

BETTY B. SATTERWHITE, M.A.

Instructor in Pediatrics and Executive Director, Child Health Advisory Group to the Department of Pediatrics,
University of Rochester School of Medicine and Dentistry,
Rochester, New York

JOHN E. SCHOWALTER, M.D.

Professor of Pediatrics and Psychiatry and Director
of Training, Yale University Child Study Center,
New Haven, Connecticut

JOHN J. SPINETTA, Ph.D.

Associate Professor, Department of Psychology, San Diego State University, San Diego, California

CAROLYN SZYBIST, R.N.

Executive Director, National Sudden Infant Death Syndrome Foundation, Chicago, Illinois

LORRAINE ANNE SZYBIST

Student, Regina Dominican High School, Wilmette, Illinois

DORIS S. THORNTON, M.S.W.

Assistant Professor and Counseling Coordinator, Central Maryland SIDS Center, Division of Child and Adolescent Psychiatry, Department of Psychiatry, University of Maryland School of Medicine, Baltimore, Maryland

PHILIP L. TOWNES, M.D., Ph.D.

Professor of Anatomy, Genetics, and Pediatrics, Division of Genetics, University of Rochester School of Medicine and Dentistry, Rochester, New York

PETER H. VILES, M.D.

Associate Professor, Department of Pediatrics, University of Massachusetts School of Medicine, Worcester, Massachusetts

MORRIS A. WESSEL, M.D.

Clinical Professor of Pediatrics, Department of Pediatrics, Yale University Medical Center; Practicing Pediatrician; Board Member, Hospice, Inc., New Haven, Connecticut

SUSAN F. WOOLSEY, R.N., M.S.

Assistant Professor and Educational Coordinator, Central Maryland SIDS Center, Division of Child and Adolescent Psychiatry, Department of Psychiatry, University of Maryland School of Medicine, Baltimore, Maryland

PREFACE

In mid-September, 1977, many of us represented by this book gathered at the University of Rochester Medical Center for a 2½ day symposium: "The Child and Death." For all those hours we, and more than a hundred others from many places and representing many disciplines, discussed, debated, challenged, and supported one another as we attempted to sort out data, clinical impressions, and personal experiences. As we struggled with our own feelings as caregivers—and some as parents—of the fatally ill child, we learned that, just as important, we are also the comforters and teachers of those who are the siblings or children or friends of someone who has died.

This compendium covers more than we could possibly have dealt with in that relatively short period of time, for it also contains the thoughts and feelings of some who could not join us then, but who agreed to add their considerations and deliberations to ours in the context of this book.

The unique thing about this book is the tremendous amount of personal sharing that many of the authors have included in their presentations, as well as the critical review to which they have subjected their particular biases. The overall impression is that there are, fortunately or unfortunately, no absolutes; instead, each individual must learn to understand the child and his family, to resolve personal issues, and to continuously support himself and those around him as each strives to find his or her own most comfortable place within the framework of coping with death.

My thanks to the contributors are incalculable.

In addition, I am indebted to Dr. David H. Smith, Chairman of the Department of Pediatrics, who eagerly provided sponsorship for the symposium and encouragement in editing this collection.

I am grateful, too, to Lyn Neary, who always maintained incredible equanimity despite all the rigors and frustrations of manuscript preparation.

To acknowledge my own family seemed almost superfluous until I realized that too often I do not actually and publicly express the thanks that I feel. And so, to Chip, who listened patiently, advised, and supported; to Brian, who taught me that toddlers can be very wise; and to Catherine, who was an integral part of me throughout the preparation of this book, arriving almost simultaneously with the galley proofs: thank you.

OLLE JANE Z. SAHLER

CONTENTS

INTRODUCTION

OLLE JANE Z. SAHLER

One of the most profound and far-reaching changes to occur in our society in recent years has been the tremendous increase in our ability to postpone, almost indefinitely in some cases, the cessation of life. What has come out of this awesome power is a new awareness of death.

It has not been to the particular credit of modern medicine that death education, the concept of death with dignity, and Right to Die legislation have, for the most part, arisen only in response to the openly and repeatedly stated needs and desires of the lay public. However, there is some consolation in the fact that, once challenged, medicine has been able to respond, meaningfully and self-critically, to the demands of those who seek better answers to the many questions that surround death. It is also understandable that the fields of nursing, social work, education, religion, ethics, economics, and law, among others, have had to join medicine in attempting to provide reasoned answers.

Despite this new openness about death in our culture, children, as a group, are precluded from expressing themselves in an organized fashion. Thus, their needs become known only by inference and only to those who go to particular trouble to discover what those needs are, for almost never are they explicit.

One of the fascinating things about children is the naive, simplistic way in which they approach the unknown. Yet it is this very naiveté that makes their questions the most difficult to answer. They usually have no prior experience on which to base their reactions, and so their earliest grief and mourning is unique to each of them, often outside the confines of socially dictated rituals of which they are ignorant. Their grief, instead, centers around the familiar: themselves, their families and friends, their daily routines. They seek comfort and acknowledgment of their own intrinsic worth.

Despite all the research that has been done on the child's concept of death, we still do not have an adequate understanding of the responses of children under 4. This shortcoming reflects the research tools that have thus far been devised, almost all of which depend heavily on verbal expression or picture drawing—impossible tasks for the infant and toddler. Behavioral observations, more appropriate to this age group, on the other hand, cannot be as carefully controlled or as easily quantitated and systematized. Yet there is great need to look more carefully at the dynamics of the very young and their families to gain better insight and by it, offer more substantial direction and consolation to the child, the family, and ourselves. Marion Barnes' careful observations in Chapter 16 offer a first step in interpreting the behavior of these children, and we learn that children under 4 are more aware and more affected by bereavement than we have speculated, although abstraction, on which we formulate norms, is not within their repertoire.

Sister Berger's comprehensive bibliography, which includes a number of books that are suitable for even the very young, offers another possible vehicle for work with children in the late toddler to early preschool age range, although here again, there is heavy reliance on verbal expression and understanding. As a general statement, however, I would like to underline one of her major tenets: the reader, even if a young child, should be allowed great flexibility in choice of books, even if, at first glance, the parent or teacher feels that the content may not be suitable. Thus is realized the intent of bibliotherapy: a working out of an emotional response to a situation, ideally in conjunction with support, guidance, and explanation from a trusted adult.

Rather than thinking, however, that the reactions of children are specific only to them, I venture that their questionings and misconceptions and feelings of guilt and magical omnipotence are pervasive throughout all ages. The major difference between a child and an adult is that the adult can usually subjugate these feelings to some higher order of thought or relegate them to the unconscious until some loss, devastating in its impact on the individual and his defenses, loosens the tight bonds that hold these forces at bay. A prime example of this adult regression to early childhood thinking is the "if only . . ." phenomenon seen, for instance, among the parents of a fatally ill child. Even when all that is rational argues emphatically that there is no, and never could have been any, "if only . . . ," this rationality gains no foothold with the parent, just as it is a fruitless argument with the child. Distance in time for the parent—perhaps—and greater maturity for the child—usually—are the only paths to eventual resolution.

Thus, the principles that apply to understanding the child's developing concept of death, managing his acute or chronic grief, helping his family, and recognizing the role of formal and informal education about death are not restricted only to the child or adolescent. Rather, they transcend all age groups, even the very old.

Throughout the following writings, some have noted the caregiver's or teacher's need to come to some realization about his own immortality before effective work with the dying can take place. My own bias probably most closely parallels that of Hal Lipton in Chapter 4, who states that this has been, for him, an impossible task. Rather, his obligation to his clients, as he sees it, is to help them sort out their feelings about dying by being an available, responsive, but nondirective sounding board for their individual deliberations. This seems to me to be the most realistic goal of any caregiver.

However, from another vantage, I am personally also a member of the team that has struggled long hours to save a life. I have experienced the exhilaration of success and the despair of failure—the most agonizing part of which is facing the family and admitting defeat. There is, undeniably, a feeling of self-incompetence, most jarring because it is usually so well hidden by complacency. I am reassured by the reflections of Peter Viles (Chapter 12) that I am not alone, and perhaps we are both reassured by John Schowalter and Bruce Axelrod (Chapters 10 and 11), who tell us that not only are we not alone, but there are many in our cohort.

Members of many different disciplines—nursing, social work, the ministry—emphasize repeatedly that work among the fatally ill is a lonely experience, sometimes very rewarding but sometimes not. When it is rewarding, we derive our support and incentive to continue from the gratitude of those we have helped. Unfortunately, that kind of gratitude is not often forthcoming when we are most vulnerable, when we perceive ourselves as having failed.

It should be noted that occasionally we rely too heavily on patients and their families to provide incentive for continued caregiving without really understanding or accepting their needs as paramount to our own. For example, we may be "turned off" by the adolescent who does not and will not share his or her deepest feelings with us, even though we accept intellectually that he or she may not need to do so because of a particular personality style or because of the presence of another support system for this kind of ventilation. We are sometimes provoked to anger when a patient becomes angry or noncompliant, morose, thankless, or withdrawn. We are personally affronted—a natural response—rather than understanding when individuals or families have no more to give, when their grief is so overwhelming that social niceties and facades are no longer tenable. Yet for the caregiver who feels deeply and who has seen himself as an emotionally supportive partner, such withdrawal is perceived as a rejection rather than as a reminder of the tremendously forceful egocentrism of profound grief: the cry, "Leave me alone. How can you possibly know my pain?"

Where do we turn? Most say that we do not turn to our peers, because admitting the need for reassurance too precisely delineates our fallibilities among the very group with which we are in constant explicit or implicit competition. We go instead to someone who is enough removed from our battles to maintain an undercurrent of admiration for us and our work no matter what the specific crisis or perceived shortcoming: to a spouse who, whether in the same field or not, can give love and understanding by virtue of the nature of the marital bond; to a professional of another discipline who "could never do the wonderful things you do"; to a confidante, a confessor, a teacher.

Lest the reader walk away with the sense that those who work with the dying or who teach or counsel about death revel in their own masochism, let me point out that the rewards are many and they are real. From those children and families whom we help, we derive a tremendous sense of fulfillment. From those innovative changes that we are able to make in the health care and educational systems that benefit society at large, we derive great personal satisfaction and public respect. From those delvings into our own minds, those struggles to comprehend what may, in effect, be incomprehensible, and from those wounds that are eventually healed, we derive a sense of ourselves, perhaps in a slightly larger context than we might otherwise have achieved.

Despite all of this, however, the battle is never completely over. It goes on through other deaths where, although the reactions of the dying and the survivors might be predictable, they are still heart-rending in their initial intensity and persistently throbbing in their chronicity. Just as no death is ever entirely erased from the memory of the caregiver who struggled to forestall it, so it is remembered all the more by the family and friends who remain, bereaved, for the rest of their lives. To "get over" a death means to be able to function adequately and appropriately despite its having happened; it does not mean to forget.

CHAPTER 1

The development of the child's concept of death

SHARON L. HOSTLER

A child growing up in America today no longer experiences many aspects of the life cycle. Grandparents live in retirement communities and nursing homes. Relatives die at the hospital or elsewhere. The media present society's image as the Pepsi generation, full of vim, vigor, and vitality. Teeth that gleam. Bodies that glow. Breath that is inviting. Death is a dirty word. This void becomes artificially filled by a death education curriculum for nursery schools and a thanatology course for high schools. A child puzzles over a graveyard. A child psychiatrist is asked to consult when a grandmother dies. A medical student views his first dead person in the anatomy lab.

Children in the eighteenth and nineteenth centuries were included in many aspects of living and dying. Siblings and relatives were born at home and died at home. Death was very much a part of the child's experiences. *The Divine and Moral Songs for Children* (1715) predicted deadly unpleasantness for disobedient children: "The ravens shall pick out his eyes and eagles eat the same." *The Children's Friend* (1830's) warned its young readers to prepare for death during an epidemic of "hooping cough."[26] Today, however, we seem determined to conspire to maintain the fantasy of a joyful childhood where there is no sorrow. We forget the many real and imaginary losses a child encounters each day in his normal development. We gather at conferences to discuss when and what to tell a child about death. We talk with great enlightenment of caring for the dying child in the security of his own home. And we concern ourselves increasingly with the dying child and forget the living ones.[25]

How can we as health care professionals help children for whom death becomes a concern (Fig. 1)? We can begin by understanding that the development of the concept of death is a gradual process that is influenced by many factors within the child's cultural and familial environment, as well as by his own unique psychologic and cognitive patterns.

The objective of this chapter then is to delineate the development of the child's death concept, recognizing its dependence on the sequences of his psychosocial and cognitive skills. The format will be the arbitrary division of childhood into: (1) early childhood, including the infant, tod-

1

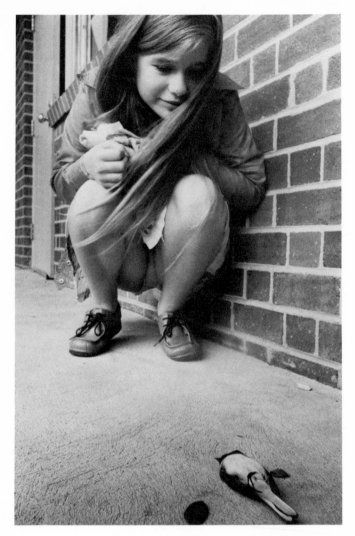

FIG. 1
Death is an integral part of the life of a child. (Photo courtesy Dan Grogan.)

dler, and preschooler; (2) middle childhood, including the primary school–aged child; and (3) adolescence. Within each grouping will be a discussion of the child's general psychosocial development, the specific peculiarities of his thinking according to Piagetian theory, the evolution of the child's death concept, and some selected clinical examples. It will become readily apparent that much of our current thinking about the child's death concept is speculative and that the literature is incomplete. Developmental sequences rather than absolute ages will be presented in an attempt to remind the reader of the extreme variability that exists in the normal population.

EARLY CHILDHOOD
Psychosocial staging

The infant in his first year is involved in differentiating himself from his environment and his caregiver, typically his mother.[10] Before 6 months, he is not aware of his boundaries. From the parent-infant bonding shortly after birth on, he is developing with his mother the primary relationship on which all future relationships will be based. From the successful meeting of his physical and emotional needs is built a sense of trust.[4] In the second half of his first year, he clearly distinguishes mother from others and manifests stranger anxiety when separated from mother or his primary caregiver. By 12 months, the child is no longer reflexively responsive to his environment but is busily exploring the world with his recently acquired gross and fine motor skills. He has a few meaningful words and is finger feeding.

The toddler no longer depends totally on his caregiver; by 2 years, he has a vocabulary of 300 words, exhibits some dressing skills, and is capable of parallel play. This is his period of increasing autonomy;[4] he is taking his very first steps in the process of separation and individuation, which will not be completed until late adolescence. Toilet training is symbolic of his increasing self-control and socialization, the prerequisite for acceptability in the neighborhood play group and nursery school. The accomplishment of toilet training may be viewed from the analytic standpoint as the resolution of the conflict between self-love and parent love. Resolution in favor of parent love, that is, the accomplishment of the expected body control, is the child's only way to maintain self-love. The rages of the terrible twos and threes probably represent the conflict in behavior between pleasing self and others. Fraiberg writes of the 2-year-old's handling of such a conflict when confronted with an unattended bowl of eggs. The child's resolution is that as she plops each spoonful of egg on the floor gleefully, she chastises herself with a very serious "mustn't do" and proceeds with the next plop of egg.[5]

The preschooler of 3 to 6 years of age makes his foray into the neighborhood, masters reciprocal play, demonstrates his sexuality with open masturbation, exhibits his active fantasy world through symbolic play (Fig. 2), displays his burgeoning vocabulary, and dreams of living forever after with the parent of the opposite sex. Nancy's brown paper bag

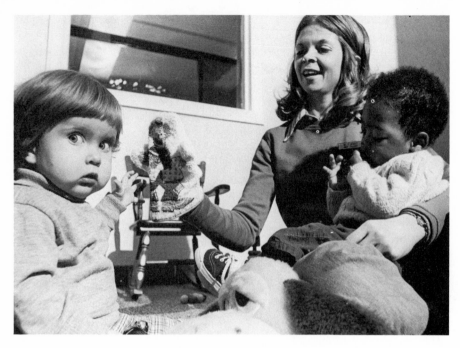

FIG. 2
Preschool children often express their thoughts through play. (Photo courtesy
Dan Grogan.)

filled with peanut butter sandwiches will happily suffice for daddy and
daughter until mother calls the family to the dinner table and reality. The
child at this age is "on the make."[4] He is actively initiating activities, in-
truding on others' conversations, and continually interrupting everyone
else. Freudian theory stresses the child's task of resolving Oedipal or
Electra conflicts with mother or father.

Although he does eventually accept the value system of those in authority, the child experiences many struggles and much anger in the process. The rages he frequently has against his parents leave him feeling
guilty. However, conscience is developing and the child does internalize
right and wrong. Preschooler activity is marked by egocentrism. This im-
plies not selfishness but the child's feeling that he is the origin of all of the
actions in his world.[18]

Piagetian cognitive development

A significant cognitive step is the infant's development of object permanence during the latter part of his first year.[18] Before this time, objects

that were "out of sight" were literally "out of mind." Now there is an internal representation of the object, or mental imagery. External objects exist independently and have forces of their own. The child begins to use symbols that represent his perception of his world. These totally internal symbols, initially unique to him, evolve into accepted symbols that are meaningful to his family and others. Thus, Piaget attributes to the toddler of 18 to 24 months the beginning of thought. By 2 years, the child has progressed from a totally undifferentiated state to a state of separation of himself and his world. His transition to symbolic thought is manifested by his abilities: "to think about a problem; to develop solutions on a mental rather than physical level . . . [to] imitate a model even though the latter may not be present . . . [and to] reconstruct a series of invisible displacements of an object. . . ."[7]

The preschool child thinks about the world from a very limited perspective, that of his own experience. The preschooler's thought process is classified by Piaget as preoperational and characterized in all aspects by his egocentrism. Even his language is reflective of such egocentrism, with much repetition of what has already been stated by others and monologues directed to no one although stated in the presence of others. Several preschoolers together may engage in collective monologues where no real attempt at communication is made. Ginsburg points out manifestations in speech of such egocentrism: (1) faulty use of pronouns and demonstrative adjectives, (2) incorrect ordering of events, (3) poor expression of causality, (4) omission of important features, and (5) juxtaposition.[7] Piaget uses the term juxtaposition to describe the placement of parts in a willy-nilly fashion without any acknowledgment of the larger issue; in other words, ignoring the whole in favor of the parts.

Magical thinking describes another aspect of the preschool child's egocentrism. The child, as the origin of all activity within his world, feels responsible for his thoughts and fantasies being enacted in the world. Thus, an external event may be interpreted by the child as a direct result of his wishes or statements, a position of an often frightening degree of power.

In describing the content of the preschooler's thought, Piaget introduced the concepts of animism, artificialism, and participation. Animism is that aspect of the child's thinking that attributes consciousness to things or natural events; inanimate things are alive in the same way people are. Artificialism refers to the child's thought that all objects are made for a purpose. Participation describes the idea that all human actions and natural processes interact.

Centration and irreversibility are two other significant obstacles to the preschool child's reasoning ability. In solving conservation problems, the child will recognize two cups of water as equal in volume (Fig. 3). How-

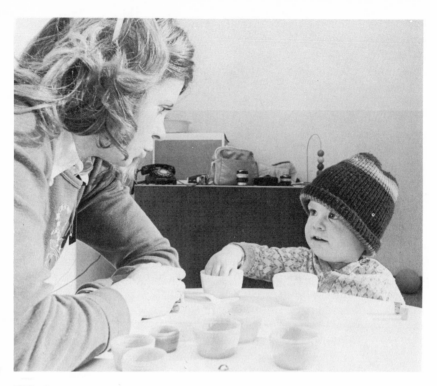

FIG. 3
The child centers on only one dimension of the problem. (Photo courtesy Dan Grogan.)

ever, if the teacher empties one of these into a different-shaped container, shorter and wider, the child will report that one or the other is larger. He has focused his thinking on one aspect of the cup's dimensions, length or width, and ignored the reciprocal relationship between those dimensions. Similarly, his thinking does not include reversibility or the appreciation of the successive changes or transformations that take place in the water as it changes containers.

In summary, the preoperational child's cognitive ability accelerates significantly with the emergence of symbolic function; however, his reasoning abilities are restricted by centration, irreversibility, and egocentrism. He may intuitively solve problems, but he cannot explain his reasoning for a particular solution. His thoughts are clearly influenced by his concepts of animism, artificialism, and participation.

Death concept

Clearly by 6 months an infant perceives differences in caregivers and the degree to which his physical and emotional needs are being met. He cannot have a concept of death until he has the beginning of thought, as evidenced by the emergence of symbolic function between 18 and 24 months. Rank suggests that the origin of death anxiety is in the traumatic separation from mother at the time of birth.[14] The delight of peek-a-boo lies in the relief of the intermittent terror of separation. The child under the age of 5 perceives death as separation, but separation from his beloved caregiver is a terrifying thought.[16]

The toddler recognizes that the puppy is alive and the high chair is not alive; his vocabulary normally includes "to die" by 2½ years and "to live" by 3 years. However, the 3-year-old asks mommy to "put the squashed caterpillar back together again" or "who murdered the garbage?" Mommy reads about waiting for the day Snow White's prince will come and kiss her back to life. The television cartoons have resilient characters who are smashed, chopped, exploded, shot, and drowned multiple times per episode. The hero shot to death on tonight's Western thrives in tomorrow's commercial. The concept of death as the permanent cessation to life and as a universal and inevitable phenomenon is not consistent with the child's preoperational thought processes.

Five-year-old Ernie, in a diary compiled by his parents, is quoted as saying lovingly to his mother: "I'll only shoot you a little dead, mummy, just a little—then you can run slowly." Ernie's death concept is less life, less running for his mommy.[24]

Nagy, in her classic study, talked with 378 children in Budapest during the 1930s concerning their ideas and feelings regarding death. Children under 5 did not recognize the irreversibility of death; they described death as a departure, a sleep, or a temporary happening. Examples are:

BJ (3 years, 11 months): "The dead close their eyes because sand gets into them."

TP (4 years, 10 months): "A dead person is just as if he were asleep. Sleeps in the ground too. . . . A dead person only knows if somebody goes out of the grave or something. He feels that somebody is there, or is talking. . . . At funerals you're not allowed to sing, just talk, because otherwise the dead person couldn't sleep peacefully. A dead person feels it if you put something on his grave."[17]

In 1967 Gartley and Bernasconi reported very similar findings among children aged 5.5 to 6.4 years* in Nova Scotia.[6] However, only 20% of 5-

---

*Throughout this chapter, decimal notations refer to years and months.

and 6-year-old midwestern children in a 1972 study saw death as reversible for their dead pets; approximately one third of the same-aged children attributed cognizance to the pet after death.[15]

In 1974 Koocher reported his discussions with 75 midwestern children between the ages of 6 and 15 years who were asked about their perceptions of the meaning of death and their expectations in regard to their own. In response to "What makes things die?" children under 8 gave answers characteristic of the preoperational child, including egocentrism, magical thinking, and fantasy reasoning. An example:

David (7.8 years): "A bird might act real sick and die if you catch it. [Anything else?] They could eat the wrong foods, like aluminum foil . . ."[11]

When asked "How do you make dead things come back to life?" eight children in the age range 6.0 to 7.1 years suggested ways to revive the dead, indicating their view of death's reversibility. Examples include: "You can't revive them unless you take them to the emergency room and get them doctored up. Then they'll be okay."[11]

The preschool child who cannot view the world from outside himself or conceive thoughts without direct experience will predictably encounter difficulty with the concept of death, for he has not died. For him, being dead is a continuum of less life or decreased function that can be interrupted like sleep. His magical thinking confuses fantasy and fact. Consequently, events such as death of a parent, pet, or friend are interpreted by the preschooler to be a result of his wishes or statements, a powerful and guilt-laden position for the young child. The question of death concept in the child may be approached by looking at what the child means by life. Piaget describes four stages of animism:

1. The child attributes consciousness and life to anything that is active, undamaged or useful.
2. The child attributes consciousness and life to anything that moves.
3. The child attributes consciousness and life to anything that moves of its own accord.
4. The child restricts his definition to animals or to plants and animals.[3]

Thus, preschool children have extremely variable ranges in their ideas of what constitutes living and, concomitantly, of what cessation of living or death entails. Death is separation, but separation from nurturing and protecting parents is abandonment. Such abandonment is a frightening thought, indeed.

Clinical discussion

The preschool child will respond to encounters with death based on his own experiences, his family's religious and cultural heritage, his own attachment with the dead person, and his developmental level. Based on the preceding sections, a likely prediction is that his response will differ significantly from those of the adults in his world.

A 3-year-old in a family mourning a beloved grandmother may distress her relatives by leaving the sorrowful gathering to skip happily out to play. The extent to which young children mourn is not resolved;[1] however, a 3-year-old's attention span is short, her time concept of forever is nonexistent, and her concept of life as well as death is not well defined.[2] It is clear that young children grieve, but cannot tolerate such painful thoughts for long periods of time. Their grief is then intense and brief, but recurrent. She most probably will require multiple and simple explanations of her grandmother's death. Evidence of her distress over this loss will most likely be manifested through her play patterns. Inclusion of this 3-year-old at the funeral would not be meaningful unless past church attendance has been a positive experience and she is accompanied by an adult sensitive to her needs.[8]

The neighbors may be distressed when a 5-year-old boy responds to his pet dog's death with an elaborate burial complete with the construction of a wooden cross, upon which sit two cans of Ken-L-Ration. However, his actions are consistent with his understanding that his dead dog "is less alive" and may still be hungry, a strong characteristic during life. His ritualistic handling of this loss provides a basis for response to future losses. The death of a pet can be a very helpful time for the child to develop his concepts of life and death, as well as the appropriate handling of grief.[13]

The 4-year-old sister of a leukemic child may respond to her sibling's death with many emotions from sadness to elation. Relief at the focus of family activity changing from the medical center to home and pleasure at increased attention provided to her may be expressed. She may have great fears and subsequent guilt for the many times she thought or wished her sibling dead as a result of suspected or real parental favoritism, days off from school, or special treats at the clinic. If parents have not accomplished their anticipatory mourning, the surviving daughter may experience the loss of not only a playmate but also her parental caregivers. Parental grief may be interpreted as distress with her or her thoughts. She may express joy over the toys, clothing, and space that no longer need to be shared. However, she may ask a week later when the sibling is coming home from the hospital. Explanations that her sister was so loved by God that she was called to live with Him may strike terror in her heart, for she imagines that she too may be called away from home and loved ones. Her dead sister portrayed as a happy angel and a discussion of joy in a mourning household only augment the child's animism and magical thinking.

The 18-month-old child whose parent dies slowly and who experiences the gradual introduction of a consistent, warm caregiver, responsive to the toddler's physical and emotional needs, does not react as strikingly as the same-aged toddler whose care is suddenly disrupted and fragmented among various caregivers. Separation anxiety clearly is manifested by eating and sleeping disturbances, followed by denial of all mothering needs and refusal to accept substitute mothering. It has been suggested that real terror for his life (or the meeting of his needs) determines his somatic reactions.[16]

The four-year-old boy, with his magical thinking in operation, "knows" his wishes that "dad stay in the office" have been enacted when his father dies suddenly in an airline crash. The power of such control is overwhelming and frightening to the child. The fantasies of having mommy to himself are equally terrifying as he witnesses his mother's grief. Anger erupts as an expression of his guilt for all the disruption and despair he has caused in his family, bringing in his mind justified punishment for his thoughts and deeds. The effective loss of both parents while the surviving parent is absorbed in her own grief is even more frightening. The 4-year-old boy may further aggravate the family and its helpers when he does not cry and refuses to talk about it. His play may take the form of building and destroying cycles. Without awareness of the child's psychologic and cognitive sequences, his helping adults may add to, rather than diminish, his anguish.

The 2-year-old child dying in a hospital has no real concept of his death, but he has a very real appreciation of the altered patterns of his care and his separation from his usual caregivers. Efforts need to be directed at supporting the parents in their grief, so that they are comfortable performing as much of the dying child's care as possible. Hospital staff providing direct care play an especially critical role in the appropriate handling and support of the mother and father.

However, the 7-year-old child on an oncology ward for his tenth and terminal admission after a 4-year course of treatment of leukemia may be mistakenly thought to be preoperational in his cognitive abilities and be denied appropriate responses to his questions and concerns. Similarly, his facility with hematologic terms and hospital routines may be misinterpreted as wisdom beyond his years, opening him to conversations and suggestions incomprehensible and terrifying to him. His request to attend the funeral of a best friend from the clinic needs to be duly considered.

In summary, health care professionals helping preschool children and their families deal with issues of death and dying have a very special role. However, to perform that role requires mastery of the preschooler's growth and developmental patterns from a psychosocial and cognitive standpoint. The child's overwhelming egocentrism and magical thinking must be understood. Although sequences seem to be constant, the ages and stages are in no way absolute. As in the studies cited earlier, the ranges are very broad. Professionals must take care not to generalize by age or size or situation, but to assess each child's developmental stage before embarking on any intervention. Each child and his developmental stage must be interpreted with an understanding of his experience and his family's cultural heritage. As always, the needs of the helper should not be confused with the needs of the child or his family.

MIDDLE CHILDHOOD
Psychosocial staging

The period of childhood from 6 to 10 years is described as latency by Freud and industry by Erikson. Piaget classifies the cognitive processes as concrete operational. The child at this age has such motor mastery that he can ride his bicycle without holding the handles while crossing his eyes and whistling "Dixie" without a second thought. The 7-year-old child begins to view the world from an external point of view; his language is becoming communicative and less egocentric. Parents become less omnipotent and omniscient and less objects of intense identification and tenderness. The child enters the world of school where the teacher and other adults become the models for identification. Sublimation of his sexual and aggressive urges are demanded by society. Magical thinking persists, but the child gains in his ability to test reality.

School work requires him to sublimate his dreams and play in order to begin to apply himself to concrete pursuits such as reading, writing, and arithmetic. Much energy is invested in intellectual activities and the development of physical skills. He develops perseverance, learns the inorganic rules of the world, and becomes an eager unit of productive or industrious situations.[4] School is not only a place of common goals but of socialization with one's peers in accomplishing these goals. School children begin to demonstrate real cooperation and reciprocity in work and play. Leaders and followers evolve.

Boys play with boys and respond with "Yuck!" if reminded of their preschool plans to run away with mommy. Social horizons are expanded beyond the immediate neighborhood. Clubs and teams are formed where cooperation and competition coexist. Multiple rules and regulations are established—the most common rule being the exclusion of the opposite sex. Girls may excel by a year or two in social and intellectual skills, cementing the separation. Teams provide outlets for competition and energy release after the restraint of the classroom.

The 7-year-old of reason continues to develop his sense of moral judgment. Initially he has very firm ideas of fairness—justice must be meted out exactly. Piaget discusses an absolutistic stage in the child's game of marbles where the rules are sacred and immutable. Gradually, the child attains an understanding that rules are of human origin and that he can participate in their origin and modification. Paralleling the absolutistic stage in marble playing, the child tends to determine culpability based on the amount of wrong done—the breaking of ten teacups is proportionately "wronger" than the breaking of one teacup. Piaget calls this moral realism, the character's guilt being determined by the sheer amount or degree of damage.[7] However, the child gradually takes into consideration the intent of the teacup breaker until the distinction between breakage by accident is distinguished from breakage on purpose.

The latency-aged child is mastering school and social skills. The boundaries of his experience are expanded from home to neighborhood to school. Increasingly, his interpretation of that experience is based on an external point of view—that of schoolmates, teachers, and other adults, as well as that depicted in his reading and the media.

Piagetian cognitive development

The child from 7 to 11 experiences dramatic changes in the characteristics of his cognition; his logical and objective abilities increase. This concrete operational period is marked by more mobility in thinking because of the transition from static to dynamic, centration to decentration, and irreversibility to reversibility.

The concrete operational child is attuned to intermediate aspects between two states. He can think about the transformation as the clay ball is rolled into the clay sausage or the water is poured into different-sized containers. He becomes capable of understanding conservation. Decentration describes the child's ability to focus on simultaneous aspects of a situation and relate the aspects; he can recognize the reciprocity of height and width of water containers, rather than centering on only one dimension. He can also classify objects according to their characteristics. However, he is still bound to his immediate world: he can only problem-solve if the elements of the problem are physically present.

Egocentrism is diminished as the child views the world from the perspective of others. Animism and artificialism persist in a diminished fashion; it is not until 10 or 11 years of age that children answer Piaget's question of "How did the sun begin?" by attributing the sun's origin to natural phenomena.

The concrete operational child has increased objectivity and logic. He can solve problems of space and time, conservation of quantity and number, and classification if objects are physically present.

Death concept

Nagy found that two thirds of the children between the ages of 5 and 9 personify death either as a separate person or as being identified with the dead person. Death is invisible, but it lurks around hidden in the nighttime, especially in those areas of dead people, such as graveyards.

BT (9.11): "Death is a skeleton. It is so strong it can overturn a ship. Death can't be seen. Death is in a hidden place. It hides in an island."

AC (7.11): "Death can't speak or move. I was often at the cemetery. It's very sad. . . . When I see a grave there's death in it. That's sad . . . . [Death] is a dead person who hasn't any flesh any more, only bones."[17]

Although Kübler-Ross writes of the "bogey man and death man who takes people away"[12] and Maurer describes the child's personification of death as a necessary defense against fear,[14] recent studies have not observed this use of personification.[6,11,15] It has been suggested that its omission may be a result of cultural differences, religious education, or different coping styles of the children studied.

Nagy's examples in this age group include some that reflect death as a contingency for bad deeds, demonstrating the child's persistent egocentrism and magical thinking.

BM (6.7): "Carries off bad children. Catches them and takes them away. . . . One night it came. I always took raisins though it was forbidden."[17]

McIntire describes 6-year-old Catholic children as saying people died "because they are bad," but not a single other child in her study attributed a known death to moral guilt.[15] School-aged children do question "why Granny was punished and died" and continue to demonstrate magical thinking in the belief that "Granny died because I was angry with her," but do so less frequently as they grow older.

At what point does the child recognize that death will happen to him? Death, in one recent study, was remote and not perceived as happening to children personally in the age groups 5.5 to 7.5 years. Children in the 7.5 to 8.4 year group did recognize death as an immediate possibility.[6]

Lillian C (7): ["Are you going to die?"]
"Yes."
["When?"]
"At the end of the world."

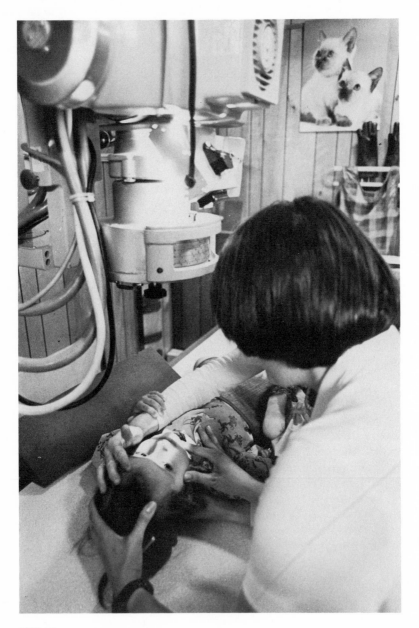

FIG. 4
The child may feel that treatment, such as radiation therapy, like death, is punishment for past bad deeds. (Photo courtesy Scott Barry.)

Elizabeth P (8):   ["Are you going to die someday?"]
"Yes."
["When?"]
"Might die now, but I hope not. I'd rather live longer."[6]

Koocher found a broad range of responses to his question of "When will you die?" from a low of 7 years by a 6-year-old to a high of 300 years by a 9-year-old. Although the averages of his preoperational, concrete, and formal groups were very similar, the preoperational group had the widest variation of responses based more on fantasy than reality.[11] Whether the fatally ill child in this age range can conceptualize his own death is widely debated; however, it is strongly suggested that the child is aware of the seriousness of his illness, although he may not be capable of talking about it.[21-23] The fatally ill child of 6 to 10 years demonstrates anxiety and preoccupation with threat to body integrity and functioning. Spinetta states that "although the concerns of the 6- to 10-year-old leukemic child may not be overt expression about death, the more subtle fears and anxieties are nonetheless real, painful, and very much related to his illness."[22]

What do children feel will happen when they die? Nagy's death man carried children off—sometimes to a "heaven" and sometimes just "away."[17] The findings among the 60 Catholic children reported by Gartley and Bernasconi, who "all understood the concepts of heaven and hell and by age 7 were speaking of purgatory with an obviously clear understanding,"[6] clearly reflect religious training. Approximately half of all McIntire's groups from 7 to 12 years stated their "dead pet knows I miss him," which was interpreted as belief in cognizance after death. However, at 10 to 12 years, 93% of Catholic children stated belief in their own spiritual continuation without cognizance after death.[15]

When asked "What will happen when you die?" another midwestern group of children aged 6 to 15 referred to: being buried (52%), heaven, hell, afterlife or judgment (21%), having a funeral (19%), specifics of how (10%), being asleep (7%), being remembered by others (5%), reincarnation (4%), and cremation (3%). Examples are:

Larry (9.5):   "They'll help me come back alive. . . . They'll keep me in bed and feed me, and keep me away from rat poison and stuff. . . ."

Mark (12.0):   "I'll have a nice funeral and be buried, and leave all my money to my son. . . ."

George (14.9):   "I'll rot. You just decay and then turn back into material like the earth. That's it."[11]

The samples are small and certainly reflect religious, educational, and family influences.

The etiology of death as conceptualized by the child at this age is not consistent. In response to "What makes things die?" concrete operational children of middle-class background suggested ways of causing death —specific weapons, poisons, or other means. Their responses addressed specific causes rather than general processes.

Todd (7.5): "Knife, arrows, guns, lots of stuff. . . . Hatchets and animals, and fire and explosions too."

Kenny (9.5): "Cancer, heart attack, old age, poison, guns, or if someone drops a boulder on you."[11]

The responses of children from age 6 to 10 to "Why do people die?" reflected their socioeconomic background. The inner-city, clinic population stated aggressive causes of death, such as accidents, violence, war, and suicide 4 times as frequently as the suburban, church-school pupils of the same age. Television-watching habits of the two groups were reported as similar.[15]

The permanence of death is apparently gradually but not completely understood by these children in middle childhood. Replying to "How do you make dead things come back to life?" children over age 7 recognized death as permanent.

> If it was a tree you could water it. If it's a person you could rush them to the emergency room, but it would do no good if they were really dead already. . . .
>
> Maybe someday we'll be able to do it, but not now. Scientists are working on that problem.[11]

Belief in personal or universal spiritual continuation after death ranged from about 20% in Jewish children to 65% in Catholic children in the 8- to 12-year-old group. Similarly, death as a total cessation ranged from 5% in Catholic to 65% in Jewish pupils in the same group.[15]

The evolution of the concept of death as a permanent cessation of life and as an inevitable and universal phenomenon occurs during the child's concrete operational years. However, the cognitive obstacles to abstract thought, namely the persistence of egocentrism, animism, and magical thinking, prevent its completion. The child's psychosocial experiences at home and in his community clearly influence the development of the death concept.

Clinical discussion

There appear to be patterns to the emergence of the child's concept of death if one looks at groups of children. It is important to note, however: (1) the very broad range of inclusion in the reported groupings, (2) the small data base from which conclusions are made, (3) the strong influences of family belief, religious orientation, educational background, and socioeconomic status, (4) the child's own life experiences, and (5) the wide normative ranges in cognitive abilities. In middle childhood, the most difficulty occurs in the application of the previous discussion, because the magnitude of change in the ability to conceptualize death is so great over such a short period of years. It is also critical to remember the differences in levels of cognition that may exist; as Spinetta suggests, there most probably exist multiple levels of death awareness before the child uses adult language to discuss the adult concept of death. States of anxiety and physical illness directly affect the child's ability to process his perceptions. Surface language, "Did you know I'm dying?" does not necessarily reflect the child's level of understanding. Communication from the child will continue to be not only verbal but symbolic through various levels of play, drawing, stories, and daily living patterns.

Seven-year-old Susie comes home from second grade each day to share her stories with Granny, who lives with the family. As Granny's health begins to fail, and she is less responsive to Susie's tales of school, Susie begins to understand her loss. When Granny dies, Susie does not need to be shuttled off to a relative's home in another town or to a neighbor's house; she can legitimately participate in mourning activities of her family and have a role assigned, if only to take the coats of the visitors to her home.[8] If she indicates a desire to attend the funeral, considerations include her previous familiarity with the church, the presence of someone who can be responsive to her needs, and her continued desire to do so. She deserves to know in advance what the ritual will entail and what the expectations of her performance are. The funeral syndrome symptomatology described by Schowalter may then be avoided.[19]

Seven-year-old Tally finds his pet dog, dead, by the side of the highway. He and the neighborhood children dig a grave and bury the beloved dog with considerable pomp and circumstance, during which Tally sheds appropriate tears. The next day Tally digs up the dog and inspects the changes of decomposition and reburies him. This ritual proceeds each day without any evidence of distress in Tally. Discussion with Tally reveals a very matter-of-fact approach to finding out what happens when something dies. The school-aged child in America seems to use mastery of detail as an effective coping mechanism.[11]

Nine-year-old Tony comes into the pediatrician's office feeling physically and emotionally miserable, but only a mild case of sinusitis is diagnosed. However, Tony remains and haltingly asks multiple questions about the seriousness of sinusitis. He is relieved when his physician recognizes that his excessive concern stems from the hospitalization of a classmate with an advanced tumor. His anxiety is readily alleviated in one subsequent visit. Similarly, surviving siblings may evidence multiple somatic complaints that require listening, not medication.

Seven-year-old Jim, who experienced the loss of his father during his Oedipal period, initially expresses his response through anger, violent symbolic play, and nightmares. In time, his nightmares become insomnia, associated with tears and sadness, as he gradually begins to be able to share some of his ideas about his father's death verbally. A definite therapeutic intervention is successfully attempted at this point.

Tammy is a fourth grader from a rural county for whom a visit to the medical center is a diagnostic workup for her advanced tumor. Over the first months of her radiotherapy she willingly seeks out the rocking chair in the physician's office to share ideas about her disease. She initially states concern about how she "caught it" from her grandmother before she died, associating death with the dead one as well as proposing a contagious quality to her disease. She becomes very sorrowful in presenting her rationale: punishment by God for having experimented with cigarettes. Magical thinking seems to color her explanations that additives in the food caused the growth. Six months later when she comes to visit she talks of the tumor as "One of these things that just happen, I guess. We all have to die. I sure wish it wouldn't have happened to me."

Nine-year-old Elizabeth with stage I Hodgkin disease is on the ward at the same time with Tammy. She cannot be reassured about her prognosis and is convinced she will die within the year. She has detailed funeral plans and has written her will. Neither repeated reassurances nor psychiatric consultation have altered her thinking.

The contrast between these two girls points out the many deficiencies of protocols drawn up with guidelines devised by age and disease rather than developmental criteria.

In many ways the child from 6 to 10 years is in a transition phase where the concept of death is evolving rapidly, as is the mastery of the rest of the world. Much egocentric and magical thinking may persist even as he is adding scientific information.[9] This group remains the most variable of any age level with respect to understanding death.

ADOLESCENCE
Psychosocial staging

Adolescence has been called a "normative crisis," a period when peacefulness is pathologic. The child experiences tremendous changes in his body over a short period of time: changes in body growth and configurations as well as the appearance of secondary sexual characteristics.

Menstruation in the girl and ejaculation in the boy commence. Sexual drives are strong and require self-control. Good health and body function are assumed. He is selfless one day and selfish the next, euphoric then depressed. Denial is his prevalent coping style. The adolescent is viewed by his family and society in general with mixed feelings.

The early part of adolescence is marked by real concern with body image and the turmoil resulting from tremendous swings in mood and behavior. In the late teen years, the adolescent's concerns become philosophical as he moves toward the assumption of his adult role in society. The achievement of identity is the adolescent's goal through mastery of the developmental tasks of achieving a stable self-concept, independence from family, an adult sexual role, and the selection of a vocation.[4]

Adolescents become increasingly distant from parents and demonstrate intense interest in the peer group and extrafamilial young adults who tend to become superheros. By later adolescence, there will be multiple falling-in-love episodes as a preliminary to his choice of marital partner. He gradually develops the capacity for self-evaluation and insight. However, the adolescent experiences episodes of regression to earlier developmental states on occasion; egocentrism, magical thinking, rages, and extreme dependency are not uncommon. His future and his mortality become increasingly evident. The denial of his mortality is manifested by the adolescent's death-denying involvement with speeding vehicles and experimentation with consciousness-altering substances.

The teenager with his clothing fads and music abhorrent to his parents eventually masters his body and its drives to assume his responsible role in the adult world. This mastery is accomplished, however, through continual conflict with himself, his family, and his immediate world.

Piagetian cognitive development

The adolescent attains formal operations with the achievement of abstract thought, although adolescents and adults of less than average intelligence may not ever attain this level of thinking. He is no longer tied to only concrete here-and-now reasoning. His mind can imagine the many possibilities inherent in a situation; he becomes able to deal with increasingly complex problems. The adolescent can consider a number of hypothetical possibilities in a problem-solving situation. He can appreciate multiple aspects of the problem rather than single aspects as in the concrete operational child. "The possible and the ideal captivate mind and feeling."[7] By the end of adolescence, the individual's thinking patterns are nearly completely developed.

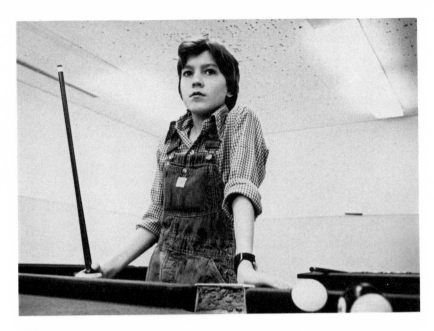

FIG. 5
By age 10, children understand that death occurs not only at the end of a full and productive life, but is possible at any point. (Photo courtesy Scott Barry.)

Death concept

The adolescent shares the adult concept of death as a universal and inevitable process by which life as we know it terminates.[9] His ability for abstract thought enables him to think about his own death. To cope with the anxiety elicited by these thoughts of his mortality, he utilizes denial.

Children in Nagy's group recognized death as the cessation of corporeal life from 9 years on.

FG (9.11): "A skull portrays death. If somebody dies they bury him and he crumbles to dust in the earth. The bones crumble later and so the skeleton remains all together, the way it was. . . . Death is something that no one can escape. The body dies, the soul lives on."

FE (10.0): "Death means the passing of the body. Death is a great squaring of accounts in our lives. It is a thing from which our bodies cannot be resurrected. It's like the withering of flowers."[17]

The recognition of death as a natural process is evident in a more recent group of adolescents asked "What makes things die?"

Dean (10.2):   "When someone gets too old. You could also die of a sickness, or
if you couldn't have enough to eat. Well, when you get old you
can wear out eventually."
George (13.5): "They get old and things, and their body gets all worn out, and
their organs don't work as well as they used to."[11]

Strong religious influences with respect to continuation after death
were found in children interviewed in church schools and in Catholic
populations.[6,15] Adolescents with frequent thoughts of suicide denied the
finality of death. In a group of 13- to 16-year-olds, 20% believed in cognizance after death, 60% in spiritual continuation, and 20% in death as
total cessation.[15] In contrast, only 7% of children in another study used
the word "god" to answer questions and only 21% referred indirectly to
an afterlife via heaven or hell.[11]

The coping styles of the adolescent in dealing with death anxiety
parallel the adults in his world; however, denial remains the most common. Concerns about one's mortality are real and must be handled if the
job of living is to proceed with some degree of comfort. From 700 essays
by high school seniors on "What comes to your mind when you think of
death?" responses varied from awareness to denial to curiosity to contempt to despair.[14]

Clinical discussion

The adolescent is full of his psychologic and physical self. The body is
all-powerful and with little modification can attain perfection. The uniform, whether it be blue jeans or patchwork quilting, is a critical part of
his identification with the peer group. The child in early adolescence
dealing with the death of an age-mate may show abnormal concern with
his own body and its function. The dying child in early adolescence often
expresses more concern over the side effects on his physical body (acne,
weight gain, hair loss) than over the disease itself (Fig. 6).

The older adolescent has resolved his self-concept conflicts by orient-
ing himself toward the future. He is establishing his educational, vocational, and marital goals. His thoughts are very much in philosophical
areas and concerned with his meaningful role in the adult world. Death
of an age-mate for him is a crashing reaffirmation of his mortality. Terminally ill adolescents in this age range have a fully developed concept
of death, as well as clearly defined goals for the future—goals that must
be truncated if not abandoned. The adult who is dying has the opportunity to review the extent to which he has met his goals in his various roles as parent, spouse, provider, and human being. The older
adolescent facing his own death is caught with goals established but

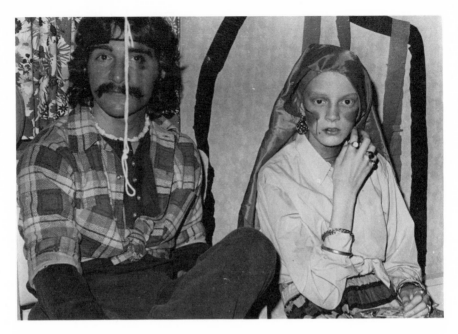

FIG. 6
In early adolescence, the visible markings from radiation therapy may have more emotional impact than the cancer itself. (Photo courtesy Dan Grogan.)

too little time to have accomplished any significant aspect of them. This conflict brings incredible frustration.

Mike is a 14-year-old with leukemia who comes in for a previously scheduled course of chemotherapy a day late. He states to the admitting resident that he doesn't understand why he is here again, wasn't it all taken care of before? Within 24 hours of admission, the staff has asked and demanded of the admitting resident on nine separate occasions that Mike "have his disease and its treatment explained to him!" Initially, the resident reacts indignantly to the hematologist's lack of communication and spends several long explanatory sessions with Mike. When by the end of the week staff concerns are unchanged, the resident is frustrated and suggests that the patient may be retarded. After a case conference, house staff and nursing staff begin to understand the nature of Mike's denial. His only communication relative to his hospitalization is the stress over acne, possible weight gain, and what his school mates will think of his tracks of intravenous sites.

Glen is a 17-year-old boy with a rapidly progressive neuromuscular disease. Discussions by staff concerning possibilities of tracheostomy, assisted ventilation, and deterioration of his blood gases are continually met with disinterest by him. His parents are concerned by what they interpret as increased anxiety at home. Hospital school teachers and therapists talk about the "strangeness" of Glen's behavior. An invitation to talk with his primary physician about his depression reveals he is not concerned directly with dying but with his virginity. Sexual fulfillment, previously a future goal, has become an immediate one "before I get hooked up on all that machinery."

An adolescent patient with a potentially fatal disease is discussed in the multidisciplinary setting at a medical center. The most frequent statement expressed will be "I've tried to talk with him several times about his disease, but he just isn't accepting it." In many institutions, staff members tend to feel rejected if the patient does not share with each individual his feelings about his disease. It becomes increasingly difficult for the staff to understand whose needs are being met and that such communication is neither necessary on a continual basis nor always appropriate with multiple individuals. The adolescent patient, although possessing a mature concept of death, remains a most difficult management problem, especially if his inclusion in decision making is attempted.[20]

CONCLUSION

The kingdom where nobody dies is and always has been fantasy. Death can occur to a child's pets, relatives, friends, parents, siblings, or he, himself, may die. The child's struggle to understand and to grieve such losses distresses adults. For professionals to help children and their parents deal with death, a clear understanding of the child's concept of death as a developmental phenomenon is important.

The young child's thinking is characterized by egocentrism, magical thinking, animism, and imperfect senses of time and causality. Thus, death may be conceptualized as gradual, incomplete, punishment, a person, reversible, or a result of the child's thoughts and deeds.

Through the middle childhood years, egocentrism, magical thinking, and animism as obligatory thinking styles diminish. Senses of time and causality are solidified. Great variability in cognitive levels, psychosocial development, and individual experiences in this age group result in a diversity of death concepts. However, most children by age 10 understand death as permanent and universal.

This chapter discusses guidelines for the health professional to anticipate the range of responses possible from a child encountering death in his environment. There are no absolute milestones; each child is very much an individual. His understanding of death depends on his cognitive

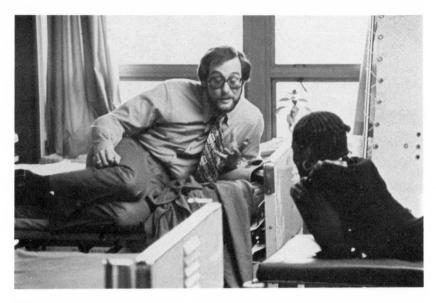

FIG. 7
The helping professional needs a clear understanding of the child's concept of death before effective intervention can begin. (Photo courtesy Scott Barry.)

ability, his psychosocial development, and his own unique set of experiences within his family's cultural and religious framework.

REFERENCES

1. Averill, J. R.: Grief, its nature and significance, Psych. Bull. **70:**721, 1968.
2. Bowlby, J.: Childhood mourning and its implications for psychiatry, Am. J. Psychiatry **118:**481, 1961.
3. Dunton, H. D.: The child's concept of death. In Schoenberg, B., Carr, A., Peretz, D., and Kutscher, A., editors: Loss and grief; psychological management in medical practice, New York, 1970, Columbia University Press.
4. Erikson, E. H.: Identity, youth and crisis, New York, 1968, W. W. Norton & Co., Inc.
5. Fraiberg, S. A.: The magic years, New York, 1959, Charles Scribner's Sons.
6. Gartley, W., and Bernasconi, M.: The concept of death in children, J. Genet. Psychol. **110:**71, 1967.
7. Ginsberg, H., and Opper, S.: Piaget's theory of intellectual development; an introduction, Englewood Cliffs, N. J. 1969, Prentice-Hall, Inc.
8. Grollman, E. A.: Explaining death to children; Boston, 1967, Beacon Press.
9. Inhelder, B., and Piaget, J.: The early growth of logic in the child, New York, 1964, Harper & Row, Publishers.
10. Klaus, M. H., and Kennell, J. H.: Maternal-infant bonding, St. Louis, 1976, The C. V. Mosby Co.

11. Koocher, G. P.: Talking with children about death; Am. J. Orthopsychiatry **44:**404, 1974.
12. Kübler-Ross, E.: On death and dying, New York, 1969, Macmillan, Inc.
13. Levinson, B. M.: The pet and the child's bereavement, Ment. Hyg. **51:**197, 1967.
14. Maurer, A.: Maturation of the conception of death, J. Med. Psychol. **39:**35, 1966.
15. McIntire, M. S., Angle, C. R., and Struempler, L. J.: The concept of death in midwestern children and youth, Am. J. Dis. Child. **123:**527, 1972.
16. Miller, J. B. M.: Children's reactions to the death of a parent; a review of the psychoanalytic literature, J. Am. Psychoanal. Assoc. **19:**697, 1971.
17. Nagy, M. H.: The child's view of death, J. Genet. Psychol. **73:**3, 1948.
18. Piaget, J.: The child's conception of the world, Totowa, N.J., 1969, Littlefield, Adams & Co.
19. Schowalter, J. E.: How do children and funerals mix? J. Pediatr. **89:**139, 1976.
20. Schowalter, J. E., Ferholt, J. B., and Mann, N. M.: The adolescent patient's decision to die, Pediatrics **51:**97, 1973.
21. Spinetta, J. J., and Maloney, L. J.: Death anxiety in the outpatient child, Pediatrics **56:**1034, 1975.
22. Spinetta, J. J., Rigler, D., and Karon, M.: Anxiety in the dying child, Pediatrics **52:**841, 1973.
23. Spinetta, J. J., Rigler, D., and Karon, M.: Personal space as a measure of a dying's child's sense of isolation, J. Consul. Clin. Psychol. **42:**751, 1974.
24. vonHug-Hellmuth, H.: The child's concept of death, Psychoanal. Q. **34:**499, 1965.
25. Wessel, M. A.: Death of an adult—and its impact on the child, Clin. Pediatr. **12:**28, 1973.
26. Yudkin, S.: Children and death, Lancet **1:**37, 1967.

ADDITIONAL READING

Schowalter, J. E.: The child's reaction to his own terminal illness. In Schoenberg, B., Carr, A., Peretz, D., and Kutscher, A., editors: Loss and grief; psychological management in medical practice, New York, 1970, Columbia University Press.

THE FAMILY AND THE FATALLY ILL CHILD

Family structure and the family's general adaptation to loss: helping families deal with the death of a child

STEPHEN W. MUNSON

To provide aid for the family experiencing the death of a child, the helping professional must accomplish two tasks: first, make careful observations of the family's response to the crisis of loss, and second, focus attempts to help by using strategies that are based on these careful observations. Medical caregivers of the dying child are frequently at a significant disadvantage in dealing with the problems of the family. They are often situated in tertiary care facilities far from the family's home and their primary physician. Even when health care is provided in a community hospital close to home, the caregivers often cannot rely on a long and intimate relationship with the family to provide information about the family's function.

This chapter will focus on families whose children have died after some exposure to hospitals and the health care system. It will outline certain aspects of family functioning that can be assessed in all families and that have relevance to those who are grieving.

FAMILY RESPONSE TO THE CRISIS OF LOSS

Research such as that conducted by Friedman and Chodoff[2-4] has produced several observations about the family's response to the terminal illness and death of one of its members. Although it is clear that every family responds to the tragedy in an idiosyncratic fashion, these studies have pointed out certain common modes of adjustment. For example, when they are told a diagnosis that has fatal implications, parents typically report sensations of either numbness and disbelief or shock. Although these experiences last for varying periods of time, they are usually displaced by other feelings and activities, such as searching for intellectual data about the illness, including its etiology, pathophysiology, and various modes of treatment. This may be accompanied by a quest for the meaning of the illness at a more philosophical level. Certain intrapsychic defense mechanisms can be observed. Many family members isolate or deny the painful affect associated with the illness and carry on activities in other aspects of their lives as if these feelings did not exist. It is clear that in the early phases of the child's illness these defense mechanisms serve a useful function.

Feelings of guilt and anger are also commonly seen. Hostility may be displaced from the unknown cause of the illness onto a spouse, the dying child's siblings, the hospital staff, or other nearby persons. A gradual acceptance of the child's eventual death with associated feelings of sadness, withdrawal, somatic complaints, irritability, restlessness, and other general signs of grief may evolve. Because these indications of grief are seldom seen with the intensity witnessed following sudden death, their appearance often confuses health professionals. This is especially true of those families who have previously used isolation and denial extensively, and therefore have appeared to be coping well.

Some investigators have focused on the development of symptoms in bereaved family members. In one retrospective study of 20 families who lost a child from acute leukemia,[1] it was found that in half the families, one or more members required psychiatric care, and in more than half, one or more previously apparently well-adjusted siblings showed altered behavior patterns that were of great concern to the parents. Generally, the symptoms occurred during the terminal illness of the sibling; however, the more severe reactions followed the death of the sibling and persisted. The symptoms covered a wide range and included enuresis, headaches, poor school performance, school phobia, depression, severe anxiety, and other somatic complaints.

Although the data are inconsistent, some studies of marital functioning indicate that divorce may be precipitated by the death of a child.[1]

FUNCTION OF FAMILY SUBGROUPS

The observations made in the above studies describe the function of individuals. It is useful for the professional interested in helping individual family members to make observations about the function of the family system as well. In making such observations one may subdivide the family into its functional components. Although many family functions are carried out by individuals working independently, many others are accomplished in subgroups of two or more family members. Membership of the subgroups can be defined purely on the basis of repeated interaction among group members. For example, there is the subgroup of mother and daughter who share cooking breakfast and another subgroup of older sons who prefer to sleep. It becomes possible to picture these subgroups as an element of the family's structure if the vignette described occurs every morning. These subgroups become a significant aspect of the family's structure if the same individuals repeatedly engage together in many activities.

It is valuable to study in some detail the function of a few such subgroups. In the classical family, the spouse subgroup originates the family. The functions of this subgroup include the attainment of sexual satisfaction and emotional and social companionship for the adults. This group, largely responsible for providing the economic necessities, must develop a system to divide the labor. Nowhere else within the family group can adults receive mutual and complementary support and nurturance. Like all other subgroups in the family, this group arranges to perform all these functions through a complex series of negotiations over time. Most of these negotiations take place at nonverbal levels, and most couples are not aware that they have entered into such negotiations.

The second subgroup that we need to examine is the parenting subsystem. The function of the parenting subsystem is to provide nurturance, guidance, socialization, and support for the children of the family. The members include the adults who parent and the children who receive the parenting. The parenting members are usually, although not always, the same as the members of the spouse subgroup. In order for this system to operate, someone must be in charge; in other words, there must be an executive class that has power over the children in the family. Typically, one member or the other of the parenting subgroup interacts with one or more children in a series of brief but often intense encounters, in order for the family to achieve its goals of teaching social values and maintaining order. It is the parent's role to determine what is safe and advisable for the children and to see that the children abide by these determinations. As with the spouse subsystem, the negotiations about the specific issues of parenting take place at both cognitive and habitual levels and evolve over time.

The third subgroup that deserves our attention is the sibling subsystem, which is made up of groups of children in the family. In a large family with children of many ages, the sibling subsystem can be broken down into several subgroups of children who have similar developmental interests and problems. Within the sibling subgroup, children learn to negotiate appropriate expression of nurturant, aggressive, and competitive impulses, and to develop and maintain contact with the peer group outside the family.

Minuchin and his co-workers[5,6] have described certain characteristics of the functioning of these subsystems that are important to observe. First there is a wide divergence among families in the flexibility of the subgroups. At one end of the continuum are families in which the boundaries and negotiations are exceptionally rigid; for example, there is the family in which the parent-child interaction is always marked by executive and authoritative function. The parents never allow themselves to participate in playful or immature behavior with the children. Similarly, they never allow anyone outside the nuclear family to act in the parenting function. Thus, the family always does everything together, and the parenting function, in extreme rigidity, severely limits the spouse function. In short, there are never any babysitters, so the parents never go out to dinner by themselves.

At the other end of the continuum are families whose subgroup boundaries are so flexible that the family approaches chaos. In such situations, the executive subsystem may include anyone at any time. Authority often rests with the person who is most vocal or obnoxious at any moment. Affiliation in such a system depends on the needs of the moment; the spouse can depend on support from his or her mate only if the mate finds it convenient or of interest to provide it.

Between the two extremes of this continuum exist subgroups that allow changes at appropriate developmental and situational milestones but still maintain predictability; thus, a father in a flexible system can play as a child with his children and become part of the sibling subgroup and still be relied upon to return to his parental role if the need arises, even if it will interrupt his fun. In another example, an adolescent may be delegated to act as a parent when mother goes shopping yet can expect to be relieved of these duties when mother returns. In an extremely rigid family, the adolescent may be expected to retain this role as a parental child when mother returns, even though the need no longer exists. In a chaotic family, mother may leave without delegating a replacement, expecting that the children will find help when and where they need it.

The second characteristic of subgroup function described by Minuchin is the permeability of the boundaries to needs of other subgroups. On one end of this continuum, all family members know everything about the business of all others. In such an enmeshed system, marital difficulties are well known to even preadolescent children, who may be allowed to participate in their resolution depending on the rigidity of the boundaries in the family. In a similar way, parents of these families are intimately familiar with the details of their young daughter's romances, reading her mail and listening to her phone conversations, often with the daughter's approval.

In some families, an enmeshed style of interaction is combined with a general attitude of extreme protectiveness. Each family member is sensitive to the feelings of others and seeks to protect the others from emotional pain of any sort. In such families, a paradoxical situation often develops in response to stress. Because all family members are sensitive to each other's feelings, the distress experienced by one person is felt by all. However, because of the family's attitude of protectiveness, the individual in distress attempts to hide his problems from others. In doing this, he prevents other family members from assisting him with his problems and also prevents the resolution of the feelings they share with him. Thus, the attempts to protect actually increase the suffering.

Impermeable boundaries are seen at the other end of this continuum. Parents disengage from the needs of their children, and only a major calamity brings a response. In such families, children are unaware of impending divorce because the parents are not sensitive to the children's need to know, and the children are totally disengaged from the parents' problems. Once again, there is a middle range in the continuum in which there is both appropriate segregation of boundaries and sensitivities to the needs of other members. The parents' involvement with their children's lives must move from the entangled and enmeshed end of the continuum when their children are infants toward the disengaged end of the continuum as children become adolescents and graduate from the family into adulthood. Learning to change in this way is one of the developmental tasks that must be accomplished if the family is to survive the adolescence of its children.

In general, the adequate function of all of these subsystems in the family depends on the ability of family members to resolve conflict with one another. The needs of each individual continually come into conflict with the needs of other family members, and there is an infinite variety of patterns available to resolve these conflicts. However, in many families, the family members are unable to resolve even minor differences. This lack of resolution can lead to severe threats to the homeostasis of the family unit. If the differences of opinion escalate, there is often no alternative but for one member of the family to leave.

PATTERNS OF DYSFUNCTIONAL CONFLICT RESOLUTION

Minuchin[5,6] has described a number of homeostatic mechanisms in families which, although not leading to resolution of the conflict, do maintain continuing integrity of the family. The patterns of lack of resolution of conflict in families tend to fall into two categories: either the family members agree to disagree, or the family members seem to agree that there are no disagreements. In the first situation, conflicts may be vociferous and even physically abusive. At the end of the argument considerable affect is spent, but the issues remain unresolved. In such families, coalitions may develop between one or more of the active participants in the conflict and other less involved family members. For example, a wife who is chronically displeased about her husband's overinvolvement with his profession and consequent inattentiveness to her will establish an inappropriately intimate relationship or coalition with her teenage daughter. As she relies more and more on the daughter for the satisfaction of her needs for companionship, she demands less and less of her husband. He, in turn, sensing his wife's withdrawal may become defensively more involved with his work. The system is thus perpetuated. As a variation on this pattern, both parents engaged in such an unresolved conflict may choose the same child as an ally. The child, needing the affection of both of her parents, is thus placed in an impossible situation. If she chooses to side with one parent, she must reject the other with whom she has a close alliance. This pattern is commonly called triangulation.

In the second pattern of dysfunctional conflict resolution, where the family members seem to agree that there are no disagreements, life seems always to be pleasant, even in the face of the crisis of death. Such families may displace the affect associated with their conflicts onto other issues. This detouring tends to take two forms. The parents may direct their affect into their concern about their children's welfare; thus, parents may focus their concern on an ill child and hide their unresolved differences under the cloak of concern for the medical management of the child's illness. Hostile affect can be discharged in a similar way by parents focusing their anger at each other onto a child's misbehavior. Because much of the hostility is displaced and is therefore inappropriate to the child's behavior, it is ineffective in stopping the behavior and, in fact, promotes further rebellion from the child.

These patterns of coalition formation, triangulation, and detouring are ubiquitous responses to stress in our culture. It is when they become rigid and repetitive that they represent dysfunction and may result in emotional and behavioral disturbances in the family members involved. It is also important to note that all members of these conflict-avoiding subgroups participate in a complementary fashion. No one is to blame, and there are no victims.

As a child with a fatal illness enters a hospital for treatment, there are many ways in which these aspects of general family function can be observed. For purposes of discussion, let us evaluate stress in the family of the child hospitalized with a chronic and eventually terminal illness.

STRESS IN FAMILIES OF HOSPITALIZED TERMINALLY ILL CHILDREN

The chronic illness itself places significant burdens on the spouse subsystem. Financial concerns may require the restriction of spouse activity with fewer babysitters and fewer trips to the movies as well as increased time spent in income-producing activities by one spouse or both. This combination of factors may reduce the amount of attention husband and wife focus on their relationship, and this in turn may lead to an increasing sense of isolation and loss of support on the part of both spouses. This occurs at a time when coping mechanisms of the spouse system are already under enormous stress. An additional burden is placed on the marital relationship of the parents when a child is hospitalized with an exacerbation of his chronic illness. Mothers frequently come to the hospital with their children and remain overnight, often for weeks at a time. An attentive mother of a terminally ill child may spend many hours of the day at the bedside. Her behavior is in marked contrast to that of her husband, who may visit as infrequently as once a week. An interested staff member may ask the ever-present mother about her husband. Often her response will be that he is very busy and does not have time to visit. The persistence of such a pattern must raise a question about the adequacy of spouse function and the possibility that a coalition has developed between the mother and the sick child, with each attending to the needs of the other. This coalition may be further complicated by a family pattern of overprotectiveness. The mother may wish to protect her husband from the intensity of guilt, anger, and sadness she feels about their child's illness. Similarly, her husband may believe it necessary to protect his wife from his quite similar feelings. In such a situation each spouse is excluded from the other.

It is possible to prevent the rigid establishment of such a coalition if the health care staff is alert to its development. Once the determination is made that an intervention is necessary to help the function of the spouse dyad, the member of the team who is both familiar with the family and skilled in couseling techniques should arrange a meeting with both parents together. The purpose of the meeting is to help both parents focus on the common aspects of their plight and to develop some practical ways to support each other in the time of stress. It is important that the counselor contact each spouse directly, rather than extend the invitation to the peripheral parent through the one who is overinvolved. Contacting each spouse helps to overcome the established pattern of exclusion and is more likely to guarantee a meeting with both parents present.

OBSERVATIONS OF PARENT FUNCTIONING

Observations of parenting function can be made directly on the ward. It is a common observation that dying children become ill tempered and hostile, particularly toward their parents. It has been suggested that this represents a displacement of anger away from the medical staff onto more familiar and in some ways safer targets.[4] The manner in which parents support each other in response to the child's abusive behavior in the hospital is worthy of note. The combination of the stress of anticipated loss and the child's attack may overwhelm the parenting system. A mother may chastise her husband openly in front of the child for being too strict. Similarly, a husband may be critical of his wife for being too protective and permissive with the ill child. When such differences are noted and persist, a thoughtful and supportive parent counseling session focusing on the difficulty of dealing with a chronically and severely ill child and the necessity of mutual parental support can often prevent solidification of a dysfunctional parenting system. It is a temptation to the ward staff to take over much of the parental function in such situations; however, there are several reasons why supporting the parents and facilitating their success in their parenting endeavors are better alternatives. It is generally agreed that the adequate care of a dying child involves maintaining as much normalcy as possible. If the child returns home in remission from an acute leukemic process, for example, it is important for the parents to maintain an adequate executive function with the child. Furthermore, successful management of their child's misbehavior provides an experience of accomplishment for parents who may otherwise feel incompetent and helpless in the face of an overwhelming medical crisis. Of course, there are times when the parents' grief may make adequate parenting function temporarily impossible. At such times, parents may welcome authority expressed by nurses and other ward staff. This is especially true with regard to painful medical procedures. It is important for the ward staff to be flexible in its approach and to consider the needs of the parents as well as the needs of the child and the organization of the ward. In any case, it is important for parents to assume more responsibility in managing the behavior of their child as the time for discharge approaches.

A family pattern of rigidity presents certain special problems for parents of a seriously ill child. Such children often regress to behavior patterns that are more immature and dependent than parents have experienced in many years. Such regression, although encouraged by many aspects of the illness and hospitalization, may be difficult for rigid parents to accept. Ward personnel should be alert to the needs of both the child and parents; thus, parents must be given an opportunity to express their dismay and frustration with the child, and should then be encouraged to develop strategies for comforting their child. At the same time, they should be helped to provide appropriate external controls for the child, since regressive behavior that is out of control produces anxiety and depression in the child as well as the parents.

EVALUATION OF SIBLING SUBSYSTEM

The evaluation of the sibling subsystem is more difficult for the ward staff, because direct observations of sibling behavior are not always available. Specific questions about the functioning of children at home should be asked of both parents on a regular basis. Information should be obtained about schoolwork, appetite, sleep patterns, discipline, peer relationships, and general mood as well as what the children understand and what questions they may be asking about their sibling's illness. The pattern of overprotectiveness discussed previously has additional implications for siblings and extended family at home. An agreement to keep secrets from children who suspect the extent of the dying child's illness leads to severe problems for the siblings, prevents their own process of anticipatory grief, and encourages fantasies of responsibility for the illness as well as concerns for their own well-being. Thus, when the health care team notices an overprotective family pattern in the hospital, it should gather information from the parents in some detail about their discussion of the illness with the children at home. If the parents feel insecure about answering young children's questions about the illness, an opportunity for the children to discuss their concerns with medical personnel should be provided.

Rigidity in the parent subsystem can lead to many difficulties with the siblings at home. A child in the hospital often means that one or both parents will be absent from the home frequently or for prolonged intervals. If the parents have never allowed other caregivers to care for the children, the arrival of a grandmother, for example, to perform that function can bring about near chaos. A thoughtful question posed to a visiting parent about how the children are getting along with the temporary caregiver may lead to the discovery of a potential problem that can be solved, again with some preventive parent counseling.

PARENT COUNSELING STRATEGIES

Every hospital staff member has experienced a family whose boundaries are on the chaotic end of the flexibility continuum. The parents visit at 3:00 in the morning and then insist on seeing the child while he is sleeping. Promises are made to the child that the mother will visit the next morning, and when morning arrives, mother does not come. Such chaotic parenting does not necessarily indicate a lack of concern for the welfare of the child. Instead it may represent a customary response that is exaggerated by the stress of impending catastrophe. Nonetheless, an extreme lack of predictability in response to the child and his medical illness on the part of the parents often results in aggravation and hostility on the part of the ward staff. This hostility must be recognized and dealt with creatively. Unusual attempts should be made to meet with the parents and help provide structure in the form of written schedules and other external supports.

The assumption behind the intervention strategies suggested thus far has been that the dysfunctional patterns observed by medical staff are transitory and in response to the overwhelming nature of the stress experienced by the family. It is possible, of course, that the dysfunctional patterns observed in the hospital represent more chronic dysfunction. If that is the case, parent counseling strategies will be of little help, and referral to more experienced psychiatric professionals is warranted.

The following case history will illustrate some of these points.

Dora P was a 9-year-old girl, the only child of upper middle class parents in their forties. She was brought to the hospital after several weeks of daily complaints of abdominal uneasiness and headaches that required her to stay home from school. At the time of hospitalization, she was noted by house officers and nurses to be a willful and often unhappy child whose mother doted on her. The combination of the mother's overprotectiveness and the child's "typical" symptoms led many, including the child's father, to the early conclusion that her diagnosis was school phobia. The child's mother was certain of a more serious illness and reported that her husband was against the hospitalization. During the diagnostic evaluation, Dora's mother, Mrs. P, stayed almost constantly at her daughter's bedside. Mother and daughter engaged often in angry exchanges with each other, each concluding that the other did not love her. Mr. P's relationship with his daughter and his wife represented a marked contrast, when it could be observed. Although he visited the hospital daily, he came only in the evenings and stayed for no more than 30 minutes. His visits with his wife and daughter were invariably pleasant although somewhat strained. Mr. and Mrs. P could be seen walking to the elevator at some distance from one another, with each telling the other that everything was fine.

Preliminary neurologic evaluation revealed the possibility of a cerebellar mass. Before the findings were discussed with the family, the health team caring for the child met together. It was decided that a special attempt should be made to include Dora's father in any discussion of the neurologic findings and their implications. The staff social worker asked Mrs. P to call her husband and arrange a meeting for later that afternoon. Mrs. P reported back to the social worker that her husband would be unavailable because of business matters. With Mrs. P's permission, the social worker called Mr. P at work. The social worker found Dora's father eager to talk with her, and he readily agreed to attend a meeting. He also requested an opportunity to meet alone with the social worker before the general meeting with his wife and the physicians. The social worker agreed. At that meeting, Mr. P stated, with much emotion, that he had been worried about his daughter. However, he had been unable to express his concern to his wife, because it would upset her if she knew he believed Dora was seriously ill. Because of this, he felt quite isolated and had invested all his energies in new projects at work.

The social worker suggested to Mr. P that she help him express his concerns and loneliness to his wife. Mr. P agreed. The social worker then met with Mrs. P alone to explore her feelings about the hospitalization and Dora's illness. As usual, Mrs. P was worried. When asked about her husband, Mrs. P stated that he was too busy to be worried about Dora's problems; it had always been her role to deal with doctors anyway. In any case, it was important that he not be needlessly harassed. His business success was important to all of them, and he did not need added stress. Mrs. P admitted that she and her husband seldom really talked about emotional issues. The social worker suggested that she meet with Mr. and Mrs. P together to help them explore their ideas and concerns about Dora's illness before the physicians met with them. In that way, she could help them formulate questions for the doctors. Mrs. P agreed.

In the meeting with the social worker, Mr. P expressed, with considerable difficulty, his fears about Dora. Mrs. P listened, at first impatiently. However, with support from the social worker, Mrs. P began to appreciate that her husband was indeed concerned, not only about Dora, but about her as well. At the end of the meeting, the couple embraced. They spent the time before the meeting with the physicians planning what to ask them.

As the neurologic evaluation progressed and contrast studies confirmed the presence of a tumor, the social worker met with the parents regularly to help them express their worries to one another. She also helped them discuss their visits with Dora and encouraged them to divide more evenly the responsibility for comforting her. She also helped them deal with their daughter's angry outbursts and her generally immature behavior.

Working together, Mr. and Mrs. P developed new ways of spending time with Dora. They also spent much more time with each other and often visited Dora together. Despite the increasing severity of her illness, Dora became more pleasant and less angry. Her outbursts ceased as her parents became able to attend to her without the added burden of their concerns about each other.

In this case example, a sensitive social worker helped a family deal with spouse and parent subgroup dysfunction that, although undoubtedly of long standing, was exacerbated by the crisis of terminal illness in a child.

FAMILY RESPONSE TO LOSS

The examples of family system dysfunction discussed above have all been responses to the stress of extended serious hospitalization. Despite anticipatory grief and the gradual changes in family structure and function that a long illness allows, the actuality of the child's death exerts a profound emotional effect on the family and its members. Wiener[7] has outlined many of the siblings' responses to death that can range from no apparent response at all to depression, nightmares, aggression, and somatic complaints. Binger[1] reports that children express a variety of feelings, including responsibility for the sibling's death, fears that they will be the next to die, resentment that the parents spent so much time with the ill child, anger at the parents for allowing the child to die, and preoccupations with fantasies about death.

A family pattern of extreme enmeshment may cause a complication in the parents' handling of such expressions of grief. Parents in an enmeshed family tend to overreact to any signs of emotional upset in their children. Thus, an unimportant argument between siblings is construed as representative of significant conflict related to another sibling's death. An innocent question posed by a child may result in a prolonged and overdetailed explanation creating more anxiety in the child than necessary. Similarly, these are families in which children are most likely to take on the problems of other family members. They may see themselves as responsible for the illness and death of their sibling. They may also insert themselves into their parents' conflicts, and in so doing prevent resolution. Thus, when the hospital staff has observed that a family operates on the extreme end of the enmeshment continuum, special attempts should be made to support the parents as they deal with the grief reaction of their other children following the death of the patient. Specific suggestions about how to answer questions may be useful. Such families often become involved with the operation of the ward and will seek continuing contact with the staff and the families of other patients hospitalized with their child. This contact can be used by an alert staff to gather information about the family's response to grief.

When a family loses a child, it may lose more than an important attachment figure. As has been noted before, the family may have used the child's illness and its complications as a means of avoiding both longstanding as well as illness-related conflicts. With the death of the child, these detouring patterns are no longer available. The family must, therefore, either face the issues, seek an alternative conflict-avoiding pattern, or disintegrate. As both Binger[1] and Wiener[7] have noted, children are often inclined to express their acute feelings of grief in ways that may not be understandable to their parents. To the extent that their responses are hostile and accusatory, they invite an angry response from their parents. Such a response will encourage more hostile behavior on the part of the children. This provides a new detouring focus for the parents, diverting their attention from the painful issues of their mutual loss, guilt, and anger. An alternative displacement is provided by another common response pattern of children: somatic complaints, withdrawal, and dysphoria. Overprotective parents in search of a replacement for the lost child may inadvertently and artificially encourage such behavior and perpetuate it. In all of these instances a temporary behavior pattern is potentially fixed with dire results for the children as well as further delay of effective conflict and grief resolution for the parents.

The potentially dysfunctional patterns that develop in families following the death of a child evolve and can become fixed over weeks and months. It is important that the health care system attend to the particular needs of these families. Follow-up interviews with the family several weeks and several months after the death of the child should ideally take place in all cases. At these times, observations and specific questions about the functioning of the spouse, parent, and sibling systems should be made. Although some families grieve without significant problems, many experience transient conflicts and problems as they attempt to adjust to their loss. When emotional symptoms persist in one individual or among several family members, appropriate counseling or referral should be made.

REFERENCES

1. Binger, C. M., Ablin, A. R., Feuerstein, R. C., and others: Childhood leukemia; emotional impact on patient and family, N. Engl. J. Med., **280:**414, 1969.
2. Chodoff, P., Friedman, S. B., and Hamburg, D. A.: Stress, defense and coping behavior; observations in parents of children with malignant disease, Am. J. Psychiatry **120:** 743, 1964.
3. Friedman, S. B.: Care of the family of the child with cancer, Pediatrics **40:**498, 1967.
4. Friedman, S. B., Chodoff, P., Mason, J. W., and Hamburg, D. A.: Behavioral observations on parents anticipating the death of a child, Pediatrics **32:**610, 1963.
5. Minuchin, S.: Families and family therapy, Cambridge, 1974, Harvard University Press.
6. Minuchin, S., Baker, L., Rossman, B. L., and others: A conceptual model of psychosomatic illness in children, Arch. Gen. Psychiatry **32:**1031, 1975.
7. Wiener, J. M.: Reaction of the family to the fatal illness of a child. In Schoenberg, B., Carr, A. Peretz, D., and Kutscher, A., editors: Loss and grief; psychological management in medical practice, New York, 1970, Columbia University Press.

ADDITIONAL READINGS

Burton, L.: Care of the child facing death, Boston, 1974, Routledge & Kegan Paul.
Cain, A. C., Fast, I., and Erickson, M. E.: Children's disturbed reactions to the death of a sibling, Am. J. Orthopsychiatry **34:**741, 1964.

Hollingsworth, C. E., Pasnau, R. O., and others: The family in mourning; a guide to health care professionals, New York, 1977, Grune & Stratton, Inc.

O'Malley, J. E., and Koocher, G. P.: Psychological consultation for a pediatric oncology unit; obstacles to effective intervention, J. Pediatr. Psychol. **2:**54, 1977.

Spinetta, J. J., and Maloney, L. J.: Death anxiety in the outpatient leukemic child, Pediatrics **56:**1034, 1975.

Spinetta, J. J.: Adjustment in children with cancer, J. Pediatr. Psychol. **2:**49, 1977.

CHAPTER 3

Communication patterns in families dealing with life-threatening illness

JOHN J. SPINETTA

This chapter will focus on two issues: (1) what the child with a life-threatening illness knows about his illness, and (2) what the child does with that knowledge. Conclusions and discussion will center on recommendations for dealing with the child and family.

AWARENESS OF DEATH IN THE CHILD WITH CANCER

The majority of authors are in agreement that the older child with a fatal prognosis, especially the adolescent, is aware of and anxious about the potential outcome of his illness.[20] For the fatally ill child under 5, it is generally agreed that anxiety takes the form of separation anxiety, loneliness, and fear of abandonment.[20] The disagreements arise with the age group in between, the child aged from 6 to about 10. There are two avenues of thought regarding the level of awareness in children in this age group. The first is that the fatally ill child under 10 lacks the intellectual ability to formulate a concept of death and therefore is not aware of his own impending death. If the adult does not discuss the issue of the seriousness of his illness with the child, the child is thought to experience little or no anxiety related to the illness.[6,11,12,19,31] The second avenue of thought is that many of the fatally ill children in the 6- to 10-year age group, if not aware at a conceptual level of their own impending death, are aware at least that something very serious is happening to them.[3-5,7,13,14,18] Both groups support their conclusions with examples, the latter group far outweighing the former in the depth and extent of observations.

Two recent studies made an attempt to deal directly with the child himself using controlled and objective measurements of the fatally ill child's response to his illness. Eliciting expression of the child's concern for present and future body integrity and functioning, Waechter[29] used a set of eight pictures, requesting stories about them from each of the 64 children in the study. She used four matched groups from the controversial 6 to 10 age range (fatally ill children, children with nonfatal chronic

43

illnesses, children with brief illnesses, and normal, nonhospitalized children). Among the fatally ill children in her study, Waechter found a higher number of overtly expressed death themes and concerns than of mutilation or separation concerns and, compared with the other groups, a greater degree of concern with threat to, and intrusion into, their bodies and interference with normal body functioning. Waechter's findings pointed to the very strong possibility that children aged 6 to 10 with a fatal prognosis not only are aware that they are dying, but can express that awareness by the use of words relating to death.

A study by Spinetta, Rigler, and Karon[24,25] was conducted in an attempt to clarify the issue of the frequency of overt expression of death concerns. The study was designed to test Waechter's conclusion about the higher level of anxiety in fatally ill children without, however, relying on overt expression about death for the measure of this anxiety. It was predicted that because of their awareness of the seriousness of their illness, fatally ill children at this age, without mentioning death overtly, would show a much greater anxiety regarding threat to their body integrity and body functioning, a higher degree of concern about hospital personnel and procedures, and a greater overall anxiety relative both to the hospital and to nonhospital-related situations than would a control group of chronically ill hospitalized children—the two groups being matched for frequency and intensity of hospital experiences. In the study, 25 children aged 6 to 10 with a diagnosis of leukemia were matched in age, sex, race, grade in school, seriousness of condition, and amount of medical intervention with 25 children with chronic (but nonfatal) illnesses, such as diabetes, asthma, congenital heart disease, and renal problems.

The children were asked to tell stories about each of four pictures of hospital scenes and about each of four figurines (nurse, doctor, mother, father) placed in a three-dimensional replica of a hospital room. Each child was also given a brief anxiety questionnaire sorting out hospital anxiety from home anxiety. The results offered strong support for the hypothesis that fatally ill children show significantly greater awareness of their hospital experience than do chronically ill children. The leukemic children related significantly more stories that indicated preoccupation with threat to, and intrusion into, their bodies and interference with their body functioning than did the chronically ill children, both in the stories relating to the pictures and the stories told about the placed figurines. The children with fatal illness also expressed more hospital-related and nonhospital-related anxiety than did the chronically ill children.

If, as the parents of the 25 leukemic children maintained, their children did not know that their illness was fatal, and if the chronically ill children generally received the same number and duration of hospital-related treatments, there should have been little or no difference between the scores of the fatally ill and the chronically ill children. Yet there was a significant difference in the level of anxiety that was present from the very first admission to the hospital. It seems that despite efforts to keep the child with fatal illness from becoming aware of his prognosis, he somehow picks up a sense that his illness is very serious and very threatening. The study established the fact that the fatally ill child is aware that his is no ordinary illness.

It seems clear both from the Waechter study and the Spinetta study that the fatally ill 6- to 10-year-old is concerned about his illness and that even though this concern may not always take the form of overt expressions about his impending death, the more subtle fears and anxieties are nonetheless real, painful, and very much related to the seriousness of the illness that the child is experiencing. Whether or not one wishes to call this unconceptualized anxiety of the child about his own fatal illness "death anxiety" seems to be a problem of semantics rather than of fact. The fatally ill child reacts to his illness in a manner exhibiting a much greater anxiety than his chronically, but not fatally, ill counterpart. This awareness is present, regardless of whether or not the family wishes the child to know. In a more recent anthropologic study, Bluebond-Langner[3] followed children with leukemia through stages in the process of learning about their illness. Her conclusions mirror those of Waechter and of Spinetta. The children eventually come to an awareness of the seriousness of their illness.

COMMUNICATION PATTERNS IN THE CHILD WITH CANCER

If it is true that a child as young as 6 is aware of the serious nature of his or her illness, what does the child do with this knowledge and awareness? Does the child talk openly with his family about the prognosis, or does the child live in silence with the knowledge? What role does the family play in the child's wishing to talk or not to talk about the illness? To help answer these questions, Spinetta and Maloney[23] studied family communication patterns around the issue of cancer in the child. To delimit the term "coping" and make it operational for the study, the authors defined the following behaviors in the 6- to 10-year-old child as successful attempts on the part of the child to master troublesome situations relative to the illness: a nondefensive personal posture, closeness to parental figures, happiness with oneself, and the freedom to express negative feelings within the family. In contrast, a child under 10 who is defensive, unhappy with self, unable to accept or express negative feelings within the family, and unwilling to express a need for parental closeness was viewed as exhibiting less effective coping behaviors. Basic to this view of effective coping is the assumption of the authors that communication of a child's thoughts and concerns, both happy and painful, is both a healthier state of mental well-being than retaining thoughts in silence[21] and a prerequisite to family support. It was hypothesized that a child whose family allows discussion of the illness and its prognosis would be able to cope more effectively with the illness. Specifically, the child whose family indicates open channels of communication regarding the illness would: (1) score as less defensive on a scale of defensiveness, (2) express closeness to family members, (3) express happiness with himself or herself, and (4) feel free to express negative feelings within the family.

The subjects of the study were 16 leukemic children, aged 6 to 10, who were being treated in out-patient clinics in three local children's facilities. The 16 children were the same ones who participated in an earlier Spinetta-Maloney study.[22] Levels of openness within the family regarding communication about the illness were measured by a questionnaire filled out by the mother. Five items, each scaled 1 to 4, questioned the mother's view of the following: (1) how much the patient-child knew about the illness, (2) what kinds of questions the child asked, (3) how the parent responded to the questions, (4) what kinds of questions the siblings asked, and (5) how the parent responded to the siblings' questions. The total score of the combined categories represented the mothers' view of levels of communication within the family. The study was envisioned as an effort to see whether or not there was a correlation among the variables; it was not intended to demonstrate a cause-effect relationship. Results indicated that the level of family communication about the illness, as expressed in the mothers' judgment of communication, was related to coping strategies in the child. Families in which levels of communication about the illness were high were those families in which the children: (1) exhibited a nondefensive personal posture, (2) expressed a consistently close relationship with the parents, and (3) expressed a basic satisfaction with self. Although freedom to express negative feelings openly within the family was not significantly correlated with level of communication, the data demonstrated a strong trend in that direction. Further studies are called for to clarify whether, in fact, the mother's judgment of openness is a valid judgment of the true situation, whether there is a difference in communication patterns as the children go through subsequent relapses,[3] and whether parents become more or less communicative regarding implications of the illness as the child nears death.[25]

It may be theorized, in accord with a cognitive-learning conceptualization,[16,17] that the fatally ill child chooses whether or not to talk about his illness based on past and present experience within the family regarding openness of communication about the illness. The child may choose silence because he is aware, even at a level preceding his ability to express it,[20] that his family does not allow communication about the illness. Or the child may choose to communicate honestly about the illness because of a family history reinforcing openness, and because he is supported by present parental attitudes. Each choice may be viewed as a different style of coping. The choice for silence can lead to excessive denial and avoidance, place distance between the child and his sources of support, and lead to a feeling of rejection and isolation and to the child's awareness of being left alone to work out his or her problems. Such a feeling of rejection and isolation comes from a level of denial supported and encouraged within the child's family. A forced openness in such a family might appear to the child as an even worse alternative than his suffering in silence. In contrast, a choice for open discussion, stemming from the sincere attempts of family members to communicate concern and support, allows overt expression of feelings. Such expressions of a child's fears relative to the illness, deriving from openness in levels of family communication, can at the child's own request lead to mutual support among family members, helping the child achieve a balanced adaptive equilibrium.

Closed communication about the illness may appear on the surface to be the simplest solution to the question of how the healthy family members are to deal with the childhood cancer—denial of a problem makes it go away, for a while. But the fatally ill child in such a family expresses unhappiness, alienation, and feelings of being left alone to work out his or her fate. In contrast, opening up levels of communication within the family is like opening the proverbial Pandora's box. A complex set of feelings emerges. Openness increases expressed levels of anxiety within the family and commits family members, as well as all others who must deal with the family members, to a confrontation with the severity of the illness. The open family may be torn apart by the confrontation,[2] or it may come through the adaptive struggle with members having grown closer together, having gained a mature ability to struggle valiantly in future life conflicts, and having achieved a level of confidence, strength, and reevaluation of basic life commitments that will make for a more effective and fulfilled life.[3,8]

A word of caution is appropriate lest the Spinetta and Maloney study be interpreted as a blanket support for open communication in all families in all circumstances. Although the study points to the generally supportive value to the sick child of open patterns of family communication, a forced openness too soon for some families can be destructive. There are parents who demonstrate a marked inability to function under the stress and others who exhibit maladaptive behavior, becoming inaccessible, withdrawn, and remote.[9,15,26,30] The goal in working with such families must be to help the family members eventually become aware of the false sense of equilibrium that may come from an excessive denial of the problem, and the harm such denial can cause the sick child. If a temporary use of denial, especially at the beginning, proves helpful in allowing the family time to pull together adaptive resources, then such short-lived denial can be useful in the overall adaptive effort.[21]

The goal of work with the families of children with cancer is to help strengthen the adaptive capabilities and coping styles specific to each family and to each member of the family, to help the family members struggle forward as best they can in a commitment to the value of the remaining months or years of their child's life, and to give them access to the intrafamilial and extrafamilial sources of support they will need to help them, both in that struggle and in the grieving after the child's death. The demonstration of the generally beneficial effects of open communication on family members and, above all, on the life-threatened child is a step toward that goal.

THE DECISION FOR OPEN COMMUNICATION

This chapter has dealt with two issues: (1) what the child with a life-threatening illness knows about his or her illness, and (2) what the child does with that knowledge. It was shown that a child as young as 6 can be aware of the serious nature of the illness. It was suggested that the child who has the personal desire and parental permission to discuss such awareness and knowledge openly within the family structure is in the best position to receive the type of support he most needs.

Circumstances of pain, reactions to medication and treatment, and the death of other children from the illness, all play a role in the child's increasing awareness of the severity of his or her illness. But above all, the parental level of willingness to discuss the illness is critical to the child's decision about what to do with the knowledge. There are those professionals who would encourage denial in order for the children to maintain mental as well as physical comfort, and, up to a point, some denial may be effective.[1,10,28] But the evidence is beginning to mount that the children, siblings, and parents would be best served by being encouraged to bring into the open their anxieties about the illness and its possible consequences.[3,8,26]

Spinetta and colleagues[27] conducted a series of interviews with families whose children had died of cancer. The most frequently discussed issue with families whose children were over 6 at the time of death was the extent to which the family had communicated with the child about the possible terminal effects of the illness. Of the families interviewed, about half felt they had talked freely and openly with their young child about his or her impending death. None of the parents who had spoken openly with their young child felt that too much had been said; on the contrary, the parents felt that a higher level of closeness was achieved with the child than might have occurred otherwise. The memory of the open discussions and exchange of family values before the child's death had sustained the families during the mourning process. The siblings in the open group reported having had time to say goodbye to their dying brother or sister, to resolve old quarrels, and to help the dying child in his or her own efforts to say goodbye as well.

In contrast, of those families whose child had died without open discussion of the illness or of the imminent death, the majority reported wishing that they had spoken more openly with the child. The parents reported feelings of incompleteness and nonresolution. Those siblings who reported unresolved feelings regretted not having been forewarned or not having had time to say goodbye and settle differences before the child's death.

In brief, the children with cancer were found to resolve the issues surrounding their diagnosis, treatment, and prognosis more effectively when allowed to speak openly about the cancer. Mothers, fathers, and siblings reported in postdeath interviews that resolution of the grief process was facilitated by their memories of having done all they could for their child, most notably by openness in levels of communication about the illness.

Certainly, further research is called for and further guidelines must be sought regarding what to say and when, taking into consideration the severity of the illness, parental and sibling readiness, and age levels of the children. Nevertheless, studies to date point to the fact that the child already knows, at some level, that the illness is serious. Allowing the child to talk about the illness can have generally beneficial short- and long-term effects on all the family members, including the life-threatened child.

REFERENCES

1. Alby, N., and Alby, J. M.: The doctor and the dying child. In Anthony, E. J., and Koupernik, C., editors: The child in his family; the impact of disease and death, vol. 2 of the Yearbook of the International Association for Child Psychiatry and Allied Professions, New York, 1973, John Wiley & Sons, Inc.
2. Binger, C. M., Ablin, A. R., Feuerstein, R. C., and others: Childhood leukemia; emotional impact on patient and family, N. Engl. J. Med. **280:**414, 1969.
3. Bluebond-Langner, M.: Meanings of death to children. In Feifel H., editor: New meanings of death, New York, 1977, McGraw-Hill Book Co.
4. Burton, L.: Tolerating the intolerable; the problems facing parents and children following diagnosis. In Burton, L., editor: Care of the child facing death, Boston, 1974, Routledge & Kegan Paul.

5. Easson, W. M.: The dying child; the management of the child or adolescent who is dying, Springfield, Ill., 1970, Charles C Thomas, Publisher.
6. Evans, A. E., and Edin, S.: If a child must die, N. Engl. J. Med. **278:**138, 1968.
7. Furman, R. A.: Death and the young child; some preliminary considerations. Psychoanal. Study Child **19:**321, 1964.
8. Futterman, E. J., and Hoffman, I.: Crisis and adaptation in the families of fatally ill children. In Anthony, E. J., and Koupernik, C., editors: The child in his family; the impact of disease and death, vol. 2 of the Yearbook of the International Association for Child Psychiatry and Allied Professions, New York, 1973, John Wiley & Sons, Inc.
9. Futterman, E. J., Hoffman, I., and Sabshin, M.: Parental anticipatory mourning. In Schoenberg, B., Carr, A., Peretz, D., and Kutscher, A., editors: Psychosocial aspects of terminal care, New York, 1972, Columbia University Press.
10. Howarth, R.: The psychiatric care of children with life-threatening illnesses. In Burton, L., editor: Care of the child facing death, Boston, 1974, Routledge & Kegan Paul.
11. Howell, D. A.: A child dies, Hosp. Top., February 1967.
12. Ingalls, A. J., and Salerno, M. C.: Maternal and child health nursing, St. Louis, 1971, The C. V. Mosby Co.
13. Kastenbaum, R., and Aisenberg, R.: The psychology of death, New York, 1972, Springer Publishing Co., Inc.
14. Kliman, G.: Psychological emergencies of childhood, New York, 1968, Grune & Stratton, Inc.
15. Koupernik, C.: Editorial comment. In Anthony, E. J., and Koupernik, C., editors: The child in his family; the impact of disease and death, vol. 2 of the Yearbook of the International Association for Child Psychiatry and Allied Professions, New York, 1973, John Wiley & Sons, Inc.
16. Mahoney, M. J.: Cognition and behavior modification, Cambridge, Mass., 1974, Ballinger Publishing Co.
17. Mahoney, M. J.: Reflections on the cognitive-learning trend in psychotherapy. Am. Psychol. **32:**5, 1977.
18. Schowalter, J. E.: The child's reaction to his own terminal illness. In Schoenberg, B., Carr, A., Peretz, D., and Kutscher, A., editors: Loss and grief; psychological management in medical practice, New York, 1970, Columbia University Press.
19. Sigler, A. T.: The leukemic child and his family; an emotional challenge. In Debuskey, M., editor: The chronically ill child and his family, Springfield, Ill., 1970, Charles C Thomas, Publisher.
20. Spinetta, J. J.: The dying child's awareness of death; a review, Psychol. Bull. **81:**256, 1974.
21. Spinetta, J. J.: Adjustment in children with cancer, Pediatr. Psychol. **2:**49, 1977.
22. Spinetta, J. J., and Maloney, L. J.: Death anxiety in the out-patient leukemic child, Pediatrics **56:**1034, 1975.
23. Spinetta, J. J., and Maloney, L. J.: The child with cancer; patterns of communication and denial, J. Consult. Clin. Psychol. in press.
24. Spinetta, J. J., Rigler, D., and Karon, M.: Anxiety in the dying child, Pediatrics **52:**841, 1973.
25. Spinetta, J. J., Rigler, D., and Karon, M.: Personal space as a measure of a dying child's sense of isolation, J. Consult. Clin. Psychol. **42:**751, 1974.
26. Spinetta, J. J., Spinetta, P. D., Kung, F., and Schwartz, D. B.: Emotional aspects of childhood cancer and leukemia; a handbook for parents, San Diego, 1976, Leukemia Society of America.
27. Spinetta, J. J., Swarner, J., Kard, T. L., and Sheposh, J. P.: Effective parental coping

following the death of a child from cancer. Paper presented at the meeting of the Western Psychological Association, San Francisco, April 1978.

28. Toch, R.: Too young to die. In Schoenberg, B., Carr, A., Peretz, D., and Kutscher, A., editors: Psychosocial aspects of terminal care, New York, 1972, Columbia University Press.

29. Waechter, E. H.: Children's awareness of fatal illness, Am. J. Nurs. **71:**1168, 1971.

30. Willis, D.: The families of terminally ill children; symptomatology and management, J. Clin. Child Psychol. **3:**32, 1974.

31. Yudkin, S.: Children and death, Lancet **1:**37, 1967.

CHAPTER 4

The dying child and the family: the skills of the social worker

HAL LIPTON

Although the work itself has been going on for a long time, writing about the poignant problems of the dying child and his family is difficult. Nevertheless, there is a small but growing literature on the subject. Some authors describe the emotional needs and struggles of the dying child,[5,15,17,18,19] his beleaguered parents, [3,6,13,19] and the staff that surrounds them.[1,2,7,14,20] Others focus, in general terms, on social work objectives, outcomes, and treatment modalities.[8,9,12,19]

An important element that is missing from the writings, however, is an examination of the skills of the social worker as he interacts with the patient, the family, and the staff. No matter how clearly one conceptualizes the inherent psychosocial problems and theorizes about desired outcomes, the questions remain: How does the professional act as he talks to parents? How are his skills realized as he interviews a dying child? How does he relate to the hospital staff?

The social worker has a unique function in the hospital division of labor. He gives no injections, takes no biopsies, and administers no medication—but he does pay close attention to the emotional reactions of patients, parents, and staff as they go through these procedures. Transactions between patient and staff are often complicated in hospitals. How much more serious, complicated, and emotionally charged they become around the tragedy of the dying child. While not responsible for informing patients or parents about potentially fatal diagnoses, the social worker is, however, available to help receivers and givers with these painful communications. Therefore, the social worker's basic interest is in advocating for both the patient and the staff subsystems as they communicate with each other. This frame of reference is partly illustrated by William Schwartz, who states:

> The general assignment of the social work profession is to mediate the process through which the individual and his society reach out for each other through a mutual need for self-fulfillment. This presupposes a re-

lationship between the individual and his nurturing group which he would describe as "symbiotic"—each needing the other for its own life and growth, and each reaching out to the other with all the strength it can command at a given moment. The social worker's field of intervention lies at the point where two forces meet: the individual's impetus toward health, growth, and belonging; and the organized efforts to integrate its parts into a productive and dynamic whole.[16]

The intent of this chapter is to focus on the social worker as he offers service to parents and patients, in particular, as part of a hematology/oncology health care team. The principles discussed, however, are applicable to a wide variety of both general and specialty care systems with modification where appropriate.

THE SETTING DESCRIBED

In 1973, I was appointed Director of Social Services at the Children's Hospital Medical Center of Akron, Ohio, a 238-bed, private, nonprofit, regional hospital that serves the pediatric needs of 18 urban and rural counties within a radius of 75 miles.

Before my arrival, the hematology team consisted of two full-time hematologists, two nurses, and two secretaries, who provided inpatient and outpatient care to children with hematologic disorders as well as cancer. The Social Services Department, organized in 1971, had not traditionally provided a specific worker for the Hematology Service, although various workers were assigned referrals periodically.

Orientation to the work—the first steps

In 1974, the Chief of Hematology, in response to parental requests, asked me to organize a group for the parents of children who had cancer. Before accepting a part in the project, I tried to look critically at the parents and myself. First, I talked with the parents and observed their behavior in the hematology clinic. While some were curious to learn how others coped, they kept most of their questions to themselves. Interactions between most parents seemed superficial: the clinic atmosphere was not conducive to sharing or mutual aid. However, many parents seemed receptive to the idea of a group.

Second, I examined my own ambivalence. Because I had not worked with the dying child previously, I wondered if I could handle the intensity of feeling that would be aroused in me by the powerful and pathetic emotions that would come out in the group. Would I become so depressed that all of my energies would go into protecting myself rather than into being emotionally available to the parents? Would I take my job home to the detriment of my own family?

On the other hand, earlier work with paraplegic patients had taught me a lot about working with the severely disabled, chronically ill patient and about mediation within hospital subsystems.[11] Work experience in other emotionally charged settings—with the parents of teenage drug abusers, with street gang members, and with groups of former mental patients—would also be valuable. Most important, I was excited about this new possibility, and deep down I felt that perhaps I could be useful to the parents and later to their children.

After searching the literature and talking with colleagues, I decided that working through my own fears about death would not be required. (I do not believe one ever completely resolves the issues involved in death. The essential perspective for the worker to maintain is that he is there to work on the client's problems, not his own.) With all of this in mind, I began to plan for an appropriate approach to the parents and to the already existing hematology team.

In an early conference with the hematologist, I outlined for him what I thought the parents' tasks were during the various phases of illness. I shared my biases about the upcoming process: there would be no final "solution," no magic phrases to erase the parental agonies. My only goal was to be as useful to the parents as possible at any given moment. I reasoned that the parents would need to feel that I was "in the struggle" with them, that understanding and kindness would be offered, and that I would try to lend my energies to theirs.

Doctor: "Good. You run this group. It's your baby. I don't want to know all the family problems."

Worker: "Fine. I like to work alone with groups and I think that the parents will feel freer to share intimate feelings without you, the medical authority, present. However, the group won't only work on deep feeling issues. They will need technical medical explanations about cancer, research, treatment, etc. When those issues arise, I'll need you to come to the group to help me out."

The doctor readily agreed to attend the group when invited.

In the above encounter, I sensed that the doctor had confidence in my ability to focus on the appropriate parental issues, was comfortable with my lack of jargon, and appreciated my limited objectives. In turn, I wanted him to know that I could not carry all the burden; I could not work in isolation. When the parents needed technical medical information, he would be the authority, I could not do this kind of communicating. What I did try to conceal from him, however, was the depth of my anxiety about leading the parent group.

After four meetings with the parents, when I began to be more confident of my skills and I knew positive feedback was going from the parents to the doctor, I approached him:

Worker: "Do you remember when I first said that I could handle this work?"
Doctor: "Yes, I do."
Worker: "Well, I lied. If you had known how scared I was, you wouldn't have let me start the group."
Doctor: (Leaning back and laughing heartily) "Don't worry. I've been at this work for 15 years and I'm still scared!"

My working relationship had now begun. At the outset, I had felt it necessary to hide some of my feelings from the clients and from the system. As my security grew, I was able to share my own feelings more honestly.

WORK WITH THE PARENTS

I received referrals from the team and also reached out myself to parents, carefully, in the outpatient clinic. In individual interviews I did not try to "sell" the group. Instead, I offered the group to those who seemed interested, and I looked for negative as well as positive feelings. The following interview with the mother of an 11-year-old leukemia patient illustrates an initial contact with a parent.

Parent: "Well, it may be a good idea to have a group for parents, but we never had a group before and my son has had leukemia for 2 years."
Worker: "Perhaps you're wondering if the group will do any good."
Parent: "What would we talk about?"
Worker: "I think we would work on some of the aggravations that parents have to face—like the strains on marriage, the energy it takes to cope with cancer, the angry and sad moments, problems around hospitalization."
Parent: "My problem is: Should I tell my son he has leukemia?"
Worker: "That must be a difficult and painful question."
Parent: "You don't know how hard it is."
Worker: "I'm sure I don't. What are you most worried about?"
Parent: "Would he give up if he knew?"
Worker: "What do you mean by giving up?"
Parent: "Would he refuse treatment? Would he stop going to school? He's getting older and I'm afraid he'll hear about it from someone outside the family."
Worker: "Would you want to talk to other parents who may be facing the same problem?"
Parent: "Who will be in the group?"
Worker: (Here I told the mother which parents were participating. When I mentioned a particular mother's name, she showed an interest.)
Parent: "I've often wondered if she's told her daughter about leukemia."

Worker: "It's hard to ask, isn't it?"
Parent: "Yes. Sometimes I think she wants to talk to me, too. But I can't talk here in the clinic. I don't want my son to overhear me."
Worker: "I don't blame you. But also the problem is so tragic and so personal that it's extremely hard to talk about it—even if the kids are not around."
Parent: "Maybe it would do some good to see how other parents stand it."
Worker: "I want you to know that neither I nor the doctor would be angry with you if you don't want to come. We know that some parents are comfortable sharing in a group and others are not."
Parent: "I'm afraid that I will cry."
Worker: "I think that you would have plenty of company."
Parent: "Would it be okay if my husband didn't come? He doesn't like to talk about our son's condition."
Worker: "If it makes you feel any better, there will be several mothers coming without their husbands."

The mother attended the group until her son died. In the above interview I reached for her self-interest and her doubts about participation. Parents may feel that participation is expected—that the doctor or the worker may be angry if they refuse a program that is "prescribed." Therefore, I tried to give the mother permission not to attend. Had she decided against participation, I would have given her the option of attending at a later date if she changed her mind or offered individual interviews as an alternative. Some parents initially refused any intervention and later asked for help; others used their own resources throughout the process.

Eighteen parents attended the first group meeting. There were six couples present; five mothers and one father participated without their spouses. All but five of the parents interviewed chose to attend.

One of my first tasks was to help clarify the purpose of the meetings—to establish the "contract" between the parents and the hospital:

Worker: "Dr. Clay [the hematologist] and the hospital administration are interested in providing the best possible service to you parents whose children have cancer. Dr. Clay, in particular, feels that more than just medical services is needed . . . . Having a group for parents gives you a chance to help each other as well as to receive help from me about some particular concerns. For example, some parents might worry about spending too much time with the child who has cancer and not enough with their other children. Tensions between husbands and wives can be severe. . . . At times grandparents and other relatives can be extremely helpful to you, and at other times they may aggravate you. When you come to the clinic or your child gets admitted, things may not always go well. You may have some gripes or suggestions . . . You may be torn about whether or not to tell your child what he has . . . . A group offers no magic, no solutions, but I think that it may help to make things just a little bit easier for you."

In this introduction I stated the hospital's stake in the work, used the dreaded word "cancer" directly, established the mutual aid theme, and gave some specific examples of the types of problems that could be shared and worked on in the group. I received encouraging feedback about my concept of purpose—parents said that I had touched on the problems they faced. Even that first day, they were ready to work:

Mrs. R: "My concern is whether or not to tell my son that he has leukemia."
Worker: "What does your son understand about his illness?"
Mrs. R: "He knows that he has a problem with his blood and he seems satisfied with that."
Worker: (In a direct effort to get the group members working) "Does anyone have any suggestions or comments?"
Mrs. H: "If he were my son, I would tell him. We like to be honest about everything."
Mrs. R: "I don't see what good telling him would do. He's doing fine. He goes to camp, he's a good athlete and a good student."
Mr. T: "What if he hears about his leukemia from an outsider?"
Mrs. R: "That's a real worry to me."
Worker: "I think telling your child about leukemia would be hard for anybody." (Many nods of assent) "But it's probably just a little different for each of you. Mrs. R, what is the hardest thing for you about telling?"
Mrs. R: "Would he give up if he knew?"
Worker: "That's a good question. Anybody want to try to answer that?" (Silence) "Has anybody told their child?"
Mrs. A: "One day my daughter told me that she thought she was going to die because they had taken out one kidney, and if the other gets bad, she could die. I asked her how she knew about losing one kidney, and she said, 'I heard, I don't remember who told me.' I told her that she lost her kidney because it had a tumor on it and if she had to lose the other kidney, her dad or I would give her one of ours. She said, 'Oh,' and then went off to play."
Worker: "How hard was it to tell your daughter about the tumor?"
Mrs. A: "Actually, I was relieved. Now I feel much more comfortable talking about it in front of her, especially when we come to clinic."
Worker: (To Mrs. R) "Has this helped you?"
Mrs. R: "I'm not sure."
Worker: "Hold onto your doubts. This is a very hard question. I'm sure we'll get back to it again and again."

In this excerpt parents were encouraged to use each other, react to one another, and share experiences. I tried to help the one mother hold onto her defenses about not "telling." She needed to deal with this problem more fully, and it was inappropriate for her to feel pressured into a decision while she was still ambivalent. In fact, this important theme was worked on many times in both group and individual sessions.

Although the parents shared many emotions at the meeting, most held back on expressing anger. In order to help the parents to be honest about their feelings, I shared mine: "When your child is very sick, you need the best of care and sometimes it might not seem that you are getting it." This enabled one set of parents to talk about their son's cancer. They described their horror, disbelief, and anguish upon hearing the diagnosis. The mother did the talking at first. When she described problems in getting proper cobalt treatments at another hospital that did not routinely deal with children, I said, "You'd think that in these days of modern medicine, they would know how to handle a simple matter like keeping a child still for treatment — boy, that must have made you mad."

The father then expressed the many angry feelings he had had about the lack of expertise in the cobalt arrangement. He had finally suggested to the oncologist that an x-ray technician from Children's Hospital accompany the child when cobalt treatment was needed, and this solved the problem. He got much positive reinforcement from the other parents for asserting himself.

At the second meeting, the parents began talking about a family that had the extreme misfortune of having two children with leukemia. They wanted some reassurance that this was a rare occurrence:

Worker: "Dr. Clay told me that it's extremely rare for two children in one family to have leukemia. But it's also very rare for one child in a family to get leukemia. You must sometimes wonder why it happened to your child."

The parents responded with a flood of personal hypotheses. One mother thought that her daughter's leukemia might be retribution for her own premarital sexual activity. Another parent discussed her child's illness as punishment for not attending church.

The theme of "Why did it happen to us?" was a pervasive and recurrent one. Perhaps if the parents could find a reason for the tragedy they could prevent it from happening to another child or to themselves. The parents, however, seemed satisfied to pose unanswerable questions and to know that others struggled with the same troubling problems.

For several months none of the parents in the group lost a child to cancer. However, the luck did not hold out indefinitely. At one meeting a mother shared her grief; her daughter was very close to death. The following interchange took place:

Jill: "My daughter will probably die in a few days."

Alice: (Amidst a general air of sadness in the room) "Don't worry, she'll make it."

Olivia: (Flatly) "Your daughter will get better."

Jill: "I'd like to think that she'll get better, but she's too far gone now."

Worker: "How sad and depressing this is for Jill and the rest of you, too." (Some of the parents were crying.) "Jill, what's your hope at this point?"

Jill: "My hope is that Betty doesn't suffer at the end."

Tina: "Is there anything we can do for you?"

Jill: "You already have. It really helps to feel that everybody cares so much." (Then, looking at me) "Just keep coming up to see me every day, Hal."

Worker: "I'll be here. The nurses have my phone number, and I can be reached whenever you need me."

In the above moments, it became clear that the denial of death was no longer useful to this mother. Yet, while death was inevitable, she still had hope—hope that her daughter would not suffer and that she would continue to receive support when she needed it most.

At one parent meeting, one of the hematologists was explaining some of the technical aspects of research that might have implications for the "cure" of cancer. After a while interest in the subject seemed to wane; the affect of the parents seemed low. Nobody in the room mentioned anything about death, yet several of the parents must have been thinking about it and the fact that research would be too late for their own children. When there was a lull in the meeting:

Worker: "This is a hard question for me to ask. Doctor, if all fails and the life of a child cannot be saved, can you keep him comfortable at the end?"

The meeting suddenly became alive, and all eyes focused on the doctor.

Doctor: "I'm glad you asked that question. There's plenty we can do."

He went on to explain various measures that could be taken to ease pain. The parents and the doctor were able to talk about other important issues surrounding the time of death.

Although it was not easy for me to ask the question about death, it was the very theme that the parents and the doctor needed to deal with at this moment in the meeting. The parents were very comforted to know more about the ending, what the doctor looks for, what the end is like, and most of all that the pain of the child could be eased or eliminated. Here it seems important to point out again that parental hopes do not entirely hinge upon whether or not the child is saved. Hope is also attached to the way the ending of life is handled and the assurance that the parents can have some control over the final event.

One morning I was notified that Alice, a 6-year-old leukemia patient, was very near death. Having helped the child's mother, a divorcee, in individual and group sessions, I knew that she was particularly concerned that her daughter's death be as painless as possible. There had been a turnover in nursing personnel on the unit, and my concern was that a nurse who was not familiar with Alice or her mother might not be comforting to them.

> Standing at the bedside with the mother and the nurse, I noticed that Alice's breathing seemed particularly labored. The child's moans were loud. The mother looked at me with tears in her eyes. Although she did not put it into words, I read her request: Please do something. I quietly asked the nurse if she didn't think that the child was too alert and needed something to lessen her pain. The nurse said that the child had been given some medication about an hour before and that the doctor would be back in another hour. Thinking that I could be overreacting, I stood at the bed for a few minutes longer. I felt that the child was getting more uncomfortable, that the end was nearing, and that the mother was becoming more anxious. Again, I said to the nurse: "I think that Dr. B is needed now. He could ease the pain." The nurse looked at her watch and said she was sure he would be back in an hour. Rather than argue with the nurse, I excused myself and went to the phone to call the doctor.
>
> Dr. B arrived almost immediately. He administered more medication, which eased the labored breathing—the child seemed free of pain. All in the room seemed a little more relaxed. Alice died about 10 minutes later.
>
> After comforting the mother and arranging with the nurses to have the mother spend some time alone with her daughter, I talked with the physician:
>
> **Dr. B:**   "I'm glad you called me. I stayed here all night because I was afraid to go home in case we had a snowstorm—I wanted to be around to do something at the end."
>
> **Worker:**   "Well, I'm glad you came. You were so kind and reassuring to Alice's mother. The way you handled things made all the difference. For a while I was worried that you wouldn't be here."
>
> **Dr. B:**   "I wish the nurse had called me. Do you know why she didn't?"
>
> I replied that I did not know why she hesitated and suggested to Dr. B that he talk to her directly. He said that he would.

The intervention was extremely comforting to the child, the mother, the doctor, and the nurse. While the mother grieved deeply at her great loss, she also had grateful feelings that her child did not suffer. The nurse told me that she had not been familiar with this child or parent and that she feared the doctor would criticize her if she called him unnecessarily. Her reluctance to call the doctor led to better communication between the nurse and the doctor and between the hematology team and the nursing service.

Unfortunately, the scope of this paper does not permit inclusion of other critical moments with the parents, for example at the time of diagnosis or after the child died. However, the basic principles of open communication whereby parents guide interventions by explicitly stating their concerns or by our getting to know them well enough so that even tacit communications can be correctly interpreted are sound ones and ones that we should cultivate with all families.

WORK WITH THE NURSES

After it was decided that a parent group would be formed, I was approached by several of the unit nurses who wanted to attend the group meetings from their inception:

Worker: "Why do you want to attend?"

Nurse A: "We need to know more about the families."

Nurse J: "We need to know what they go through and how we could be more helpful to them."

Worker: "I'm not so sure it would be a good idea just now. What would you want to do at the meetings?"

Nurse A: "We just want to listen and observe."

Worker: "I think that it's going to be very hard for the parents to share some of the painful problems they have. They will have to test me and learn to trust each other, too. The more professionals there, especially if just listening and observing, the harder it will be for them to open up. My hunch is that they will feel 'experimented with' if there are too many of us."

The nurses were obviously disappointed and angry with me.

Worker: "I know that you are angry with me. I think it is very important that more communication between parents and nurses take place. Just give me some time. The parents will want to talk with you—when they are ready. In the meantime, I will keep you posted about the issues that the parents raise."

It was difficult to turn the nurses down. However, professional observers, no matter how concerned, can inhibit parents. I knew that the parents would eventually find it in their self-interest to communicate directly with the nurses. Bringing the nurses and parents together could be mutually beneficial but only when both subsystems were ready for it as full partners in participation. Meanwhile, I assumed the role of liaison. With that role came increased communication with the nurses, who became more comfortable asking me for both formal and informal consultations about particularly difficult cases.

One of the most effective and easily used tools for transmission of information about parents to nurses (and other personnel) is the medical chart. Actually writing down an impression of concern in a brief, sharply focused note that could be referred to at change of shift, for example, helped the staff to understand and respond to a patient or parent more sensitively. The following chart entry was made soon after a dying patient was admitted:

> On the surface the mother of the patient appears to be calm and self-sufficient. On the inside, she feels panicky and lonely and would appreciate the staff reaching out to her. I am very familiar with this family and can be reached at (phone no. _____) any time if needed.

After the chart entry, the mother told me that the nurses were much friendlier than usual, that they were around to talk with her, offer her coffee, and spend time with *her* as well as her daughter.

Succinct notes are likely to be read. Rambling notes tend to obscure the essence of the worker's facts and feelings and hinder, rather than enhance, understanding and responsiveness on the part of the staff.

BRINGING THE NURSES AND PARENTS TOGETHER

During the parent meetings, the participants shared very good feelings about the treatment that their children received at the hospital. Beneath the surface, however, was an undercurrent of dissatisfaction about certain nursing procedures. I pursued the theme in the fifth parent meeting:

Worker: "You know, I think it must be awfully frightening to complain or speak up about problems with nurses when you feel that your child's care— even his life—depends on them. On the other hand, if you don't assert yourselves, the nurses can't help you. As you know, I talk with the nurses all the time. They would be willing to meet with you so that things could be a little smoother when your kids are admitted."

Mr. J: "Do they really want to meet with us?"

Mr. D: "I think we should meet with them. I know I sometimes get angry and nervous when my son is admitted. I'd like to talk with them when I'm calm. I want them to know that they shouldn't take my anger personally."

After a full discussion, the parents decided to invite the nurses to a meeting. The parents and the nurses were thus primed to meet about mutual efforts to improve communication. There were 14 nurses and 12 parents present when I began the meeting.

Worker: "The purpose of our being together is to work on some of the problems that exist between parents and nurses. While I can honestly say that the parents feel that nursing care is excellent and that there is a comfortable relationship most of the time, sometimes there are problems. From what the nurses tell me, things are usually fine between them and parents, but sometimes things don't go well. So, we are here to try to work on some of the issues that might make communication a bit easier. Is there an issue someone would like to start with?"

Nurse: "Sometimes, I would like to ask parents to do some things for their children during hospitalization, but I hesitate to ask because I'm afraid parents might think I'm trying to get out of doing my job—like feeding or diapering. What I'm really trying to do is keep the parent and the child as close as possible."

Worker: "Can you think of a time when you wanted to make such a request but hesitated?"

Nurse: "Yes. Once there was a child on the unit who was really sick—in fact, it was soon before he died. I thought the child would be comforted if his mother did the things she normally did for him at home."

Worker: "Did something stop you from asking the mother?"

Nurse: "Yes. She was a very quiet person. I really didn't know what she liked or didn't like—I was afraid that she might be angry."

This led to some very fruitful nursing-parent work on relationship problems.

It was useful to begin the meeting by making it clear that the communication gap was certainly not total—that generally the atmosphere was congenial. This had the effect of reducing, on both sides, the defensiveness that could have been mobilized. It also seemed important to help the nurse to be specific about the particular difficulties she faced in dealing with the mother in question. Bringing out the details served to deepen understanding and responsiveness between the nurses and the parents.

Important issues were shared by the parents: their anxiety when IVs run out or become blocked; their desire not to have a student nurse, unless unusually skilled, when their child's condition was critical; and their concern about coming across as too angry with the nurses on the wards when they really were angry at the cruel fate that had been imposed upon them.

The nurses, in turn, shared their own particular difficulties in reaching out to parents. They were all concerned about the children and their families and appreciated the fact that better communication between parents and staff led ultimately to more successful closure after a child's death.

Perhaps most important, as the parents and nurses grew to understand one another better, it became clearer to the staff that individual parents progressed through the stages of grief, as outlined by Kübler-Ross,[10] in very different ways. As a result, the nurses became much more flexible in their approach to the parents' distress and reactions. Our work together underlined the fact that there were numerous individuals to whom the parents could ventilate and to whom they could look for support. Thus we all learned to be less demanding and intrusive and to listen more carefully to the parents, respecting their decisions about those with whom, if anyone within the hospital system, they wished to share their grief.

WORK WITH THE CHILDREN

Work with the children began shortly after the start of the parent group. I established relationships with each of the children soon after diagnosis and continued contact during clinic visits. Permission from the parents was obtained, formally or informally, before any counselling with a child was undertaken.

My approach to the children was similar to that taken with the parents: no hidden messages, no "shoulds," no goals of changing them from one psychologic state to another. Rather, I would listen, show concern, offer help in the communication process, and tolerate negativism. Could I solve anything? Certainly not the big problems. But helping the dying child, even just a bit, would be satisfying to me and, ideally, useful to him and his family.

One of the ways of showing concern for the children was to provide craft supplies for them in the clinic waiting room. Siblings, often resentful of the attention that their afflicted family member received, were also given supplies to use.

At times, the atmosphere in the clinic was very lighthearted. At other times, when one or more children were not responding well to treatment, the atmosphere was sad. On one such negative day, the doctor gave me bad news: Tom, a 12-year-old with a chest tumor that had initially responded well to cobalt therapy, had just been found to have a recurrence. Tom's mother was concerned about her son's reaction to this setback. The mother and doctor asked me to see the boy.

> I entered the room in the clinic where Tom was receiving some IV medication to prevent nausea caused by the chemotherapy.

Worker: "Hi, Tom, I hear you're feeling lousy."

Tom: "I feel rotten. I've been throwing up all the time.

Worker: "You sound disgusted."

Tom: "I am. They found the tumor growing again."

Worker: "I'm very sorry to hear that. You look worried."

Tom: "I won't go through another operation. Last time I almost died from my operation."

Worker: "Who said that you need another operation?"
   Tom: "Nobody told me that I would need another operation."
Worker: "Well, don't scare yourself. Maybe you won't need one."

Tom went on to describe his absolute terror, both before and after his previous surgery. I reached for his anger. Tom was furious about his hair falling out again from chemotherapy and his constant nausea in recent days. He was angry with himself and God. He was terribly discouraged by his physical deterioration and the blows to his self-image.

I began to feel that Tom perceived his situation as totally hopeless and that he might wish to discontinue treatment. The parents and staff had many of the same impressions.

Worker: "Tom, your life sounds very discouraging. Do you feel like giving up?"
   Tom: "Sometimes I do. It's not worth it."
Worker: "When do you think about giving up?"
   Tom: "When I get so nauseated and when I start worrying about another operation. I would rather die than go through that again."
Worker: "I'm sorry that you have to go through such terror and misery. Do you have any way of distracting yourself from your troubles, or is there no way to shut them out of your mind?"
   Tom: (beginning to brighten) "Oh yeah, I do have a lot of fun. I like school and I watch football on television. Boy, that Penn State game was great on Saturday!"
Worker: "Did you see the long touchdown pass?"
   Tom: "That was a great pass."

       He was beginning to look much more calm, and I felt that he was completely distracted by his talk about sports. We then talked about recent satisfactions in school. After listening for a while, I ventured:

Worker: "Tom, your life sounds rotten at times but satisfying at other times."
   Tom: "I think that I'll feel a lot better when the nausea stops. Then I'll be okay and get back to school. . . . Hey, Hal, don't forget that when I feel better I want to go bowling with you."
Worker: "Whenever you're ready, Tom, I am."

       I realized that Tom still had a lot of hope and energy left.

In the preceding exchange, it was clear that the boy needed to talk to somebody about his discouragement, panic, and anger. By getting close to his near despair, listening, and encouraging further elaborations of his problems, I helped Tom get many of his negative feelings out of the way, so that he was able to get in touch with the satisfactions he still derived from life.

One afternoon, I visited a 3½-year-old child who had a recently discovered tumor. I had met the child and the parents on the previous day and had helped this verbal child with a picture puzzle. The following interchange occurred when I stopped to visit her again:

Jody: "How come they have to do all these things to me? Why do they have to stick me so much?"

Worker: "They're trying to help you get better, but those needles sure must hurt a lot sometimes."

Jody: "They do hurt a lot, *all* the time."

Worker: "I'm sorry they hurt so much, Jody. Do you cry when they hurt you?"

Jody: "Sometimes, I do."

Worker: "I think if I had to get stuck so much I would cry and I would be angry, too."

Jody: "I get very mad."

Worker: "I don't blame you. Well, as soon as you're well enough, you won't have to get stuck so much and you can go home."

Jody: "I want to go home soon."

Worker: "The doctors and nurses and your mom and dad want you to go home as soon as possible."

Jody: "Good. Will you help me make another puzzle now?"

Worker: "Sure."

The child needed some adult to listen to her complaints without minimizing them. The "keep a stiff upper lip" approach would have been useless and insensitive. If sad and angry feelings are tolerated, the child is less likely to feel isolated and depressed. In my contacts with phlebotomy technicians, nurses, and parents, I often explained the child's need to have acceptance of negative expression. Additionally, I suggested that whenever possible the child be given some choice—some control—over procedures. For example, if blood had to be drawn, a question like "which finger should I use today?" gives the child some control over his frightening treatment and usually results in a more cooperative patient.

Very young children were often fearful when unfamiliar adults entered their room in the hospital. Many patients feared yet another painful procedure—another separation from their parents. The following occurred when I visited a newly diagnosed leukemia patient, aged 20 months:

I entered the room and smiled at Mrs. S, who gently rocked her daughter Sally in her arms. Sally began whimpering apprehensively as I approached. She gripped her mother tightly.

Mrs. S: "This is Hal—he's a friend."

Sally: (Crying)

Worker: (Moving quickly to a chair) "I won't hurt you, Sally. I came to visit with you and your Mom."

I gave the child the space she needed and allowed her to keep an eye on me. I began talking softly with the mother. In a few moments the child, feeling secure again, fell asleep in her mother's arms.

At times the child and the parent need each other's undivided attention. The time they have together is extremely precious. The lack of privacy adds considerably to the strain of hospitalization. The professional needs to use his judgment about when interventions are necessary immediately and when they can wait for a more appropriate time.

I entered the room and saw that Terry and her mother were working on a puzzle together. The child, a 3-year-old lymphoma patient, was obviously enjoying playing with her mother. The mother was very pleased with the good interaction between them, because the child had recently been extremely irritable.

Mother: "Oh, hello. We were doing a puzzle together. Why don't you sit down?"
Worker: "I'm glad to see that Terry looks more comfortable today. You two seem to be enjoying yourselves. I think I'll come back later."
Mother: "Thank you. It's really a pleasure to see Terry so energetic again."
Worker: "I'll see you later, Terry."

In another situation, which looked similar to the above at first glance, I acted differently.

I greeted Arlene and her mother, who were looking at a coloring book together. The child seemed listless and disinterested. The mother looked frustrated. Nothing the mother could do sparked any enthusiasm from the 4-year-old, who was lethargic from her chemotherapy.

Worker: (To the mother) "You look frazzled."
Mother: "I'm worn out. She's been in a foul mood all day long."
Worker: "Can I do something for you?"
Mother: "I'd love to take a coffee break. But the nurses are short-handed today, and I want somebody to stay with Arlene because she's been so sick."

The child made no protest at the prospect of her mother leaving.

Worker: "I'll be glad to stay with Arlene." (The mother was delighted with the break. She left quickly). "Arlene, I can read you a story or I can just stay here and sit with you if you want to go to sleep."

The child smiled and soon fell asleep.

The parents of the fatally ill child are generally encouraged to treat the patient "normally." Since there is nothing "normal" about a child dying, it becomes very difficult for most parents to avoid indulging him—especially during hospitalization. While it is certainly beneficial for the child to receive some extra attention during periods of illness, some children will exploit parental concern and guilt. They can become almost tyrannical toward parents, siblings, and staff. At times the professional needs to help the parent deal directly with the child who becomes too demanding.

> I entered the room and greeted 6-year-old Jerry. His father and I were scheduled to talk about some problems over coffee.
>
> **Mr. M:** "Jerry, I have to go now and talk with Hal about something. I'll be back soon."
>
> **Jerry:** "No, you stay here."
>
> **Mr. M:** (Pleading) "Please, Jerry, I need a break. I've been here for hours."
>
> **Jerry:** (In an angry tone) "No, you stay right here."
>
> **Worker:** "Jerry, your dad and I are going for coffee. Would you like me to try to get a nurse to stay here with you or would you rather stay here by yourself until we get back?"
>
> **Jerry:** "I want Ellen [a nurse] to stay with me."
>
> **Worker:** "I'll see if Ellen can stay with you. If not, I'll try to get somebody else."
>
> **Jerry:** "Okay."
>
> **Mr. M:** (As we were leaving) "Thanks. I guess you do have to put your foot down sometimes."

Working with the dying child is an enormous challenge. Although there is no fixed formula, I found over and over again that the old skills of listening, partializing, allowing for negative expression, setting limits, giving choices, and paying close attention to details were always useful.

The siblings of the dying patient usually received reassurance and support around their own fears, guilt, anger, sadness, and resentments. This support was provided by parents and staff. In the following instance, however, these necessary communications apparently did not take place:

> I received a call from one of the inpatient units. Ned, an 11-year-old with osteomyelitis, was becoming completely withdrawn. For no obvious reason he would not come out from under the bed covers, refused to talk, and would not eat. I called Ned's mother and discovered that Ned's 13-year-old brother had died about 6 months before of leukemia. Feeling that there could be some connection between the brother's death and Ned's withdrawal, I approached Ned, who was lying under the covers, with an IV inserted in his arm.
>
> **Worker:** "Ned, my name is Hal Lipton from Social Work. I came up to talk to you. The doctors and nurses are worried about you."
>
> **Ned:** (No reply)
>
> **Worker:** (Loudly) "Ned, come out from under the covers—I think I can help you."
>
> **Ned:** (No reply)

Worker: (Loudly) "Ned, look at me. I won't hurt you."
 Ned: (Peeking from under the covers)
Worker: "I understand your brother died several months ago."
 Ned: (Nodded)
Worker: "I heard that you visited your brother before he died."
 Ned: (Nodded)
Worker: "Did he have an IV—just like you have?"
 Ned: (Nodded)
Worker: "Well, you just might think that you have the same thing that your brother did and that you're going to die, too."
 Ned: (Nodded)
Worker: "Ned, you aren't going to die. You have osteomyelitis of the knee, and your brother had leukemia. Your condition is completely different from your brother's."
 Ned: (Eyes wide open)
Worker: "I know you don't know me, and it's probably hard to trust me. But I did talk to the doctors and nurses, and they tell me that you'll be fine. I think you might want them to tell you what I just said."
 Ned: (Nodded and began smiling)
Worker: "I'll ask the doctors and nurses to talk to you as soon as possible."

> I informed the nurses and the resident physician about what had just occurred with Ned. The patient was reassured by the medical staff. Within the hour, he was out of his shell.

Ned's case exemplifies how important it is to counsel parents about both immediate and late-appearing problems that might arise among siblings of a child who dies and to offer either direct service or appropriate referral when necessary. This boy's hospitalization offered us an opportunity to help him and also reminded us of our ongoing obligation to these families.

CONCLUSION

Before beginning my work with fatally ill children and their parents, my concerns were personal ones: Was I emotionally ready for the work? Would I be able to help? After actually beginning, I needed to build up my professional authority and self-confidence. This required reaching out, sometimes in the face of resistance, to the patients, parents, and staff. It soon became apparent that the various subsystems needed to communicate more effectively with each other and I, in my social work role, needed to facilitate that process. As I became better able to perform my function, I became a member of the team.

In this chapter, little has been said about the interdisciplinary teamwork involved. In fact, formal team meetings were not held on a regular basis by the hematology staff. Collaboration did occur when needed—in the clinic, on the units, and in the doctor's office. I appreciated the fact that long meetings, merely for the sake of meeting, did not take place. There was a lot of work to be done, and time was precious. The team members had tremendous faith in one another and knew that essential communication would take place. Perhaps the most important contribution that I made was in deepening that communication among those involved in work with the dying child.

My greatest frustration was that other job responsibilities did not allow for more practical and research work with the patients, parents, and staff. For example, more needs to be known about the skills required to respond appropriately to the dying child and his siblings. More work needs to be done with the family *after* the child has died. Additionally, we need a greater understanding of how personality factors affect the course of hospital treatment.

Those who would venture into this kind of social work need not only good technical supervision but emotional support as well. This work calls for courage—the courage to get as deeply involved as is therapeutically appropriate with people in severe difficulty.

I learned, from repeated intervention, that kindness and effort on the part of all staff are tremendously important—even if the life of a child cannot be saved. One mother whose child died after a long illness, put it this way:

> . . . the only thing, when the chips are down, that really matters is kindness. . . . To you who are professionals, to you who have been in the hospital all day long with sick kids and dying kids, I know you have to go home at night and live with yourself and your family, and it's hard. I know you have to turn it off but, please, in educating yourself to turn it off so you can carry on functions that you have to do, please don't stifle your compassion or your kindness. . . .[4]

When kindness is disciplined, functional, and built into the system, it becomes visible as professional skill.

REFERENCES

1. Artiss, K. L., and Levine, A. S.: Doctor-patient relation in severe illness, N. Engl. J. Med. **288:**1210, 1973.
2. Binger, C. M., Ablin, A. R., Feuerstein, R. C., and others: Childhood leukemia; emotional impact on patient and family, N. Engl. J. Med. **280:**414, 1969.
3. Bozeman, M. F., Orbach, C. E., and Sutherland, A. M.: Psychological impact of cancer and its treatment. The adaptation of mothers to the threatened loss of their children through leukemia, part 1, Cancer **8:**1, 1955.
4. Fischoff, J., and O'Brien, N.: After the child dies, J. Pediatr. **88:**140, 1976.

5. Freud, A.: The role of bodily illness in the mental life of children, Psychoanal. Study Child **7:**69, 1952.
6. Friedman, S. B., Chodoff, P. Mason, J. W., and Hamburg, D. A.: Behavioral observations on parents anticipating the death of a child, Pediatrics **32:**610, 1963.
7. Green, M. Care of the dying child, Pediatrics **40:** 492, 1967.
8. Heffron, W. A., Bommelaere, K., and Masters, R.: Group discussions with the parents of leukemic children, Pediatrics **52:**831, 1973.
9. Knapp, V. S., and Hansen, H. H.: Helping the parents of children with leukemia, Soc. Work **18:**70, 1977.
10. Kübler-Ross, E.: On death and dying, New York, 1969, Macmillan, Inc.
11. Lipton, H., and Malter, S.: The social worker as mediator on a hospital ward. In Schwartz, W., and Zalba, S. P., editors: The practice of group work, New York, 1971, Columbia University Press.
12. Mann, J. K., and others: The social worker on the critical care team, Nurs. Supervisor September 1977, p. 62.
13. Orbach, C. E., Sutherland, A. M., and Bozeman, M. F.: Psychological impact of cancer and its treatment. III. The adaptation of mothers to the threatened loss of their children through leukemia; part 2, Cancer **8:**20, 1955.
14. Rothenberg, M. B.: Reaction of those who treat children with cancer, Pediatrics **40:**507, 1967.
15. Schowalter, J. E.: The child's reaction to his own terminal illness. In Schoenberg, B., Carr, A., Peretz, D. and Kutscher, A., editors: Loss and grief; psychological management in medical practice, New York, 1970, Columbia University Press.
16. Schwartz, W.: The social worker in the group, The Social Welfare Forum New York, 1961, Columbia University Press.
17. Solnit, A. J., and Green, N.: The pediatric management of the dying child; part II. The child's reaction to the fear of dying. In Solnit, A. J., and Provence, S., editors: Modern perspectives in child development, New York, 1963, New York International Universities Press.
18. Spinetta, J. J., and Maloney, L. J.: Death anxiety in the outpatient leukemic child, Pediatrics **56:**1034, 1975.
19. Travis, G.: Leukemia. Chronic Illness in Children, Stanford, Calif., 1976, Stanford University Press.
20. Wiener, J. M.: Responses of medical personnel to the fatal illness of a child. In Schoenberg, B., Carr, A., Peretz, D., and Kutscher, A., editors: Loss and grief; psychological management in medical practice, New York, 1970, Columbia University Press.

CHAPTER 5

The primary physician and the family during the terminal illness and afterwards

MORRIS A. WESSEL

Most pediatricians function as primary physicians, initiating their relationship with a family when a first infant is born. They assume responsibility for preventive health care and for the majority of illnesses and psychologic crises that occur during infancy, childhood, and adolescence. A major component of pediatric care is the provision of support for families as they experience life's developmental tasks, cope with illnesses and, at times, with the death of a loved one.

A primary practitioner often serves as the initial contact with the health care system for the family. The extent of his professional service varies. In the first few weeks of parenthood when parents experience exhaustion and discouragement, the physician's role includes a great deal of reassurance and support. During an acute illness, the psychologic stresses may demand as much consideration as do the specific symptoms of the illness. The primary physician's contact with a family over many years often builds a mutual relationship of trust, which is a great asset when he assumes responsibility for care during a serious illness.

The primary physician usually arranges for consultation with appropriate specialists when a patient has symptoms suggestive of serious disease. The extent of his responsibility depends on the illness, his working relationship with colleagues, and geographic factors. He may arrange for consultation and laboratory studies and assume responsibility for the continuous care of the patient, or he may decide to recommend that a colleague take on the responsibility for definitive treatment. There is greater possibility for a primary physician to maintain active involvement when a patient is hospitalized at a nearby medical center than when the hospital is located in a distant community. However, even when geographic factors prevent a primary physician from assuming a daily role, he can be supportive by maintaining telephone contact with his patient and members of the immediate family. He can be helpful in either case by meeting with the family and patient after initial studies are completed in order to share with them the clinical impressions and make recommendations for further evaluation and plans for continued care.

Most parents suspect when a child's symptoms reflect a serious illness. The immediate response when they discover their worst fears to be true is to be dazed and numb.[7] They may deny, at least verbally, the seriousness of the illness. They may say, "I hear you, but it can't be. I know he doesn't have what you say he does. I am certain he will be all right."

This initial denial is normal. It makes an intolerable situation tolerable. Parents and children, too, need to know that their doctor understands and accepts their behavior and that he and his colleagues will continue to provide care and support as they cope with the overwhelming nature of the illness. Parents are usually bitter and angry at this moment. They are seized with powerlessness as they realize their inability, even with their doctor's help, to protect their child from harm.[2,4,11] The doctor who has a long-standing relationship with a family can offer valuable support through this critical life crisis. No matter how dedicated, conscientious, thoughtful, or caring hospital-based consultants and house officers may be, they are likely to find it difficult to establish the trusting relationship that exists between a family and the primary physician. The consultant is often responsible for a number of critically ill patients. He can involve himself only to a limited degree with each family. The primary physician, who may request that the consultant assume definitive responsibility for the care of his patient, nevertheless has a unique base from which to offer ongoing support.

COORDINATING CARE FOR HOSPITALIZED PATIENTS

Any hospitalized patient should have one doctor designated clearly as the responsible physician who oversees the patient's care and coordinates recommendations for treatment. A primary physician or a hospital- or community-based consultant may assume this role. This physician should visit with the patient and family frequently; he should be the one to answer questions raised by the patient and relatives. There are many advantages when a primary physician with a long-standing relationship with a family can assume this coordinating role, because his relationship, developed over the years, may serve as a bulwark of support during a critical illness.

The responsibility for coordinating a patient's care and communicating with relatives is all too often delegated to house officers, who are overburdened with other duties and likely to be reassigned to other services at critical moments in a patient's illness.

It is unfortunate that communication between consultants, house officers, and primary care physicians is so often minimal and that the family's physician becomes isolated from the hospital-based team. The more critical the decisions become, the more vulnerable family, patient, and doctors are to misunderstanding. Lack of active involvement of the primary physician deprives a patient and family of the sustaining and comforting relationship of their personal doctor.

Even when a hospital-based consultant assumes the role of the responsible physician in charge of a patient's treatment, the primary physician still has an important role. Families do not expect a primary physician to provide total care of a patient. They realize that a serious illness demands the skills of many specialists. However, families and patients do have the right to expect that their primary physician will support them during the complicated crises and the moments of anguish that occur when one experiences a critical or terminal illness.

When care takes place largely on an ambulatory basis, as is the case with many individuals with leukemia, hospitalization may occur only a few hours before death, or death may take place at home. Ida Martinson of the University of Minnesota reports satisfying experiences with leukemic children whose parents preferred to have their children die at home.[8] The primary physician should be notified immediately at the time of death. His prompt appearance at the hospital or at the home offers great comfort at this tragic moment. When geographic factors make this impossible, an immediate telephone call from the primary physician to a family member is comforting. The family needs to know that their personal physician is available to help them cope with their loss. The primary physician is too often prevented from functioning at this critical moment because he is not notified of the patient's death.

A brief daily visit with the family and patient during the terminal phase of life is important. Whenever decisions are made concerning the use of respirators and other support systems, family members need to know that their doctors and nurses do care about them and the patient who is dying. The collaborative role of the primary physician and his hospital-based colleagues is illustrated by a recent conference that took place in a newborn intensive care unit. The patient, a critically ill, 1400-gram infant who had survived two pneumothoraces and seemed to be doing well, suddenly suffered a massive intracranial hemorrhage. The primary physician arranged to meet with the parents, the neonatologist, the social worker, and several nurses. The neonatologist presented the hopelessness of the situation, stating that if the baby did survive he would be severely damaged neurologically. Death appeared to be imminent. Life could be prolonged by the use of a respirator but only for a few days.

The question was whether or not a respirator should be used to maintain life if death appeared to be imminent. The mother turned to her primary pediatrician saying, "We have known you for 10 years; you took care of our other child. We trust you to do what's best for us and our baby." The primary physician, after further discussion with the parents, decided that when it appeared as though the baby was about to die, a respirator would not be used. The infant died quietly 14 hours later. There was no feeling among the nurses or the house officers that they should institute heroic measures to prolong life. When the primary physician telephoned to notify the mother of the baby's death, she responded that she had been expecting the call and finished the conversation by saying, "You all loved him so much."

The parental response at this tragic moment reflects the superb, sensitive attention of the staff of the newborn intensive care unit. Several house officers and nurses remarked later that even though death did occur, they felt a sense of personal and professional satisfaction in the care of this infant. A primary physician, when involved as in this instance, is uniquely able to perform an important supportive role, though he may not have the direct responsibility for the care of the patient.

Every medical and psychologic skill must be used constructively to care for a patient and to support a family through the terminal phase of life and afterwards. This includes frequent and open communication between health care givers, family members, and whenever possible, the patient. Neither the patient nor relatives should ever feel alone as they begin to grieve in anticipation of death.

The unique manner in which a health care team that was transported from China to Switzerland provided a community of suport in the final weeks of Edgar Snow's life is portrayed eloquently in Lois Wheeler Snow's memoir.[10] Health care workers reading this book will gain valuable insight into the extensive therapeutic benefits that can accrue when supportive roles receive high priority during the terminal phase of life.

Hospital staff members, physically and psychologically exhausted by the unending demands of the critical illnesses in many of their patients, often have little energy left to meet the needs of relatives coping with the imminent death of a loved one. Wende Bowie portrays vividly her husband's and her own feelings during their baby's short life in a newborn intensive care unit. What is sad in this experience is that although the staff obviously worked diligently to the point of exhaustion, poor communication between doctors, nurses, and parents created confusion, intensifying the parents' anguish unnecessarily.[1]

I do not wish to imply that hospital-based specialists fail to put human values in command—far from it! However, I do believe that when the end is imminent or when a death occurs, a family faces the fact that specialized skills of the hospital-based physicians can no longer offer a cure. No matter how compassionate consultants and house officers may be, it is too much to expect that they can take on single-handedly the task of tending to the needs of the family at this tragic moment and during bereavement.

All physicians feel a sense of helplessness when a death occurs. They must deal with the fact that medical skill and knowledge have failed. This is difficult to accept, because doctors are so largely motivated in their choice of profession by the wish to cure illness and prevent death.

Another factor that has limited many physicians in being helpful at this critical moment has been the lack of descriptive material dealing with normal manifestations of grief. Fortunately, recent publications by Colin Murray Parkes[9] and Erna Furman[5] present clinical studies that are helpful for physicians seeking to understand this important syndrome.

How much anyone—professional, friend, or relative—extends help to a bereaved family depends on the magnitude of the grieving person's distress, the confidence one has in one's ability to bear this distress, one's understanding of the grief process, and how worthwhile one thinks it is to be of service at this time.[5] When geographic factors allow cooperative relationships between the primary physician and the hospital staff during the last days of life, at the moment of death, and afterwards, these relationships offer opportunity for mutual participation in the difficult task of professional comfort and support of a family. The presence of the primary physician at the hospital or at the home at the time of death or shortly afterwards demonstrates that he cares about the family.

Most families work out their own arrangements for funeral services reflecting their own needs and beliefs. One must realize that there can be no "nice" funeral. However, the gathering of relatives and friends and the ritual of the service provide an opportunity for human beings to support one another as they grieve in a socially prescribed manner.

HELPING CHILDREN COPE WITH GRIEF

The primary physician may on occasion be asked to suggest ways of helping a child when a loved one dies. All too often adults are so preoccupied with their own grief that little consideration is given to the needs of a child. We all wish that a child could be spared the pain of losing someone he loves. The intensity of this wish may impede one's ability to provide appropriate support. The professional, relative, or friend who assumes that a child is too young to understand may really be feeling that the anticipated poignancy of the child's reaction will be so heart-rending that he would rather avoid the task of trying to help the child at all. This common avoidance by adults of this difficult task demonstrates little consideration for the child, who is then left alone to struggle with the loss. A bereaved child needs explanation, comfort, and support just as a bereaved adult does.

Children often grasp the meaning of death at an earlier age than many people realize. The previous experience of losing a pet through death, for example, can provide a child with the basis for beginning to comprehend the death and loss of an important person. There is, of course, an enormous difference in a child's capacity to understand the death of an animal pet as compared with the loss of a close family member—particularly a parent or sibling. However, the value of having previously lost a pet was demonstrated quite vividly when I was asked by a school principal to meet with a class of first grade children whose teacher had died the day before. The children asked me to take them to see their teacher. They were openly critical of me because I could not fulfill their demands. While I struggled to find an appopriate explanation of why their demands were impossible to meet, a seven-year-old girl raised her hand saying, "I don't think it would do any good if we could see Mrs. Smith. My dog was hit by a car last week, and he was stiff and cold. When I tried to pet him, he didn't even know I was there. I don't think Mrs. Smith would know we were there either."[12] Thanks to this little girl's comments, it became easier for me to discuss with the children the inaccessibility of a deceased person.

A primary physician can help a family achieve open communication when the death of a loved one is imminent. It is inevitable that a child feels left out and deserted by members of the family who are preoccupied with grief. It helps, even when a child is as young as 3, to be told, "Mommy is upset because Grandpa is sick. He's very sick and may die." This explanation helps the child know why adults are acting in a strange manner; it frees the child to some degree of the belief that his parents' withdrawn attitude is caused by anything he may have done to incur wrath.

The palpable gloom in a house at the time of death is frightening to a child. When he is whisked away to the home of a neighbor or relative, or sent to his room with no explanation, he can only be bewildered and deeply hurt. Health professionals, teachers, and clergymen should intervene at this critical moment, helping adults to be cognizant of children's needs during this crisis.

Parents often ask whether or not a child should attend a funeral. A child of 4 or older should make this decision for himself. One can discuss the type of service to be held and the fact that everyone will be sad and may be crying. An appropriate way of presenting the option is: "We will all be very sad because we miss him so much. I will be sad, too. There will be some music and prayers. Our minister (rabbi or priest) will talk about Grandpa or read some psalms. If you would like to come with us, I'll ask (a relative, close friend, or a babysitter) to join us. If you would rather stay home, that's all right, too. He (she) will stay at home with you." A child may find the gathering of grieving relatives and friends and the ritual supporative. On the other hand, he may sense that the experience is more than he can cope with and decide to remain at home.

Careful choice of words is important when one is explaining to a child what happens after death. The discussion should reflect honestly the philosophic and religious beliefs of a family. The concept of life hereafter is difficult for a child to comprehend until the second decade of life. When this belief is consistent with the family's philosophy, it is wise to present the idea in forthright terms such as, "The body of a person who dies is placed in a special box in a cemetery; I'll show you where that is. I like to believe that part of the person—the spirit and things we love him for—rests in a place called heaven, far, far away, where there is no pain, hunger, or suffering. He will remember and we must, too, all the nice times we had together."

Explanations involving a description of how God needs the deceased to work in heaven or God's coming down and taking him to heaven may offer adults comfort and solace. This is little help to a child, however, who wants his beloved person to return at once. This conceptualization of death is likely to encourage distrust and hatred of a God who swoops up a beloved adult, leaving a child deserted. The "I like to believe" presentation allows a child to accept or reject this point of view. The use of the word sleep in reference to death is unwise, for it creates undue anxiety. A child is likely to fear that he too may die while asleep and God might carry him off to heaven. "No longer living" or "absence of life" is a preferable way of describing the concept of death.[5,6] A child is quick to sense dishonesty and insincerity. An adult who presents a concept of life hereafter, hoping that even though it is alien to his own convictions it will somehow be helpful to a child, only creates confusion and engenders a serious distrust.

Hope for the return of a beloved deceased person is present in all bereaved human beings. A child may assume that a person who dies disappears voluntarily. He feels deserted; he wonders what he may have done to cause someone he loved to leave him. He recalls angry feelings he once had toward the deceased, or a refusal to honor a request, wondering whether these thoughts or actions might in some magical way be responsible for the person's disappearance. To allow a child to assume responsibility for the absence of a loved one is a heavy burden. It can be diminished somewhat by saying "I know you wonder why he died. He was very sick (or hurt very badly or was very old and weak); there was nothing you did or said that could have caused him to die."

Adults who wish to help a bereaved child must appreciate the limits of what can be done to alleviate sadness. They must be able to respect a child's feelings and need to be sad. The best adults can offer is to comfort and support a child grappling with the meaning of death and the loss of an important person he loved and who loved him. Adults must recognize that the initial moment of sadness may be replaced by a return to normal behavior as a denial that anything has happened. This short sadness span is a protection against having to deal with the reality of the loss all at once. Most children, particularly when they are well cared for by an understanding adult, will sooner or later begin to discuss their loss and express their feelings of sadness.[5,6,12,13]

TREATING THE BEREAVED

Many physicians find it appropriate to offer bereaved family members the opportunity to confer a few weeks after the death. Indeed, as Colin Murray Parkes points out, bereaved individuals often spontaneously consult doctors to discuss their own physical and psychologic states.[9] Early in my pediatric practice, several families sought opportunities to meet with me some weeks after the deaths of their children. They wanted to know more about the particular diseases, to learn about autopsy findings, and also to share with me their feelings of grief. Since this initial experience 25 years ago, I have made it routine practice to telephone a family a few weeks after a death, suggesting that they might like to confer with me either in my office or at their home. Parents invariably accept this offer to meet. They seem grateful for the opportunity to talk about their problems and feelings.[3]

One may ask whether grief and bereavement represent illnesses and if bereaved individuals need to see a doctor. Grieving individuals do experience physical and psychologic symptoms. They suffer with exhaustion; they move slowly; they have overwhelming episodes of loneliness accompanied by outbursts of intense sobbing; they have a decrease in appetite and lose weight; they have difficulty sleeping and are likely to experience nightmares. Symptoms related to underlying cardiovascular, rheumatic, or gastrointestinal diseases may become intensified. What is less well known is that the death rate among widows and widowers during the first 6 months of bereavement is 40% higher than that in a comparable population who have not experienced a recent death of a loved one. Most of the deaths during bereavement are due to cardiovascular disease.[9] A physician should take careful notice of symptoms presented by individuals suffering a recent loss and consider carefully the need for a medical examination.

Grieving individuals are often frightened by the intensity of their reactions and the degree of their exhaustion. Hallucinatory experiences, which commonly appear during the initial phase of bereavement, can be unnerving, even though they represent a common coping mechanism early in the adaptation to a loss. These normal reactions may cause a bereaved individual to wonder whether he might be "crazy."

Bereaved individuals may bear a great deal of guilt, wondering if the patient might have lived had they done something differently. Their bitterness, expressed toward the hospital, nurses, doctors, relatives, clergymen, and even God, can be overwhelming. A physician must realize that, although this anger may be focused on him, these intense feelings are a general reaction to a devastating loss and are not personally directed.[9]

The loss of a child is a particularly severe blow because parents see in their children the promise of their own unrealized hopes and achievements.

UNDERSTANDING ADOLESCENT REACTIONS TO PARENTAL LOSS

Adolescents who lose a parent have unique problems because of their stages in development.[14] The predominant task in adolescence is the difficult struggle to free oneself of the close dependence on parents. The normal family structure allows young people to break away repeatedly and try a variety of activities outside the immediate family. Yet during these phases of independence when an adolescent is often critical of and at times openly hostile to parents, there always remains the comforting option of regressing and being taken care of like a child as in former years. Even during intense bursts of independence, an adolescent often remains at home, or if living away, returns home periodically where his parents will be available to provide basic care.

These vacillating ways in which adolescents normally relate to adults must be kept in mind when one is analyzing the adolescent's reaction to the loss of a parent. It is one experience to struggle to be independent, knowing that both parents are available when needed. It is quite a different experience when death removes a parent in the midst of an adolescent's struggle for emancipation. A parent is so necessary for healthy development that adolescents are likely to cling with great fervor to the idea that the dead parent is still very much alive and available. Teenagers talk incessantly about the sterling qualities of the deceased parent, forgetting characteristics that only a few months ago were the basis for intense criticism. This idealization occurs even in families where in reality the deceased adult may have been an ineffective parent.

The bereaved adolescent may seek an appointment with a doctor because of concern about a pain or rash or other discomfort. He actually may be looking for reassurance about his health; he also may be seeking a replacement for the deceased parent.

The physician should perform a thorough examination even though the symptoms appear to reflect the mourning process. One must remember, however, that underlying conditions such as malabsorption syndrome, regional ileitis, peptic ulcer, and asthma may become clinically symptomatic during the stress of bereavement.

The relationship between an adolescent and the remaining parent needs consideration. The living parent is usually grief-stricken and preoccupied. The adolescent is thus doubly deprived; he experiences the loss of the deceased parent and the loss due to the inaccessibility of the remaining parent. Many adolescents attempt to comfort the grieving parent, only to be rebuffed and feel a sense of failure. On the other hand, the comforting may be so successful that the adolescent and the parent develop a close relationship that interferes with a healthy grieving process in both individuals. The institution of temporary sleeping arrangements with a parent and adolescent in the same room, or in the same bed, is a common adaptation to loneliness during bereavement. This comforts both generations for the moment. However, these arrangements, once initiated, may extend for months and years and limit the possibility of either person mourning and adjusting in a healthy way to the loss. Even in the absence of these intimate sleeping arrangements, the relationship following the loss of a parent can become so intertwined that it inhibits the adolescent's emancipation.

Adults often mourn at a faster pace and more completely than do children and adolescents. They gradually detach themselves from the beloved spouse who has died and are ready to seek new alliances and remarry.

Because the two generations may be out of phase in their grieving, a sensitive physician should be alert to the confusion children and adolescents often experience when a parent remarries. If the remaining parent and a proposed marital partner seek an opportunity to discuss their concerns with a physician as they anticipate the new family relationship, the physician can offer guidance and reassurance. When a new spouse offers sensitive parental care, a bereaved child or adolescent, because he is being well taken care of, may proceed with mourning more freely than before the new marriage. He may openly express for the first time his sadness over the death of his parent. This freedom to mourn is a reflection of successful care by the new parent. It is not a sign of parental failure. Explaining this phenomenon can be very reassuring and helpful to husband and wife.

The physician who feels defeated following the death of a patient may find personal and professional satisfaction in continuing his relationship with the family as he helps them grieve, mourn, and regain equilibrium.

Bereaved adults and children need to know that their doctors care about them. The suggestion that the physician's role is "to cure sometimes, to relieve often, to comfort always" is as true now as when enunciated by Edward Trudeau more than 50 years ago.

REFERENCES

1. Bowie, W. K.: Story of a first born, Omega **8:**1, 1977.
2. Burton, L.: Tolerating the intolerable; the problems facing parents and children following diagnosis. In Burton, L., editor: Care of the child facing death, Boston, 1974, Routledge & Kegan Paul.
3. Fischoff, J., and O'Brien, N.: After the child dies, J. Pediatr. **88:**140, 1976.
4. Friedman, S., Chodoff, P., Mason, J., and Hamburg, D.: Behavioral observations on parents anticipating the death of a child, Pediatrics **32:**620, 1963.
5. Furman, E.: A child's parent dies; studies in childhood bereavement, New Haven, 1974, Yale University Press.
6. Furman, R.: The child's reaction to death in a family. Schoenberg, B., Carr, A., Peretz, D., and Kutscher, A., editors: Loss and grief, New York, 1970, Columbia University Press.
7. Futterman, E., Hoffman, I., and Sabshin, M.: Parental anticipatory mourning. In Schoenberg, B., Carr, A., Peretz, D., and Kutscher, A., editors: Psychosocial aspects of terminal care, New York, 1972, Columbia University Press.
8. Martinson, I., editor: Home care for the dying child; professional and family perspectives, New York, 1976, Appleton-Century-Crofts.
9. Parkes, C. M.: Bereavement; studies of grief in adult life. New York, 1972, International Universities Press.
10. Snow, L.: A death with dignity; when the Chinese came, New York, 1974, Random House.
11. Solnit, A., and Green, M.: Psychological considerations in the management of deaths on pediatric hospital services, Pediatrics **24:**106, 1959.
12. Wessel, M.: Death of an adult—and its impact upon the child, Clin. Pediatr. **2:**28, 1973.
13. Wessel, M.: A death in the family; the impact on children, J. A. M. A. **234:**865, 1975.
14. Wessel, M.: The adolescent and death of a parent. In Gallagher, R., Heald, F., and Garrell, D., editors: Medical care of the adolescent, New York, 1976, Appleton-Century-Crofts.

CHAPTER 6

Alternative environments for care of the dying child: hospice, hospital, or home

IDA M. MARTINSON

In this chapter, background material will be given on three alternatives for care of a dying child: (1) a hospice, (2) a special unit for the dying within a hospital, and (3) home care. The hospice, hospital, and home care will be examined from the viewpoints of the child, of the family, and of the health care professional, especially the nurse. In these alternative environments for the dying child, there is an underlying assumption that there is consideration for the whole individual—his emotional, physical, and cognitive stresses—and equally important, for the social unit in which he is most intimately involved: his family.

The stress from the death of a child causes the parents to be particularly vulnerable to both physical and psychologic disease.[1] At the same time, appropriate care management has the potential to decrease or prevent the occurrence of such postdeath family problems. Such care is not only a legitimate concern of health professionals as preventive health, but is also a responsibility.

HOSPICE CARE

The hospice is a relatively new concept in American health care delivery systems.[5] The term hospice originally indicated an open door and hospitality for weary travelers. The modern use of the term hospice as a terminal care center has come into being during the past decade and recognizes the need of the travelers, not only for physical care, but for spiritual and emotional care as well. Its aim is to help a person feel a part of ongoing life and to be allowed to do what is especially significant to him before life comes to an end. Together patients and their families are seen as an integral whole, the well-being of each member affecting in some way that of the others. Patient care services are available both at home and in special facilities where individual life styles can be respected, accepted, and supported. Because the need for help can occur at any time, services must be available around the clock. Care under the hospice concept does not end when the patient dies; help is afforded parents and other family members in the mourning processes as well.

The hospital I am most familiar with and the one most generally known is St. Christopher's Hospice in London. It was founded by Cicely Saunders, who is also its medical director. The goal of St. Christopher's is to welcome and to help the family, in the wards and in their homes, both before and after the death of a patient. Family members, including young children, are a part of hospice care, and they spend a great deal of time with the patient and talking to the staff, other patients, and visitors. The usual supply of medical apparatus is lacking, but human warmth is abundant.

In the United States, Hospice, Inc. in New Haven, Connecticut, which was modeled after St. Christopher's, is recommended as a model for all new hospice groups throughout this country. Although it is limited at present to home care services, construction is progressing, and the intention is to include an in-hospice care program.

The New Haven hospice team consists of professional staff members, including nurses, ministers, social workers, and physicians as well as volunteers who act as surrogate friends, relatives, and homemakers to the dying. These people make up teams who consult with the attending physician and evaluate individual family needs. They provide care at home for both the patient and his family. Besides medical and nursing care, the hospice program includes psychologic support, such as listening to the patient and his family members talk about the impending death. The medical director, Dr. Sylvia Lack, states, "We see ourselves as helping people live."[3]

HOSPITAL CARE

Concern for the holistic approach to the dying child and his family is increasingly evident in the contemporary hospital situation. Consider a hospital unit at the University of Minnesota, where day beds are available for parents' use. Here parents and siblings are given unlimited visiting privileges, and if desired, parents may stay up nights with their child. Hospitals on the whole are changing their admission procedures. In many hospitals, the child is settled in his room before the parents are asked to fill out the lengthy forms in the admission room. In hospital units, when the staff and family are aware that the child will die, there is a growing tendency for increased attention to be given to the child and the family.

At the Royal Victoria Hospital in Montreal, Canada, special emphasis is placed on providing care for the family of a dying patient.[4] A task force on grief was formed in 1973. This then became the ad hoc committee on thanatology. This multidisciplinary group studied the defects in the delivery of health care to the dying and their families at the Royal Victoria Hospital. They spent time pursuing what needs to be done, and from this a palliative care service was established as a separate unit within the general hospital. This unit is concerned primarily with comfort care of patients and support of their families. This hospital service has regular department rounds for the continual education of staff and students. Bereavement follow-up of the families recently involved with the ward is now routinely done and reported to the staff.

Another hospital-based approach to special care of the dying is in St. Luke's Hospital in New York City. It is also adapting the hospice approach within an acute hospital setting. Within the metropolitan area of St. Paul–Minneapolis, several hospitals are actively studying the feasibility of such care. At least one of these hospitals is planning to include dying children in their service population.

HOME CARE

When a family is able to participate in the life of the patient, particularly if the patient is cared for at home, perhaps the separation that takes place in death is easier to bear. It has been observed that family members who are involved in the care are less prone to self-criticism and guilt after the death. Reports from the hospice also show that if the patient and family relate as a unit with humanistic support, both can learn to cope more effectively with death.[3]

The same regard for the wholeness and integrity of both the individual and his family unit has characterized a research project entitled Home Care for the Child with Cancer,* which is currently under way at the University of Minnesota School of Nursing. Varying family reactions to crisis and differing home environments and life styles may preclude universal recommendation of home care for all dying children. Nevertheless the home needs to be seriously considered as an alternative to the hospital for the dying child. The following background material from this study is included so that the reader may evaluate the feasibility of home care.

During a 12-month period, 32 families from Minnesota, North Dakota, and Wisconsin were involved in the Home Care project and experienced the death of a child from cancer. All but 5 of the 32 children died at home. The children's diagnoses included leukemias, lymphomas, and solid tumors. The families were involved in the project for 2 to 104 days before their children died.

To aid a given family in home care, the project staff located a primary

*This study is supported by DHEW, National Cancer Institute, Grant CA 19490.

nurse who resided within a short distance of them, and she was given intensive preparation, including guidelines for care and a packet of written material. The project staff served as on-call consultants to this primary nurse.

Home care has proved to be a feasible alternative to institutionalized care; there are no insurmountable obstacles to its application. In each of the 27 cases in the present study involving death of the child at home, the child has either expressed the desire to remain at home, or the parents of the younger children decided their child's behavior indicated that he was frightened of the hospital and wished to be at home. A possible factor in the acceptance of the home care alternative may have been that either the child, the parents, or both had experienced a trying hospital situation.

Separation of a child from his family and home environment during this crucial event—the process leading to death—is traumatic. During hospitalization the child and the rest of the family have limited control over what happens. With home care, the parents have an opportunity for direct care of their child during the dying process. Of the children who died at home, only one child was comatose; the rest responded to their parents. Death occurred during sleep for five children. Twenty children died in the living room or the dining room, close to the center of family activity. One or both parents were present at the child's side at the time of death, with the exception of two children: a teenage boy and a $2\frac{1}{2}$-year-old girl, both of whom died at 4 AM. In these two cases, the parents were resting in a nearby room.

One of the most salient variables identified in applying home care was the effective control of pain, which was present in all but three of the children in this study. According to findings thus far, it seems that pain can be as well controlled at home as in the hospital. This may indicate that the hospital is perhaps not essential in providing the comfort care needed by a dying child. If so, this fact must be recognized by all four major participants—the physician, the nurse, the parents, and the child. The physician will need to allow some flexibility in pain management for the nurse and the family. The nurse must be knowledgeable regarding pain control, for she appears to be a major factor in the maintenance of pain control in the home. The parents must realize that pain can be as well controlled at home, or they will unnecessarily take the child to the hospital. When two children were admitted to the hospital for pain control, the treatment given was injectable morphine sulfate. This could have been administered at home. Finally, the child needs to know that pain can be controlled at home. Pain control at home appears to be particularly important at night in order to provide uninterrupted sleep for the family. Pain medication that is effective for a 6- to 8-hour period is therefore preferred.

Another important variable identified was rapid availability of nursing services. That is, the first contact with the family needs to be immediately after referral, and thereafter services must be available 24 hours a day, 7 days a week. Providing remote paging systems for the primary nurse facilitates family-nurse communication.

Conditions supporting home care

Preliminary analysis of the data suggests that home care may be considered as an alternative to hospitalization when the following conditions are met:

1. Cure-oriented treatment has been discontinued.
2. The child wants to be at home.
3. The parents desire to have the child at home.
4. The parents recognize their own ability to care for their ill child; the fact they can care for the child until death is frequently not recognized until later.
5. The nurse is willing to be available 24 hours a day to facilitate care.
6. The child's physician is willing to be an on-call consultant.

A question has been raised: "How does one determine which families will be able to manage home care for their children with cancer?" The following are typical responses from health professionals and lay persons we have interviewed regarding their own ideas about which families should be offered home care.

Frequently, the first suggestion given was that there needs to be a stable family unit. There must be love between father and mother. If there is not a stable unit, many believe home care is too much of a strain on the marriage. Second, many think that the support systems of the family should be taken into consideration. For example, there needs to be more than one person available. Several other guidelines were agreed on by those interviewed. They concurred that health professionals can assess what the parents do for their child in the hospital and from this predict their ability to cope at home. Many responded that the parents need to have considerable technical knowledge. They agreed that there needs to be an acceptance of the impending death by the family and consideration of the child's attitude toward the hospital. Does he want to be at home, or does he want to be in the hospital? Siblings of the dying child need to accept home care with the qualification that if siblings are traumatized by the child's presence and death at home, home care is of no use. Finally, they cautioned that one should be concerned about financial considerations. Home care is less costly than hospital care, but may not be covered by insurance, whereas hospital care is covered.

In our home care study, we have encountered situations that disputed almost all the preceding suggested criteria. Families with only one parent present have cared for their dying children at home. Also, all families with whom we have worked have reported that there was extreme strain on their marriage before involvement in the home care project. Some families have had no support network outside the family. There has been no apparent correlation between what the parents did in the hospital and their ability to cope at home. With the exception of three families, the technical knowledge that parents have needed has been minimal. The key seems to be family acceptance of the impending death and the child's wish to be at home. Our preliminary data indicate that siblings were initially frightened to have their brother or sister at home, but after the death they were no longer afraid of death and reported that the experience itself was not frightening. In fact, they related the positive things they had done for their sibling before death. The financial considerations by the parents and the cost of having the child at home have been minimal.

BENEFITS AND LIMITATIONS OF HOME CARE, HOSPICE, AND HOSPITAL CARE

Let us contrast some of the benefits and limitations of home care, hospice, and hospital care according to three categories: the child's point of view, the family's point of view, and the nurse's point of view.

Beginning with the child's point of view, the benefits of home care are the intimate family contact and familiar surroundings, which lead to a greatly increased sense of security. Home care permits constant opportunity to provide an individualized approach, for example, special foods. One mother stated, "There was so much more to do at home." The parents give the kind of care that is consistent with their parental role from the child's point of view. The limitations, possibly, of home care from an older child's point of view could be that he feels the burden of guilt for his parents' additional responsibilities. Also, he might feel insecure being away from hospital-level care or sense that the neighbors and family do not know what to do regarding dying and death at home.

The benefit of the hospice from the child's perspective is the relative ease and acceptance of family members, including pets, within an institutional setting. In contrast to the hospital, where rules and regulations may preclude such acceptance, the hospice is structured to encourage family participation. The possible limitation with respect to hospice care is whether or not there is a sufficient population of dying children to support such an independent institution. If there is not, then a hospital with a special unit may be more logical.

One of the benefits of hospital care from the vantage point of the child is peer group support. That is, there are other children in the hospital in similar situations with whom to interact. Other benefits include the protection of the parents from the pain and death process. (Ultimately for the parents, this protection might be a limitation.) The professional staff is there to care for unanticipated medical needs. The child becomes the center of attention of hospital personnel. If the home is not a secure place, the hospital can replace the home as a source of comfort for the child. The limitations of the hospital include changes in the child's perception of home, for example, "When you get better you can go home," as if you can go home *only* when you are better. The hospital limits the opportunity to have familiar things present, such as toys, hobby items, and pets. Certainly a major limitation of hospital care is that it is a structured, more institutional, approach.

The advantages of home care from the parents' viewpoint are several. They are in control of giving the care. Death becomes a family experience.[2] The family has more hours with the child. Because the parents are able to do everything they can for the child, this may minimize guilt following the death. Home care is less costly. Finally, the family structure is maintained within a more normal environment. The family is not separated by taking turns visiting in the hospital. Limitations include the possible physical and emotional strains. People in the community may reject the child because of their own discomfort concerning the child's changes in appearance, and this may in turn hurt the parents. Others may make parents feel guilty for not doing enough, implying the child should be in the hospital. Another possible limitation is that the siblings, grandparents, or other relatives may not support the parents in their effort at home care.

Looking at hospice care from the parents' perspective, the hospice would welcome them and would give support to them. Nevertheless the hospice, although more like the home, cannot be a substitute for the home where there is almost limitless opportunity to individualize the care for the child.

Hospital care, from the viewpoint of the parents, can have some definite advantages. Parents come in contact with other parents of sick and dying children. They can give each other emotional support. Parents can temporarily get away from the situation. There is professional support from nurses, doctors, and other health team members. Parents may feel reassured that they have in no way neglected their child when he is in the hospital. The hospital is a culturally acceptable place to die. There is more often insurance coverage. Conversely, limitations to hospital care include the disruption of family structure; parents and other family members are unaware of their right to protest—they sometimes submit to measures because they do not know the alternatives and because they have not learned to evaluate the need for procedures, and they are not in control of the situation. At times the hospital may appear as a locus of people who are merely interested in the dying process of the child.

The third category involves benefits for the nurse. In home care there is opportunity for a new kind of service. Creativity is tapped, and she develops a new sense of responsibility and independence. The physician is a consultant, and a new relationship with the physician and other health team members results. An intimate experience with the family may occur. The limitations of home care include the fact that the nurse gives up direct control. Closure may be difficult for the nurse, and the nurse may be uncomfortable in the home. There is less support, less equipment, and at the same time more responsibility for her. She also may be on call 24 hours a day.

One advantage for the nurse in the hospice program is certainly the emphasis on and commitment to staff support. All the professionals are committed to the hospice philosophy, so coordinating efforts follows smoothly. Because the hospice includes a home care component, the limitation for the nurse is minimal.

The advantages of hospital care from the nurse's point of view include the support system of other nurses as well as other staff, many of whom are committed to improving the care of dying children and their families. The scheduling of time allows her to get away without jeopardizing 24-hour coverage for the child. She gets exposure and experience, and there is security in having consultation and equipment available. A limitation of hospital care for the dying child from the nurse's point of view is that there is the temptation to hide behind equipment and other tasks and to avoid or isolate the dying child and the family.

An additional consideration is the involvement of the interdisciplinary team in the three settings. The hospital provides the easiest access to a full team, facilitating involvement of all disciplines, even when not necessarily essential to provide quality care. The hospice interdisciplinary team is generally more selective. However, it tends to insist on having physician involvement regardless of the documented needs. Home care, as presented in the study mentioned earlier, utilizes a nurse as the coordinator of care. The nurse then includes the interdisciplinary team members as necessary. While the physician is kept informed, he does not become involved in the day-to-day experience. This approach provides potentially a much greater cost effectiveness and better use of medical expertise. The child's physician is the nurse's consultant, especially in matters related to symptom control.

In conclusion, alternative environments are being developed, and continued research must be encouraged so that in the future there will be an opportunity for all families of dying children to be better informed in order to make a choice most appropriate for their children and themselves.

REFERENCES

1. Kaplan, D. M., Smith, A., Grobstein, R., and Fischman, S. E.: Family mediations of stress. In Moos, R. H., editor: Coping with physical illness, New York, 1977, Plenum Publishing Corp.
2. Keyser, M.: At home with death; a natural child death, J. Pediatr. **90:**486, 1977.
3. Lack, S.: I want to die while I'm still alive, Death Educ. **1:**165, 1977.
4. Mount, B. M.: Palliative care service, October 1976 report, Montreal, 1976, Royal Victoria Hospital, McGill University.
5. Plant, J.: Finding a home for hospice care in the United States, Long-Term Care **51:**53, 1977.

ADDITIONAL READING

Sauer, S.: The hospital setting for the child with cancer. In Martinson, I. M., editor: Home care for the dying child; professional and family perspectives, New York, 1977, Appleton-Century-Crofts.

CHAPTER 7

The effect of neonatal death on the family

ROSE GROBSTEIN

Losing a child brings the worse grief we'll ever feel in our lives. You can only know if you've gone through it.

Doreen Bodycombe
San Jose News, August 9, 1977

Many in our society do not understand that the death of an infant has as great an impact on the mother, father, and siblings as does the death of an older member of the family. It is thought that because the life of the infant has been so short, there is not enough time to form the same strong bonds that one forms with the longer-lived members of the family. And, after all, it is always possible to have another child.

In discussing the development of a mother's attachment to her infant, Klaus and Kennell[7] emphasize that attachment frequently begins to develop when the mother first feels the movement of the fetus. It appears that not only the mother but also the father begins to attach. The father places his hand over the mother's abdomen, feels the movement, and frequently expresses a feeling of awe that their child is a "real being." "Parental nesting behavior" begins. Long discussions are held about the possible sex, about the proper name for this new individual, and about their hopes and aspirations for him. Often a pet name is concocted, and the father will ask, "How is Bozo today?"

Is it any wonder then that the death of this being has a great impact on the family?

Some other, perhaps most primitive, cultures have been aware of the devastating effects a neonatal death may have, sometimes even leading to the death of the mother. Thomas H. Lewis quotes a mother of the Trio tribe of Brazil who was in a severe depression; she was not eating and becoming weaker and weaker after the loss of her infant. Urututu, the mother, explained that "an infant who dies goes beyond the trees, to the circling horizon, to the sky where the souls stay. It has an invisible cord attached to the umbilicus and extending to the mother. The cord functions to nurture both until the child can care for itself, until it can walk and talk and eat by itself. If the child dies before this, it misses its mother and keeps pulling on the cord. She misses the child and responds by giving up that which keeps her on earth."[13]

Many observers have reported on the reactions of families to the loss of a newborn.[1-3,6,13,15] All state that both mothers and fathers respond to their infants' deaths with typical grief reactions as described by Erich Lindemann[14] and Kübler-Ross.[11] They progress through the stages of somatic distress, anger, guilt, resignation, and finally acceptance of the death of their child.

Mothers frequently express guilt over the fantasized cause of death, such as coitus during pregnancy, a fall, continuing employment, moving, or not taking iron pills or vitamins.

Seldom is it mentioned that fathers also have strong guilt feelings. At Stanford, parents whose children are in the intensive care nursery have the opportunity to meet with each other, a nurse, and a social worker on alternate Sunday afternoons. The purpose of the meetings is to share feelings and experiences related to having a sick infant. Many fathers have told us of the guilt that they have felt after the birth. Some have said they did not feel ready for parenthood and had urged their wives to have an abortion. Others said that they felt they had not spent enough time with their wives and had not responded adequately to their needs. Others wondered whether there were genetic reasons or "something wrong" with them.

Anger is expressed in many ways. There is anger at the failure of medicine. There is anger at nursing care. There is anger at the loss of their hopes for the future. The anger is directed both at themselves for their failure to have a healthy child and at others for not helping them to avoid this failure.

The most common physical complaints are those of fatigue, a feeling of emptiness and numbness, and a lack of motivation and direction in one's activities. One mother stated that she really did not want to do anything except sit. However, she forced herself into activity but felt as though she was not really experiencing anything. She felt "dead inside." A father told us how he would just sit in his office staring out the window for minutes at a time. Many fathers grieve longer than mothers, particularly if the child had been transferred from another hospital and he had acted as a go-between for the mother.

Giles[2] mentions that Freud in 1917 observed that grief itself is not pathologic. It is a normal process that cushions the impact of the loss and leads toward an acceptance of what has happened.

How then can parents be helped to experience and resolve their grief and arrive at a healthy outcome?

TASKS OF CAREGIVER AT DEATH OF A NEWBORN

Klaus and Kennell[7] state that the caregiver has three major tasks at the time of the death of a newborn. These are: (1) help the parents digest the loss and make it real, (2) ensure that normal grief reactions begin and that both parents go through the entire process, and (3) meet the individual needs of the specific parents.

To help the parents accept the death of their child, many observers suggest that they have some contact with the infant. If the child has lived for a time, it is wise to help them visit the child and to participate in his care in any way possible. While an intensive care nursery is an extremely frightening place at first, with preparation and assistance parents can become accepting of all that goes on there. However, there will be many different reactions. One mother told us that she just walks in and does not look at any of the other babies. She goes directly to her baby. On the other hand, her husband said that he looks around and sees how the others are doing as he walks toward his baby's isolette. Very important, parents should always be informed in advance about their child's condition and what to expect should anything be changed from their last contact.

After the child dies, the parents should be permitted to see and hold their child if they wish. They should, of course, be prepared for the altered skin color and the stiffness and coldness of the body. I remember sitting with a mother who was holding her dead infant. This infant had weighed less than 700 grams at birth and had subsequently lost weight. The mother held the baby in the palm of her hand, stroking him with her fingers. She talked to the child, saying, "You really didn't have a chance. You were really only half-done." She cried, and talked, and at last gave the child to the nurse with a final kiss and "good-bye."

I think the reason for this is best summed up in a quote from Nanette Neuman's "Lots of Love" as quoted in Dr. Jolly's article.[5] "When my daddy was driving, we saw a fox lying in the road and nobody stopped. You should always stop and say good-bye to dead things." Saying good-bye is an important step in the acceptance of a death.

Also, part of saying good-bye and achieving a closure is to have some type of formal ceremony. This promotes grieving and does not leave the family with the feeling that the life and death of their child were unimportant events.

Young parents in particular who have not had much experience with death may rely heavily on the caregiver for advice and support. When their child dies, all parents need some very practical help because even minor decision making can take on crisis proportions. They need help in contacting those who are close to them and who can be supportive at this difficult time. They need help in making funeral plans. They need help in deciding whether or not to have an autopsy. They need help in explaining the death to other children and, perhaps, to other relatives.

Klaus and Kennell[7] indicate that there is a continuing role for the caregivers. They see the parents three times after the death. The first time is immediately after the death of the child. Besides the helping tasks detailed above, the purpose is to explain the mourning process in simple terms and the normality of the feelings they will experience. It is explained that at times they may imagine the baby is still alive. I remember one mother telling me that about 2 weeks after the death of her child, she woke up one morning and thought she had to go to the hospital to see her baby. These are not unusual feelings or thoughts.

The second contact takes place 2 or 3 days later. At this time the grieving process is reviewed again with the parents, and it is emphasized that grieving is a normal process. It is important to emphasize the sharing of emotions and thoughts between the parents so that they can be mutually supportive. Also, it should be explained that some friends and relatives will not really understand their grieving. I talked with a couple at one of our group meetings, and they were feeling bitter about the support given by friends. They said that some had said, "If you want to talk, just call on us." When this was done, the friends did not have time to talk. This, of course, does not always happen. Other couples have told us of particular friends with whom they have spent hours talking about the events surrounding their infant's birth and death and about the infant himself, the way he looked, the way he felt, and the things that he had done.

Parents need reassurance that sudden bouts of crying or feelings of sadness for 6 to 9 or more months after the death do not mean that they are losing their minds.

Many parents do not know what to do about other children in the family. They need to know that it is helpful to the children to be truthful and to share their grief with each other. Just as adults have feelings of guilt about some behavior that caused the death, so do children. They may have been jealous of the time spent at the hospital, or they may have had thoughts about not wanting the sibling to come home. They need reassurance that they did not cause the death. Some children show their disturbance by having nightmares, enuresis, acting out, or school problems.[3] Parents should be encouraged to listen to and talk with other children about the death. The topic should not be taboo in the household.

The third meeting occurs 3 to 6 months after the death. The purpose of this meeting is to discuss the autopsy findings if one has been performed and to answer the many questions the parents have about the causes of their infant's illness and death. These questions can be difficult ones for the professional. Many times there are no answers, but unfortunately many people still believe that medicine is a very exact science and has all the answers.

This meeting is also used to determine if the parents are progressing through the mourning process, reaching the time of acceptance of the death, and beginning to plan for the future. Acceptance does not mean that the parents feel the death is fair and reasonable. It means that they have accepted the reality of the death and have so integrated it that they can plan for the future.[17]

Signs of pathologic grieving should be noted, such as excessive crying, inability to plan for the future, excessive concern with the dead infant, and so on. A referral for psychiatric help should be made if indicated. This can be a difficult process, because many times the person concerned does not recognize the need for such help, and several additional contacts may be necessary to accomplish the referral.

STILLBIRTH

Stillbirths occur in about one in 80 deliveries.[12] After such a birth, there is usually a conspiracy of silence. The mother is discharged as soon as possible. There is little follow-up on the part of most physicians and other health professionals. On everyone's part—friends, relatives, and caregivers—the conspiracy of silence is continued.

Dr. Lewis[12] quotes Bourne as stating that a stillbirth is a nonevent, in which there is misery, guilt, and shame. There is no joy after a stillbirth, only a sense of complete failure on the part of the mother.

According to Dr. Jolly,[5] many people have the concept that the stillborn has never lived; therefore, many of these bereaved families suffer from a lack of understanding, and many of their needs are not met. When Dr. Jolly became interested in studying the reactions to a stillbirth, he received many letters from women describing their feelings. One woman wrote that only now after 34 years has she been able to ask her husband where their son was buried. The vast majority wrote saying that they wished they had seen the baby, even if it was malformed.

Wolf and colleagues[18] studied 50 patients who had experienced a stillbirth, and 40 of these were followed for 1 to 3 years. He found that in dealing with this loss, one half blamed themselves or projected blame on others, one fourth said that it was "God's will," and a fourth consciously or unconsciously avoided dealing with the event. All reacted with typical grief reactions, and none developed other significant psychiatric difficulties. Fifty percent planned to become pregnant again. Of those who did not plan to become pregnant, 50% chose sterilization.

As Klaus and Kennell detail it, attachment of the mother and father begins during pregnancy and grows with each month that the pregnancy continues. It is important then to help parents mourn the loss of a stillborn as well as the infant who lives, either for hours, weeks, or months.

The woman feels shame because she has the sense of having failed as a woman who can give birth to a live baby, and feels guilt about what she may have done to cause the stillbirth by either thought or action. Both parents feel an acute sense of loss for their hopes for the future.

All those who have looked at the event of stillbirth recommend that parents be encouraged to see and touch the dead baby.[4,5,9,10,12,16,18] It is agreed that most mothers, at first, do not wish to see and touch. With some assistance, however, they do so, and the mourning process is facilitated because now there is an actual person to mourn. Lewis[12] cites some vivid case histories that support this approach.

It is further suggested that a name be given to the infant and that parents plan some simple burial event. Other children in the family find the stillbirth frightening and incomprehensible, and a burial makes it more understandable to them. Also, friends and relatives can more readily understand the mourning of the parents and can be of more support to them, and thus avoid the "conspiracy of silence."

As in any crisis that a family experiences, open communication between the parents and between parents and other children is extremely important in resolving grief. The sharing of feelings and thoughts leads to the acceptance of the event so that one can be free to begin to plan for the future.

MISCARRIAGE

Neither in this chapter nor in the literature does one find much discussion about the effects of miscarriage. It is only logical to think that many of the same processes apply. Certainly attachment, while it may have begun, has not had the opportunity to fully develop in an early miscarriage. However, the same feelings of guilt and shame do appear, and hopes for the future are destroyed. It is important, therefore, to have open discussion between parents about causes, feelings, and hopes for the future, so that blame, guilt, and inadequacy do not become overwhelming and cause difficulties in the relationship.

SUBSEQUENT PREGNANCIES

In all of these events (neonatal deaths, stillbirths, and miscarriages), the subsequent pregnancy causes great anxiety, and the parents need a great deal of support from their physician. Seitz and Warrick[17] state that during labor and delivery the mother's tension is increased, and she sometimes needs to review the events of the last labor in order to reassure herself that events are proceeding normally.

At the time of delivery the mother and father may need more time to be with their newborn in order to be reassured about his viability.

Sometimes mourning for the previous loss recurs during the first postpartum days. If the previous infant lived only a few hours, a mother may not wish to have close contact with the new baby until the baby has lived past the magic hour. She then slowly initiates mothering. If successful mourning for the previous infant has taken place, the mother and father can begin to see this new infant as an individual who will have his own identity and needs either immediately or very shortly after this normal birth.

CONCLUSION

As mentioned above, professionals can be helpful to parents during these times of stress: (1) helping them to digest the loss and make it real, (2) ensuring that normal grief reactions begin and that both parents will go through the entire process, and (3) meeting the individual needs of the specific patients.

There are some very specific don'ts for all professionals who work in this area of neonatal deaths.

1. In supporting the parents, don't do all the talking. The best support is to listen to the feelings and needs expressed. The parents are the ones who have experienced the greatest loss, and they need to talk about it. The support given is probably inversely proportional to the amount the professional talks.

2. Don't use the reassurance of saying, "You can always have another child." William Kotzwinkle[3] in his novel expresses this so beautifully in describing the thoughts of Laski, the father of an infant who has just died, while a physician tells him there is no reason why he and his wife cannot have another child. "Laski listened numbly. He thinks that's what has been at stake, our wish for a child, any child, not this particular child who swung down the road between us. They can't know how special he is. They point to the future. But we're here, forever, now."

3. Don't offer tranquilizers to soften the impact. This just delays the mourning reaction and is not really helpful to the individuals experiencing the loss. As Proust has said, mourning is the transition from grief to memory. This memory is important.

4. Don't impose your feelings about viewing and holding the dead infant. Some parents may not be able to do this. If they do wish to hold or touch their dead infant, give them the opportunity to do so without the feeling that they are strange or abnormal. If, however, they do not wish to, they should not be made to feel guilty because of this reaction. Everyone should honor individual differences.

The impact of neonatal death on families is a very complex subject.

Ideally, as we become more aware of its importance to a family's emotional health, more help can be given to families so that the effect will not be so devastating.

In concluding, I should like to quote Lewis.[12] "With stillbirth or neonatal death, it is partly the loss of what might have been, the loss of experience in the future which makes for such heart-rending and deeply frustrating experiences."

REFERENCES

1. Benfield, D. G., Leib, S. A., and Rentor, J.: Grief response of parents following referral of the critically ill newborn, N. Engl. J. Med. **294:**975, 1976.
2. Giles, P. F. H.: Reactions of women to perinatal death, Aust. N. Z. J. Obstet. Gynecol. **10:**207, 1970.
3. Gilson, G. J.: Care of the family who has lost a newborn, Postgrad. Med. **60:**67, 1976.
4. Grief and stillbirth, editorial, Br. Med. J. **1:**126, 1977.
5. Jolly, H.: Family reactions to stillbirth, Proc. R. Soc. Med. **69:**835, 1976.
6. Kennell, J. H., Slyter, H., and Klaus, M. H.: The mourning response of parents to the death of a newborn infant, N. Engl. J. Med. **283:**344, 1970.
7. Klaus, M. H., and Kennell, J. H.: Maternal-infant bonding, St. Louis, 1976, The C. V. Mosby Co.
8. Kotzwinkle, W.: Swimmer in the secret sea, New York, 1975, Avon Books.
9. Kowalski, K., and Bowes, W. A., Jr.: Parents response to a stillborn baby, Contemp. Obstet. Gynecol. **8:**53, 1976.
10. Kowalski, K., and Osborn, M.: Helping mothers of stillborn infants to grieve, Maternal Child Nurs. **2:**29, 1977.
11. Kübler-Ross, E.: On death and dying, New York, 1970, Macmillan, Inc.
12. Lewis, E.: The management of stillbirth; coping with an unreality, Lancet **2:**619, 1976.
13. Lewis, T.: A culturally patterned depression in a mother after loss of a child, Psychiatry **38:**92, 1975.
14. Lindemann, E.: Symptomatology and management of acute grief, Am. J. Psychiatry **101:**141, 1944.
15. Morris, D.: Parental reactions to perinatal death, Proc. R. Soc. Med. **69:**837, 1976.
16. Saylor, D. E.: Nursing response to mothers of stillborn infants, J. Obstet. Gynecol. Neonat. Nurs. **6:**39, 1977.
17. Seitz, P. M., and Warrick, L. H.: Perinatal death; the grieving mother, Am. J. Nurs. **74:**2028, 1974.
18. Wolf, J. R., Nielsen, P. E., and Schiller, P.: The emotional reaction to a stillbirth, Am. J. Obstet. Gynecol. **108:**73, 1970.

ADDITIONAL READINGS

Feifel, H.: New meanings of death, New York, 1977, McGraw-Hill Book Co.
Goodman, M. B.: Two mothers' reactions to the deaths of their premature infants, J. Obstet. Gynecol. Neonat. Nurs. **4:**25, 1975.
Moos, R. H., editor: Coping with physical illness, New York, 1977, Plenum Publishing Corp., Chapter 2.
Steinfels, P., and Veatch, R. M., editors: Death inside out, New York, 1974, Harper & Row, Publishers.

CHAPTER 8

Sudden death

SUSAN F. WOOLSEY
DORIS S. THORNTON
STANFORD B. FRIEDMAN

> Today, even more than in the past, parents expect their children to survive to adulthood. Such an assumption is, of course, not universal, in that many parts of the world do not benefit from modern practices of medicine and public hygiene. However, in this country, the sudden, unanticipated death of an infant or child represents to parents a direct confrontation of their belief that their child would "grow up," and requires a major psychological adaptation by them to cope successfully with their loss. Yet, families experiencing such a loss rarely benefit from professional counseling, although a physician known to the family can assume a significant role in this crisis situation.[11]

Literature discussing sudden, unexpected death is, for the most part, related to sudden death in the adult. Adequate research has not been done on the process of adaptation to the unanticipated loss of a child. Some descriptive information related to the reactions of parents to such a loss are available from studies of families experiencing the loss of an infant from the sudden infant death syndrome.[3]

There are a few accounts of the behavior of children after the death of a sibling.[6,36] Most of the literature describes children in psychotherapy who apparently have been greatly influenced by the death of a loved one. These data are not representative, because those referred for psychotherapy represent a distinct minority of children. Frequently, it is noted that adolescent and adult patients being treated for depression, delinquency, sociopathy, or other psychopathology experienced the death of a loved one when they were children.[1,2,15,16]

Most studies have dealt with situations in which death has been an-

We wish to gratefully acknowledge the insights provided by parents of infants who died from sudden infant death syndrome, many of whom are directly quoted in this chapter. We also wish to thank Stanley E. Weinstein, M.S.W., for his administrative support during the time of its preparation.

ticipated. They have not been concerned with the more difficult problem of unanticipated death nor have they attempted to describe what happens when compared with situations in which death was anticipated. The purpose of this chapter is to begin to identify those characteristics that are generic to families who experience the sudden, unanticipated death of a child and to suggest a plan for management.

ANTICIPATED LOSS OF A CHILD

The feelings and experiences commonly shared by parents of fatally ill children and their patterns of coping with such a crisis have been described in detail.[4,12,18,27] Characteristically, when told the diagnosis of a fatal illness in their child, parents describe initial feelings of shock and disbelief, even though they may have already strongly suspected it. A few parents will use almost complete denial to cope with their feelings and may refuse to give permission for the child's treatment, acting as if their child were not ill. However, despite feelings of unreality, most parents accept the diagnosis at the cognitive level and are able to comply as the prescribed medical regimen is initiated. As time passes, they gradually accept the diagnosis in a feeling way and typically communicate their feelings by using phrases such as: "It finally hit me," or, "It seems real now." Thus, an acute emotional impact usually follows the more intellectualized acceptance, beginning what has been described as "anticipatory grief."[24]

As the child's condition deteriorates, many parents progressively adapt to the anticipated loss. This may be reflected by their renewed interest in routine activities typical of their lives before the diagnosis was made. The death, when it occurs, may then be described as "just the final step," because it has been anticipated. In a sense, adaptation to the loss takes place in a step-wise fashion. The grief process that follows the anticipated loss of a child may be viewed as both a continuation of adaptation (or maladaptation) that has occurred during the child's illness, and a response to the death itself.

If anticipatory grieving has not taken place, the parents experience acute emotional pain comparable to that described by parents whose children have died unexpectedly. They are confronted with these intense feelings related to grief at a time when they are emotionally and physically exhausted as a result of their investment in the child's illness. During that time, the parents often rely on the health care team for support and loosen their reliance on support from friends and family. However, when the child dies, supportive relationships developed within the health care system usually are terminated. This occurs at a time when their needs are greatest for such support and when they are least able to renew their reliance on relatives and friends.[10] In addition, they may attempt to have a "replacement baby" to help eliminate their feelings of abandonment.[6]

Because of individual differences, the mourning period varies both as to length and characteristics. In general, the acute mourning period is thought to extend over 3 to 4 months; however, mourning may never be complete. Surviving family members will be reminded of the loss on anniversaries and other occasions, and some aspects of mourning may be renewed, especially during the first year after the death.[19]

UNANTICIPATED LOSS OF A CHILD
Sudden infant death syndrome

It is estimated that one in every 350 to 400 live births end in death due to sudden infant death syndrome (SIDS), or 6,000 to 8,000 deaths per year in the United States. It is the leading cause of death of infants after the first month of life. Because none of the proposed theories of etiology has been proved, there can be no definitive medical explanation to give to the question, "Why did the baby die?" The aftermath of guilt and blame is often intense. That the baby was apparently healthy and is suddenly dead is illogical. This leaves many unanswered questions in the minds of the parents as well as relatives, friends, and others in the community. "The parents of SIDS victims are often young and may be experiencing the death of a loved one for the first time. It is often the first major stress on their marriage. They have waited nine months for the birth and were just sampling the joys of parenthood when the infant died."[35] Such a loss is particularly difficult for the mother, because she has been both physically and psychologically attached to the baby, and it takes considerable time to neutralize the intensity of the loss, as illustrated by these typical remarks made by parents:

> For weeks I would find myself in her room wanting to crawl into the crib and curl up there. I guess it's because I missed her so much, and she always looked so cuddly when she was sleeping there. I wanted so to be close to her. At first, I thought I was losing my mind to feel that way, but now I know such feelings are normal since she was such a big part of my life.

> When I hear another baby cry I experience "let-down" of my milk. Being able to breast feed was so important to me and now it causes such agony!

Accidental deaths

Fifty percent of the deaths of children between 1 and 14 years of age are due to injuries. In 1976 in the United States, 12,000 children died in this manner.[26] In retrospect, it often appears that an accident could have been prevented; consequently, parents, siblings, peers, or others responsible for the child's safety may feel they have contributed directly to the death. It also has been reported that members of the health care team may overtly blame the parents for the child's death.[33]

When an accident occurs, usually both intrinsic and extrinsic causative factors can be identified.[22] The children may have common personality traits, there may be coexistent social problems, or other family members may have identifiable physical or psychologic pathology.[20,28] A high percentage of fatal accidents involve automobiles or motorcycles, indicating that social and economic conditions also can play a role in causing accidents.

This kind of crisis may bring more closeness within a family, but it also may become the focus for dissolution, as portrayed in this extreme example:

> My wife blamed me for what happened, and whenever we would have a disagreement, she would bring it up again as though I had purposely run over our son. We finally got a divorce.

THE GRIEF PROCESS IN UNANTICIPATED LOSS

In contrast to families of children who die from anticipated causes, parents of children who die unexpectedly describe a sudden surge of intense, disruptive, and almost intolerable feelings. As there is no time to psychologically prepare for the loss, parents experience the death as a major insult, resulting in extraordinary, strong feelings of shock and disbelief that may persist for several weeks or months:

> When I touched her, she was stiff and cold; I just dropped her back in the crib and ran screaming through the house.

> She was so cold I put another blanket around her and held her tightly to try and warm her. I really knew she was dead, but she was *so* cold.

> After the funeral I had almost uncontrollable urges to go to the graveyard and dig him up to be sure he was really dead.

In their attempts to comprehend the total nature of the loss, parents often choose isolated facets about the death and deal with them selectively over time:

> Being able to pass her room and either look in or go in and touch her things was very important to me.

> I got the SIDS information out and read it and reread it, and went over it in my mind to be sure it checked out okay.

If the child was young and had not been ill, friends and relatives may think the parents will not require long to recover from the loss; however, the grief process for parents of babies and children who die unexpectedly occurs over time and may take longer to resolve than in families who have experienced anticipatory grieving.

Coping behavior is not only intrapsychic but may involve motor activity or actual avoidance. For example, a father relates the following:

> I just got on a bus and rode as far as my money lasted. I kept going over what I knew about what had happened. Finally, after a couple of weeks I decided it was foolish to blame my wife or myself, so I came back home.

Extreme sadness, depression, and desperate loneliness are common feelings after the death of a child. The bereaved person may feel empty and worthless, lack energy, become extremely restless, or be unable to concentrate. These feelings may be accompanied by loss of appetite and insomnia. The mother may experience physical pain around the heart or abdomen, or her arms may "ache to hold the baby."

Anxiety is always present. The death of someone close reminds one of his own mortality, and further anxiety may arise from feelings of helplessness. If the parents have not experienced the mourning process before, they may feel that the pain will never disappear, or that such intense reactions are abnormal: "Am I going crazy?" The level of anxiety may be increased considerably by the insensitive responses of friends, relatives, the health care team, or others in the community. They may, in fact, directly or indirectly, accuse the parents of negligence or murder.

In response to their extreme loneliness, thoughts about having another baby usually occur, and parents may react in opposing ways. The fear that this could happen again may lead them to decide they never want to have another baby, thereby depriving themselves of the opportunity for future satisfying parenting experiences. Or, almost paradoxically, others respond by wanting to have another baby as soon as possible, thus not allowing themselves to resolve their loss and taking the risk that the next child may be expected to replace the dead child.[34] Neither approach is optimal.

Well-meaning people often try to persuade parents that the best solution is to have another baby as soon as possible, not realizing that healthy resolution of grief takes time. If parents are able to incorporate the death into their lives before having another child, their ability to parent subsequent children will be greatly enhanced.

During the acute grief period, parents need to be comforted themselves, and consequently their ability to care for and comfort the surviving siblings is greatly impaired. The surviving siblings may experience the death as a double deprivation. They have lost the brother or sister who died, and they may think their parents no longer love them, because they do not understand the meaning of their parents' mourning behavior. In addition, neighbors or relatives may take the children away from home until after the funeral, thus depriving them of the opportunity to say good-bye to the dead brother or sister. The future relationship a child will have with his parents will certainly be altered if he perceives his being sent away as a rejection by them.

Because coping patterns are individual, bereaved persons will utilize those behaviors that in the past have helped them deal with their anxiety:

> I get out my tools and putter with some really insignificant task.
>
> The house is clean, but I keep cleaning anyway.
>
> I sit and rock and turn the music on loud and cry.

Anger is commonly experienced when a child dies suddenly. The circumstances surrounding the death may provide a focus for anger, as in the case of accidental death, or the parents may express anger in a way that seems inappropriate. For example, the medical profession is often blamed: "The doctor just examined our baby and said he was fine. He should have seen something." Anger may be directed at God: "I've done nothing to deserve such punishment." Ambulance personnel may be blamed for not coming sooner or not being able to revive the child. In some cases the dead child may even become the focus of the anger: "How could he do this to me after all I've done for him?"

A surviving sibling may be selected as the focus of anger: "Why did it have to be Sue and not John?" In this situation the surviving child may be expected to "make up" to the parent in years to come. During a time of crisis, the parent may say, "If only Sue had lived, she would have been able to help me," thus contributing to the surviving child's feelings of helplessness and low self-esteem. Or the parent may become overprotective with a surviving sibling: "After Sara died, we just couldn't allow Joan to go away to school." In such cases the surviving child may never be allowed to become independent.

One parent may blame the other or fear that the other blames him. It is not unusual for parents to report that even after several years they have never discussed the child's death out of fear that they will not be able to handle their feelings. However, as time passes, most parents are able to gradually neutralize the intensity of their feelings of anger by finding appropriate outlets for it. Many report that being able to talk it out was extremely helpful. Often parents report: "I poured myself back into my work." Some will use energy generated from their anger to provide impetus for establishing research funds or campaigning to bring about congressional hearings: "We had to bring some meaning to what happened—

at least she didn't die for nothing." However, some parents are not able to resolve their anger:

> The minister told me that he didn't know why God did this to us, and we have never been back to church. I can't believe in a God who would punish people so severely.

Self-blame and guilt are normal feelings. One of the first responses to the death may be overwhelming guilt:

> I had let her cry for about ten minutes before she fell asleep, and when I found her she had a little bloody spot on her nose [characteristic in many SIDS babies]. I thought she had ruptured a blood vessel from crying and that's what caused her to die. I started screaming "I killed my baby!"

In the case of sudden death, most states require a police investigation, which may intensify the guilt feelings. If another child was present at the accident, the shocked parents may demand to know why he was unable to prevent the accident. Such an accusation may cause serious retardation in the child's emotional development and even result in later psychiatric illness.[1]

During the months that follow, parents have many thoughts that are "if only" in nature:

> I got up to go to work at 5:30 and I could have easily gone in to check on him, but I didn't. Then, when my wife woke up and went in to him at 7:00, he was dead. Why didn't I go in at 5:30? Maybe he wouldn't have died if I had.

> I keep remembering the times I was cross with her and sent her out to play to get her out of my way. If only I could have her back, I'd never yell at her again!

The long-term ill effects of unresolved grief are well documented.[1,5,31,32] When grief feelings are delayed or repressed, they tend to find expression in maladaptations that may persist for many years.

It is assumed that maladaptation may be prevented; however, little is known about the mechanism required for successful resolution of grief. Incorporation, substitution, and denial have been identified as useful mechanisms in the working-through process of grief.[21]

Incorporation is a device in which the survivor turns feelings of the deceased inward: "Jenny was such a happy child; I know she wouldn't want me to cry all the time." In the case where the death was caused by obvious physical symptoms, the survivor may even acquire the symptoms of the dead loved one. While working through the loss, the mourner may move beyond the need for this mechanism.

The bereaved may choose to *substitute* somebody or something outside himself to, in a sense, replace the dead person. Strong attachment may occur to the clothing or a toy of the dead person: "I hold his teddy bear and rock it for hours. I sometimes pretend that it is really my son." Substitution can perform a useful function in assisting the mourner to gradually relinquish attachment to the loved one.

Shock and disbelief that occur immediately after the death may be viewed as a form of *denial*, and its use is helpful during the months that follow. Various types of searching behavior may occur,[29] which allows those grieving to gradually disengage from attachment to the dead loved one: "I find myself going out on the porch to watch for him when I hear the school bus," or, "Occasionally, I tiptoe into her room as though to check on her."

The tasks of mourning have been summarized as including the full realization and acceptance of the loss, the resolution of anger and irrational guilt related to the loss, significant withdrawal of emotional investment from the deceased, and a redirection of interest and involvement with the environment of the bereaved.[6,23,24] However, even after many years have passed, parents who have lost a child say that such a loss leaves "a hole in the house" that can never truly be filled again: "We've been told we have to accept her death, but how does one *accept* the death of one's child?"

Families vary greatly in their makeup and functioning. The coping behavior of family members depends on such factors as the size and complexity of the family constellation, the communication patterns within the family, the roles played by each of the family members, and the age and developmental stage of the dead child. In all cases, the loss of the child will have a different meaning for each of the survivors. Special consideration should be given in the case of the single parent or the teenage mother; the grandmother may have been the primary caregiver of the child, and the parent's relationship to the child may have been like that of a sibling. In cases where the child had been legally placed in a foster home, the needs of the natural and foster parents must be considered.

SUGGESTED MANAGEMENT PLAN

The procedures carried out by the emergency room staff at the time of the child's sudden death are not as important as the attitudes and underlying philosophy they communicate to the family. Those who experience such a death need immediate, sympathetic, and active intervention.

Accidents and sudden death seldom happen at "convenient" times. SIDS deaths are usually discovered at night or early morning when emergency rooms have minimum coverage, and accidents often occur at the busiest times. The family members accompanying the child may be in various stages of dress and cleanliness, depending on what they were doing at the time of the discovery of the child. They may have no money or identification, and they may need help in order to meet their basic human needs (food, drink, rest, communication with significant others).

During the emergency, if the medical staff is engaged in resuscitative or other life-saving procedures, the family may be left unattended for what, to them, seems an eternity. Some hospitals are beginning to recognize the opportunity for preventive intervention afforded in the emergency room's waiting room by assigning one member of the health care team to stay with families of critically ill patients.[8,14] This individual can elicit the recent events that will provide essential health history data, and at the same time support the family by giving them brief and accurate information and allowing them to talk about their feelings.

When death occurs, the health care team should determine an appropriate and sensitive approach to the family. The family should be provided a place where there is a degree of privacy, because expression of strong emotions often is difficult in the presence of others. Both parents should be informed together if possible, and efforts should be made to contact any individual whose presence is important to the well-being of the parents (friend, relative, clergyman, grandparent, the family's private physician).

Acceptance of the reality of the death has been described as the first step toward resolution of grief.[23] Family members should be given the opportunity to touch and hold the dead child if they wish. This, in fact, may be difficult for the staff, but it will allow the family members to have a feeling of closure. Some physicians also state that touching the dead child in some way is helpful to them: "I usually need to rumple the child's hair or something like that if he's been my patient."

Most states now have laws requiring a postmortem examination in cases of sudden death. A simple statement to the family that such an examination will be done can help the parents understand that death has occurred. During the acute stage, a statement as to the cause of death, as well as a brief description of the grief process, will provide them with a framework with which to put their feelings into perspective and allay some of their unfounded concerns.

The matter of a funeral must be handled with sensitivity. Klaus and Kennell[23] suggest that in most cases a simple burial will help the family deal with the reality of the death; however, this is not true for all:

> We told them [the hospital] to give her body to the medical school to do research with her tissues and then have her cremated. We were so wounded by what had happened it seemed we could not have tolerated the pain of going through a funeral.

In a nationwide survey of parents of SIDS victims, Bergman and associates found that parents tended to be most grateful to those who were able to extend them sympathy as human beings rather than those who maintained professional distance.[3]

FOLLOW-UP

Of primary importance for the health care provider is the realization that even though the death was sudden, the adjustment by the survivors will take time. In the emergency room, parents are usually so overcome by their loss that they may only comprehend that their child is dead. For that reason, a follow-up interview in 2 or 3 days is recommended.[23] A physician, public health nurse, or social worker, preferably already known to them, can play a significant role in assisting the family during this acute stage and in the difficult months ahead. If they have a pediatrician or family physician, he should be notified and his help solicited. If not, an appointment might be arranged with a clinic that has had a relationship with the family.

The family may need to have the tasks of mourning reviewed during the follow-up interview, because many young parents have had no previous experience with death and are extremely frightened by the intensity of their feelings of isolation and loneliness.

Frank and sympathetic verbal communication should be facilitated. Occasionally, a meeting involving extended family members, friends, or interested community representatives may prove invaluable. Unresolved issues or unanswered questions discussed in an open and frank manner may serve a double purpose: the health care provider can demonstrate that open communication is helpful to the bereaved, and the presence of a group of people who are concerned about them may alleviate the parents' feelings of loneliness.

It is important to note that parents may need help in their communication about the death to surviving siblings.[13,17,30] Children are quick to notice changes in the behavior of their parents, and part of the parents' denial behavior may be to believe the other children are too young to know what has happened. If the situation is not explained to the children, they will place their own meanings upon what is happening. This may lead to isolation, intense loneliness, and distorted images, which may cause severe and unnecessary long-term suffering.[25]

The primary health care provider should plan further, periodic contacts with the family to ascertain whether or not their grief is being resolved—perhaps 2 or 3 months after the death, and near anniversaries and holidays for the first year. Certainly, contacts should be intensified if there is indication of dysfunctional behavior for an extended period of time.

Reactions of the health care team

People who enter the health professions tend to envision themselves as dedicated to a life of helping others recover from illness. They seldom are aware that eventually they will be faced with situations in which, despite their efforts, their patient will die.

The literature of the 1970s is abundant with demands that people have the right to die with dignity. Yet curricula for medical schools provide little opportunity for the young physician to learn the skills to help others with humane and dignified dying. In 1976, it was reported that only seven medical schools had a full-term course on death and dying, some had a "lecture or two" or a "minicourse," and fourteen had no course at all.[7]

The manner in which the physician reacts to death and deals with his own feelings, affects how the patient and family respond. Studies indicate that physicians often have an increased fear of death and may have become doctors to control that fear.[9]

The house officer, in particular, may feel overwhelmed if faced with the sudden, unanticipated death of an infant or child. He is already under stress because of his expectations of himself and his perception of the expectations of others. He may have had no previous experience as a professional with death and perceive it as his failure to cure. Possibly this is his first confrontation with the conflict between the high value placed on curative activities and the need to help a family cope with grief.

In order to play a supportive role with the family, the physician will need to be aware of and understand his own reactions to the situation. If he can accept his feelings and those of the family, he will come to realize the important contribution he can make to them. He is in the position of being able to ease suffering at the time of the death and, in addition, prevent possible dysfunctional resolution of grief:

> When our baby died, the doctor came over, took my shoulder firmly and said, "Now see here! There was nothing you could have done that would have made any difference. Your job now is to pick up the pieces. Talk to each other and be strong for each other. The other children will need you even more than ever now!" When I fall back into searching for things I should have done, I remember what he said, and that's a great source of strength to me.

It should be noted that other members of the health care team will experience similar feelings to those of the physician, particularly the members who are parents and who have not, as professionals, had responsibility for helping another deal with the death of a child. As a result of their anxiety, they may direct their anger at the physician because the rescue efforts he directed ended in failure. Where the work involves intense, emergency situations, it is important to have regular team meetings where feelings can be openly expressed and discussed, thereby establishing an environment of mutual trust and support. Tolerating another's pain and distress is not easy, and without an effective support system within the health care setting, staff members find long-term employment difficult if not impossible.

> The physician's duty is to heal sometimes,
> to relieve often, to comfort always.
>
> *E. L. Trudeau*

REFERENCES

1. Archibald, H. C., Bell, D., Miller, C., and Tuddenham, R. D.: Bereavement in childhood and adult psychiatric disturbance, Psychosom. Med. **24:**343, 1962.
2. Beck, A. T., Sethi, B. B., and Tuthill, R. W.: Childhood bereavement and adult depression, Arch. Gen. Psychiatry **9:**295, 1963.
3. Bergman, A. B., Roy, C. G., Pomeroy, M. A., and others: Studies of the sudden infant death syndrome in King County, Washington. III. Epidemiology, Pediatrics **49:**860, 1972.
4. Bozeman, M. F., Orbach, C. E., and Sutherland, A. M.: Psychological impact of cancer and its treatment. III. The adaptation of mothers to the threatened loss of their children through leukemia, part 1, Cancer **8:**1, 1955.
5. Buhrmann, M. V.: Death—its psychological significance in the lives of children, S. Afr. Med. J. **44:**586, 1970.
6. Cain, A. C., and Cain, B. S.: On replacing a child, J. Am. Acad. Child Psychiatry **3:**443, 1964.
7. Dickinson, G. E.: Death education in U. S. medical schools, J. Med. Educ. **51:**134, 1976.
8. Epperson, M.: Families in sudden crisis, Soc. Work Health Care **2:**265, 1977.
9. Feifel, H.: The meaning of death, New York, 1959, McGraw-Hill Book Co.
10. Fischoff, J., and O'Brien, N.: After the child dies, J. Pediatr. **88:**140, 1976.
11. Friedman, S. B.: Psychological aspects of sudden unexpected death in infants and children, Pediatr. Clin. North Am. **21:**103, 1974.
12. Friedman, S. B., Chodoff, P., Mason, J. W., and Hamburg, D. A.: Behavioral observations on parents anticipating the death of a child, Pediatrics **32:**610, 1963.
13. Furman, E.: A child's parent dies, New Haven, 1974, Yale University Press.
14. Green, M.: The family and the first critical hour, Report of the Sixth Round Table, Ross Laboratories **5706:**53, 1976.
15. Greer, S.: Study of parental loss in neurotics and sociopaths, Arch. Gen. Psychiatry **11:**77, 1964.
16. Gregory, I.: Anterospective data following childhood loss of a parent, Arch. Gen. Psychiatry **13:**99, 1965.
17. Grollman, E.: Explaining death to children, Boston, 1967, Beacon Press.
18. Hamovitch, M. B.: The parent and the fatally ill child, Duarte, Calif. 1964, City of Hope Medical Center.
19. Hilgard, J. R.: Anniversaries in mental illness, Psychiatry **22:**113, 1959.

20. Husband, P., and Hinton, P. E.: Families of children with repeated accidents, Arch. Dis. Child. **47:**396, 1972.
21. Jackson, E. N.: Grief and religion. In Feifel, H., editor: The new meaning of death, New York, 1965, McGraw-Hill Book Co.
22. Kastenbaum, R., and Aisenberg, R.: The psychology of death, New York, 1972, Springer Publishing Co., Inc.
23. Klaus, M. H., and Kennell, J. H.: Maternal-infant bonding, St. Louis, 1976, The C. V. Mosby Co.
24. Lindemann, E.: Symptomatology and management of acute grief, Am. J. Psychiatry **101:**141, 1944.
25. Mills, G. C., Reisler, R., Robinson, A., and Vermilye, G.: Discussing death, Homewood, Ill. 1976, E T C Publications.
26. Office of the Chief Medical Examiner, Balitmore, Personal communication, December 8, 1977.
27. Orbach, C. E., Sutherland, A. M., and Bozeman, M. F.: Psychological impact of cancer and its treatment. III. The adaptation of mothers to the threatened loss of their children through leukemia, part 2, Cancer **8:**20, 1955.
28. Padilla, E. R.: Predicting accident frequency in children, Pediatrics **58:**223, 1976.
29. Parkes, C. M.: Bereavement; studies of grief in adult life, New York, 1972, Basic Books, Inc., Publishers.
30. Parness, E.: Effects of experiences with loss and death among preschool children, Children Today, DHEW Publication No. (OHD): 76-30088, 1975, U.S. Department of Health, Education and Welfare.
31. Pollock, G.: Anniversary reactions, trauma and mourning, Psychoanal. Q. **39:**347, 1970.
32. Poznanski, E. D.: The "replacement child"; a saga of unresolved parental grief, J. Pediatr. **81:**1190, 1972.
33. Schowalter, J. E.: Death and the pediatric house officer, J. Pediatr. **76:**706, 1970.
34. Szybist, C.: The subsequent child, DHEW Publication No. (HSA): 76-5145, 1976, U.S. Department of Health, Education, and Welfare.
35. Weinstein, S. E.: Sudden infant death syndrome; its impact on families and a direction for change, Am. J. Psychiatry **135:**831, 1978.
36. Weston, D. L., and Irwin, R.: Preschool child's responses to death of an infant sibling, Am. J. Dis. Child. **106:**564, 1963.

CHAPTER 9

Genetics and death in childhood

PHILIP L. TOWNES

Death of a child as the result of a genetic disorder introduces complications beyond those encountered in death from nongenetic causes. In childhood death from nongenetic diseases, such as leukemia, pneumonia, infection, and sudden infant death syndrome (SIDS), the parents are at least able to cope with their loss without the threat of loss of yet other children and without identification of themselves as the biologic source of the fatal disorder. Moreover, there may be considerable solace in the knowledge that there is negligible risk of recurrence, and "replacement" of the lost child may prove to be an important adaptive mechanism. Alleviation of parental guilt with the explanation that no one is to blame is also an important aspect of parental adaptation and adjustment to their loss.

Regrettably, these important mechanisms of adjustment are not available to parents of a child who died of a genetic disorder. The contrast may be clearly seen if one compares sudden infant death syndrome with cystic fibrosis (CF). In SIDS, parents are concerned with questions of "Why did my baby die?" "Was I responsible for the death?"[4] One can reassure the parents that SIDS is not a hereditary disorder and that there should be no significant risk for subsequent children.[1] In contrast to this situation, parents of children with CF are generally informed that CF is an autosomal recessive disorder and that there is a 25% recurrence risk for a subsequent child to have the disorder and ultimately become a victim of it. To have a child slowly die of CF is a tragedy of enormous proportion; to recognize that future children may do so also is tragedy compounded.

When death is due to CF, the prolonged period of severe chronic illness may provide opportunity for gradual parental adjustment to the ultimate death of the child. In other forms of genetic disorders, the period of chronic illness may be reduced to weeks, days, or even hours. In these instances, stresses on the family may prove to be extreme. For example, we recently saw a young couple whose firstborn child proved to have a severe form of congenital polycystic kidney disease. The child died of renal failure on the second day of life. The parents were informed of the diagnosis

113

and prognosis on the day of birth of the child because of impending death due to renal failure. The parents were also informed that the condition was hereditary and that it could occur again in a subsequent child. Genetic consultation was immediately requested and provided to ensure that the unfortunate parents had a clear understanding of the etiology of the disorder. After obtaining a detailed pregnancy and family history, the parents were carefully informed, with the aid of diagrams, of the autosomal recessive inheritance of congenital polycystic kidney disease. This was accomplished in a long discussion in a quiet room near the intensive care nursery. The parents were understandably extremely upset about the tragedy that had befallen them, for they had already been informed by other physicians that the child would certainly die within the first few days of life. The added knowledge that they would have a 25% risk for recurrence in any subsequent pregnancy was no less devastating.

As is usually the case in autosomal recessive disorders, the family history of both parents was entirely negative, and they had no reason to suspect (before the birth of the child) that they would be at risk for this very serious genetic disorder. The fact that they had no other living children was an additional complication for this young couple. In the course of the discussion, emphasis was placed on the fact that both parents were single-dose (heterozygous) healthy carriers of a gene for congenital polycystic kidney disease. With the aid of diagrams, the parents were shown how, on a random basis, a homozygous (affected) child may be expected in one of four pregnancies.

In order to provide some basis for optimism, the parents were repeatedly informed that there was a 75% chance that any child they might have would not have congenital polycystic kidney disease. Emphasized was the fact that all individuals are carriers of the genes that cause genetic disease. Indeed, many couples have a 25% risk for recessive disorders such as CF, phenylketonuria, or congenital polycystic kidney disease, but are unaware of their carrier status simply because their children are among the 75% of progeny who are free of the disease. This emphasis is important in helping parents view themselves as not very different from others whom they consider to be healthy and more fortunate. The unstated but implicit recognition that there would be no risk for a child with this disorder if it were not for the fact that they happened to marry carriers like themselves may introduce marital stress. There is regrettably no way to avoid this recognition, and so the situation proves overwhelming in several respects: first, a totally unexpected neonatal death, then awareness that there is a 25% recurrence risk for other children, and finally the recognition that their plight results from the fact that their marriage involves a union of two healthy carriers of the same disorder. Indeed, their entire outlook on life, family, children, and so on, had been dramatically changed during the preceding 24 hours.

One may question the timing of the genetic advice in this particular instance. It might have been better to have concentrated on supporting this family in terms of the loss of the child and defer to some postmourning period the discussion of their genetic prognosis. In this particular instance the genetic consultation was provided immediately, because the parents had been informed on the day of birth that the condition was hereditary. To have deferred genetic counseling might have conceivably subjected them to even greater stress, for they might have assumed that their risk was 100% because they had no living, normal children to dispute that misconception. Because the parents were under enormous stress, arrangements were made to meet again 2 weeks later. This lengthy meeting differed from the first meeting in that the parents had overcome their initial mourning and were better able to focus more specifically on the genetic prognosis. The parents were assured that the original diagnosis had been confirmed by postmortem study, and the original advice was thereby substantiated. The autosomal recessive pattern of inheritance was again reviewed and discussed to ensure that they understood the basis and meaning of the 25% recurrence risk.

There are many additional complications to parental adjustment when death of a child is caused by a genetic disorder. Foremost are the threat of recurrence and the parental guilt that may result from the recognition of oneself as the biologic source of the fatal disorder. These complications to parental adjustment may vary considerably, depending on the specific mode of inheritance and the recurrence risk.[5]

CHROMOSOME ABNORMALITIES

Chromosome abnormalities comprise a well-defined group of genetic disorders, including trisomy 21 (Down syndrome), trisomy 18 (Edwards syndrome), trisomy 13 (Patau syndrome), 5p deletion syndrome (cri du chat), and the sex chromosome abnormalities (Turner, Klinefelter, and related syndromes). Except in rare instances involving familial translocations, recurrence risks are low, usually less than 1%. This enables the genetic counselor to provide considerable reassurance to the parents. However, while the recurrence risks are generally low, the cytogenetic diagnosis may indicate a dire prognosis. For example, survival beyond 1 or 2 years of age is rare (less than 5%) in individuals with trisomy 13 or 18. Consultations for these disorders are frequently obtained during the neonatal period in order to establish the diagnosis, because it may become a major factor in the subsequent management of the patient.

Physicians may be less aggressive in medical support efforts if they know that the ultimate prognosis of the child is early death.

When genetic studies are completed, it is generally desirable to review the findings and the prognosis with the parents. One may not choose to explicitly indicate the expected length of survival, but one cannot avoid the necessity of informing the parents that survival will not be greater than 1 or 2 years. In this setting, it is highly desirable to explain the etiology as one of random nondysjunction, to assure the parents that they are normal, that they do not have any cytogenetic disorder, and that the disorder was caused by an accident of cell division, that is, segregation of chromosomes in the formation of egg or sperm. It is advisable to avoid the specific identification of mother or father as the source of the aneuploid gamete, even though identification may be possible with chromosome-banding studies. Particularly beneficial to the parents at this crisis point is the reassurance that the recurrence risk is low (1% or less) and that it may be reduced even further through prenatal diagnosis if they choose to have such studies in subsequent pregnancies.

POLYGENIC ABNORMALITIES

Included in the polygenic abnormalities are many of the more common congenital malformations. Fortunately, relatively few result in death of the child; most are correctable, such as pyloric stenosis, congenital dislocation of the hip, club foot, and cleft lip and palate. The more serious, life-threatening defects include spina bifida, anencephaly, hydrocephaly, and congenital heart disease. Recurrence risks are less than 4% to 5%, and there is good reason to be reassuring to the parents. With prenatal diagnosis, such as $alpha_1$-fetoprotein levels in suspected recurrence of spina bifida, the risk in some instances can be reduced even further. Again, there is benefit in the explanation that neither parent is really a carrier of any unusual defect-causing genes. The genetic factors responsible for these birth defects are common, and many couples have the same genetic potential but on a random segregation basis are unaware of their risk. Indeed, 95% of couples with the same genetic endowment remain unaware of their risk. Confirmation of this assessment can be convincingly provided by emphasizing that the risk for the recurrence is less than 5%.

AUTOSOMAL DOMINANT ABNORMALITIES

Inherited forms of autosomal dominant traits are fortunately not a frequent cause of death in childhood, because if the disorder were one that resulted in child death, there would be little likelihood of affected individuals achieving reproductive age. Therefore, if death is due to an autosomal dominant trait, it is generally due to de novo (gametic) mutation, and the recurrence risk is thus, fortunately, negligible. This is well exemplified in Apert syndrome (acrocephalosyndactyly). A few individuals with Apert syndrome have reached adult years and become parents. The risk to their progeny is 50%. However, the vast majority of cases of Apert syndrome are due to new mutation, which accounts for the fact that the incidence at birth is approximately 1 in 200,000, but in older individuals the frequency is 1 in 2,000,000. The vast majority die during childhood years.

Of note is the variable expressivity that may be encountered in some autosomal dominant traits. For example, the death of a child due to optic glioma may lead to the diagnosis of von Recklinghausen disease (neurofibromatosis) in a parent. The manifestation in the parent may be nothing more than a small number of cutaneous lesions (cafe-au-lait spots), and other members of the family may be similarly affected. The recurrence risk for the disease in children of an affected parent is clearly 50%, but one can be moderately reassuring in that the severe expressions (optic glioma, acoustic neuroma) are fairly uncommon complications of this disorder.

AUTOSOMAL RECESSIVE ABNORMALITIES

Of the several different modes of inheritance, the autosomal recessive is undoubtedly the most threatening. The initial occurrence is invariably unexpected, and the recurrence risk is unfortunately high (25%). The family histories are usually negative, and the parents are completely ignorant of their risk until the birth of the affected child reveals their carrier status and their 25% recurrence risk. This situation is exemplified by the family with congenital polycystic kidney disease already discussed. Although the art of syndrome identification has been expanded in recent years, a specific diagnosis is frequently not achieved in many infants with multiple congenital malformations and/or mental retardation, and/or failure-to-thrive syndromes. Fortunately, in most instances these poorly defined dysmorphic syndromes prove to be nongenetic with negligible recurrence risk. However, one occasionally encounters a family in which the birth of a *second* affected child establishes the genetic etiology. For example, the firstborn daughter of a young married couple died at 3 months of age as the result of a progressive neurologic disorder. The infant spent her entire life in the hospital, was evaluated by many consultants, and underwent innumerable diagnostic studies. The parents were informed that although an autosomal recessive disorder with 25% recurrence risk could not be excluded, it was considered unlikely, and the overall risk might be 5%. Their second child, a son, was born 2 years later and had an identical course. The family was again referred for genetic advice and informed that their recurrence risk was probably 25%. They have been understandably reluctant to have further children.

We have also recently seen a family whose firstborn child died of renal agenesis. They had been assured by their physician that there was no appreciable risk for recurrence. With the birth of their second affected child, they were referred for genetic counseling. They were informed that renal agenesis is usually of sporadic etiology, and only a few families have been reported to have a second affected child. Despite the rarity, the recurrence in their family suggests autosomal recessive inheritance with a 25% recurrence risk. As in the family with the progressive neurologic disorder, the recurrence risk was not recognized until after the birth of a second affected child, truly an instance of tragedy compounded by tragedy.

X-LINKED RECESSIVE ABNORMALITIES

In contrast to the mutual sharing of carrier status in an autosomal recessive disorder, the situation in an X-linked disorder is potentially even more difficult to manage. In an inherited X-linked recessive disorder, genetic counseling ultimately identifies the mother as the source of the mutant allele. The identification of the mother as the progenitor of the mutant allele may evoke strong feelings of guilt and may render her subject to subtle or overt accusation and indictment by her "healthy" husband. While the situation in this respect is worse than in an autosomal recessive disorder, there are, for some couples at least, choices that may allow them to have other children without the 50% risk of an affected male. With prenatal diagnosis, for example, one may determine the sex of the fetus, abort the males, and allow pregnancies of female fetuses to continue. By this means, parents can be assured that there will be no other affected sons. Obviously, these alternatives peculiar to X-linked recessive diseases are viewed differently by different parents. To those parents who may have had one or more sons and are wishing to have a daughter, the carrier status of the mother may provide an unexpected opportunity for selection of the desired sex. On the other hand, some couples are, for a variety of reasons, totally unaccepting of the possibility of terminating a pregnancy, and for them the overall risk remains 25% as in the autosomal recessive disorder. Occasionally, selective abortion is viewed as deferring the problem to the unborn daughters and is rejected for that reason. In some instances, the marriage may be dissolved, the husband deciding that he can avoid the threat by remarriage. While that decision may "solve" the problem for him, it leaves the wife in an unenviable situation.

NONGENETIC DISORDERS

Paradoxically, most individuals seeking genetic advice prove to have no genetic disorder. Indeed, genetic evaluation is frequently sought in order to determine whether or not the disorder is genetic. The determination that the disorder is not genetic and that there is consequently no increased recurrence risk is a very important aspect of genetic counseling. In these instances, genetic counseling provides reassurance and a better understanding of the cause of the disorder, alleviates guilt, eliminates misconception, and promotes better parental acceptance and adjustment.[3,5]

With the current emphasis on public education and the consequent high level of public awareness that genetic factors may cause disease, it has become a matter of importance to provide, when possible, a positive statement that a given disorder is *not* genetic. This need is well reflected in the disclaimer "SIDS is not hereditary," which appears in the SIDS brochures.[1,4] Until recently, such disclaimers were rarely included in literature directed to the lay public. The disclaimers serve an important function in reassuring families of the low probability of recurrence of the tragedy that has befallen them. This reassurance can be an important factor in their adjustment to their loss.

SUMMARY

In general, all parents of children born with major birth defects deserve some form of genetic advice, whether the etiology proves to be genetic or nongenetic.[5] Such advice is particularly important if the disorder proves to be fatal. However, while death in childhood may be viewed as the ultimate tragedy, it is important to recognize that some parents may equate severe morbidity with death. A severely retarded or grossly deformed child may be viewed by parents as a death equivalent. Parents may occasionally verbalize their wish for death of the child and in some instances refuse permission for lifesaving surgery. Most families receiving genetic advice can be assured that the disorder is not genetic, no one is to blame, and there is negligible chance of recurrence. Unfortunately, in some instances the disorder will prove to be genetic, and there will be an appreciable recurrence risk. For these families it is, unfortunately, not possible to provide the same reassurance. On the contrary, the clarification of the genetic etiology, including the threat of recurrence and the guilt that may be evoked or augmented by parental understanding of the hereditary basis of the disorder, may have significant negative effects. Fischoff and O'Brien[2] have recently noted that parents may perceive the loss of a child as a loss of a part of themselves. Through genetic counseling, further recognition of self as progenitor of the fatal genetic disorder may consolidate and amplify these feelings and result in overwhelming complications in parental adjustment to the death of a child.

REFERENCES

1. Facts about sudden infant death syndrome, DHEW Publication No. (NIH) 76-225, Rockville Md., 1972, U.S. Department of Health, Education, and Welfare.
2. Fischoff, J., and O'Brien, N.: After the child dies, J. Pediatr. **88:**140, 1976.
3. Reynolds, B. DeV., Puck, M. H., and Robinson, A.: Genetic counseling; an appraisal, Clin. Genet. **5:**177, 1974.
4. Szybist, C.: The subsequent child, DHEW Publication No. (HSA) 76-5145, Rockville, Md., 1976, U.S. Department of Health, Education, and Welfare.
5. Townes, P. L.: Preventive genetics and early therapeutic procedures in the control of birth defects, Birth Defects **6:**42, 1970.

THE CAREGIVER AND THE FATALLY ILL CHILD

The reactions of caregivers dealing with fatally ill children and their families

JOHN E. SCHOWALTER

To understand caregivers' reactions to dying children, one must examine at least three major factors that influence those reactions. The first is the psychologic makeup of the caregivers: who are they, and how did they become what they are? Second, one must know some of the variables involved in the task, including the general circumstances, how well the patient is known, whether the caregiver is of similar age to the patient, and so on. Third, one needs to be aware of what is available to aid caregivers to work better with dying children, with their families, and with each other.

THE CAREGIVERS

The psychologic makeup of the caregivers is undoubtedly the most important variable in giving good care. Almost everyone nods confidently when they hear Francis Peabody's well-known quote that "the secret of the care of the patient is in caring for the patient."[10] What, however, can be said about those who become the caregivers? Much has been written about the reactions of physicians to death, and nurses' reactions are commonly discussed, but there is much less in the literature about the background and training of chaplains, dieticians, physical therapists, psychologists, child care workers, and social workers. This differential probably has more to do with who needs to write to be promoted than who has more or fewer feelings.

Vaisrub in a *JAMA* editorial, "Dying is Worked to Death,"[19] suggests that the paucity of hard data makes articles on death and dying easy to write and therefore increasingly common. He goes on to state that he does not believe the dying are really ignored and that he is convinced that more people lose sleep over the thought of their taxes than over the thought of their deaths.

Such bold declarations are a natural lead-in to a discussion of physicians' attitudes toward death. What are the feelings about death exhibited by students who choose medicine? One cannot, of course, speak for every student, but there have been some studies on this matter. One suggests that premedical students have more concern about death than other undergraduates,[8] while another showed that concerns about death increased for medical students during their clinical years.[7] The latter finding is consistent with other studies that show that those physicians who see death most are the most reluctant to face the fact of death with their dying patients.[5]

In the literature, much is made of the fact that physicians *do* seem, more than other caregivers, to avoid the implications of death and dying. They are the least likely group, for example, to attend a lecture on thanatology given at a medical school. Why might this be? For one thing, too much is expected from physicians. They are consistently identified in polls as the most trusted professional group, and expectations begin early. Playing doctor is a popular children's game, because from the child's point of view, doctors are allowed by society to take off other people's clothes, to look without shame, to know the mysteries of sex and elimination, and to deliberately cause pain; but because physicians cure people they not only are not punished for such indulgences, they are respected and extremely well paid.[16] Society will give much to stay alive and well.

Unfortunately, death is a maddeningly common problem, and in spite of the huge advances in medical science the death rate remains at 100%. Medical students should therefore obviously learn to face death as well as to fight it, but for some professors, the discussion of death seems defeatist and therefore distressing. Of 121 medical school deans and department chairmen who responded to a survey by The Foundation of Thanatology in the early 1970s, 89% stated that the majority of their faculty would agree that students in their institution were not adequately prepared to care for the dying patient's family.[6]

Most beginning medical students divert the high expectations they have of the profession to themselves. In this, of course, may be the wish to take care of others as they wish or wished to be cared for themselves. There is good evidence, for example, that physicians who had difficult childhoods are more likely to have alcohol and drug problems than other physicians or nonphysicians matched for socioeconomic backgrounds.[18] This may be because these physicians are greatly disillusioned by not finding the self-help or the omnipotence that they had hoped to find in the profession.

Much has been written about the stresses that face physicians. It seems at least likely that an important component of this stress is the impossible expectation. In most medical schools, it is very rare to have lectures on what to do when you cannot do anything more for the patient's disorder. In fact, specialties having to do with chronic illness or rehabilitation medicine traditionally suffer low prestige and limited exposure in the medical education hierarchy. So, through societal expectation, self-expectation, and training, the young physician expects perfection.

The initial tendency of the beginning medical student is to overidentify with patients. This may lead to adopting their symptoms and often leads to feeling depressed when they are not cured. "Cured" is a word certainly heard more from the young than the old. In response to the psychic pain and the disappointment caused through identification, there may evolve a different but more protective perspective in the student: dehumanization. This is not a universal defense, but it is an effective one. If patients are not persons, they have no relevance to the physician's own vulnerability, either as a physician or as a mortal. Dehumanization is seldom a conscious defense, which is too bad, because it is more easily modifiable when it is.

A corollary to the implied omnipotence of the physician is that he or she must feel, or at least appear, energetic and competent at all times. It is, for example, surprisingly common for doctors to believe they cannot catch their patients' diseases, and physicians are notoriously poor at looking after their own health.

Studies on the incidence and prevalence of illness, especially mental illness and suicide, among physicians compared with the general population are conflicting and difficult to sort out. Although it does seem that except for a much higher rate of drug abuse, physicians are probably not more likely than their chronologic and socioeconomic counterparts to commit suicide or become mentally ill,[20,21] they are more reluctant to seek help when they are troubled or sick. There is too often a tendency to follow the admonition of that ancient colleague, St. Luke, "Physician, heal thyself."

Death is often accepted as the opposite of success in regard to the treatment of a patient. As already suggested, some students enter medicine in order to conquer their own death fears through others. Although it is probably true that the field of medicine is the best approach available to study how to thwart death, medicine not only does not always work but eventually always fails. And, even if a physician is not more fearful of death than is usual, he or she will have to deal with it and its stresses much more often than will the average person. Indeed, with the increasing substitution of science for religion during this century, doctors more than clergymen are now looked to for answers and comfort.

Medical training has not kept pace. Feelings and empathy are seldom discussed except in psychiatry; and psychiatry, which is not biologically based, is often considered impractical by medical students and by the scientific investigators on the faculty, who represent the students' most powerful role models.

Being around death brings up thoughts and feelings about past and future deaths for the medical student. Medical students are often especially vulnerable to the threat of death. Having come so far, having worked so hard, and having so much that is good and exciting poised just ahead of them make the thought of their own deaths an especially macabre possibility. Indeed, I have been consulted by medical students who, because their position in life is so enviable, have developed a fear that some catastrophe would occur and through death destroy all that they were about to attain.

A final possible factor in regard to the emotional makeup of the physician as a caregiver is a general change in medical treatment approaches. There has been a burgeoning of the field of medical engineering and of favoritism shown medical school applicants who possess training or degrees in the "hard" sciences. As medicine has become more sophisticated technically, "things" have tended to supplant concern for people. These changes have caused medicine to become more complicated morally as well. It is not always taught that we should be concerned with ends as well as means: just because a thing can be done, we are not obliged to do it, and the more we can do the more we have to think about what we wish to do.[2]

Although a physician's professional life is arduous and experiences with the dying are particularly stressful, the death of a child is especially painful. In one study of events that cause doctors anxiety, the death of a child was ranked considerably higher by the physician respondents than was the death of an adult.[1] In another study, in which English and American adults were asked to scale 61 life events as to how upsetting the event would be to them, the death of one's child was rated first by the populations on both sides of the Atlantic.[9] It seems as though the belief that only old people die develops early in one's life and remains forever. There is also a common belief that children are "simpler" than adults, and therefore those who work with them require less training, skill, and compensation than those who work with adults. This myth is even believed by some caregivers. When a child patient does not respond to therapy, the novice may feel especially bad that he or she could not even cure a child. Solnit has noted that some health workers choose to work with children because they wish to avoid the deteriorating in favor of the developing and to avoid the end of life in favor of the beginning.[17] Such individuals may find a dying child impossible to care for.

Because there are more data available on the subject, I have emphasized the factors that are involved in the development of the physician as a caregiver. The discussion also acts as a baseline, because many of the psychologic components noted are similar to those found in other caregivers. One difference is that the physician has the stress of ultimate responsibility for the patient, whereas other members of the staff often suffer by not having responsibility. For example, nurses spend a relatively large amount of time with the dying child while often having little say in or little knowledge of the treatment regimen. Although nurses may not make policy, they are often asked to answer for it. Because the patient and family often believe it is unsafe to attack the doctors, for the physicians seem in charge of their fate, they deflect their anger and dissatisfaction onto the safer and more readily available nurses. Young female nurses may be additionally affected because they are at or approaching the peak age for child bearing. Their identification with dying patients' mothers often raises the question for them of whether or not they should have children.

Other caregivers, such as chaplains, social workers, child life workers, psychologists, and physical therapists, are generally more peripheral to decision making than the physicians and nurses. They each also have a special skill that is their interface with the patient and family and that can lead to specialized stresses.

Child life workers and recreational therapists are often requested to work with seriously ill and dying children in order both to keep the patients' minds off their plight and to encourage them to express their feelings through various expressive techniques. Such a challenge is a difficult balancing act, and it requires great tact, skill, and maturity to maintain the necessary close physical contact while coping with massive denial, anger, depression, and/or anxiety. In addition, because of their close relationships, child life workers often see things that should be changed in the rest of the staff's approach to the patient and family, but because of their relatively low status in the hospital, they are often not listened to as much as they should be.

It is not unusual for physical therapists to be asked to work with dying children. Their task is usually a very specific one. Problems arise, however, because often the child is deteriorating, and the work is more to maintain skills than to improve them. It takes unusual sensitivity and dedication to work under these conditions, especially when, as is so often the case, the patient is not motivated, other staff have given up, and there is a great likelihood of exacerbation.

Most hospitals now have psychiatrists, psychologists, and/or social workers available for consultation. These caregivers are usually expected to provide emotional support to dying patients and their families. Although they may work closely with the pediatrician in charge, these caregivers may be forced to perform their task in relative isolation. Pediatricians too often abdicate too much responsibility for emotional care when others are available to fill in. Psychologists, social workers, and psychiatrists work best when in constant touch and coordination with the pediatrician. This coordination is crucial not only to allow a reciprocal flow of information, but also to provide the pediatrician's imprimatur on the importance of the work and the reassurance to patient and parents that the pediatrician is aware of and does care about the emotional stresses they are under. When surveyed following their child's death, parents remember their caregivers' skill or .lack of it in terms of personal care much more than in terms of technical care.[3] An added service often provided by the social worker, psychiatrist, or psychologist is support of other staff. Often, however, there is no one to support the supporters.

The chaplain may be deeply involved as an important caregiver on the ward. This may be the family's rabbi, minister, or priest from home or a hospital chaplain. A dying child is one of the severest tests possible for one's religious faith, and the chaplain must try to comfort the family while often having to deal simultaneously with religious doubt and the expectation of a miracle. He also often must withstand the rage and frustration that are the reactions of not knowing why the tragedy occurred. This frequently comes not only from patient and parents but also from nonreligious hospital staff who may experience and resent, often unconsciously, the chaplain's presence as a mystical intrusion into their scientific environmnet. This may not be a common reaction, but it is not a rare one. Indeed, it seems likely that one reason for the recent increase in the general interest in death is the decline of religion and the substitution for it of science.

Parents, siblings, and grandparents are often important caregivers and are often forgotten as such by the hospital staff.[4] These individuals are crucial for the care and the support of the dying child, and full expositions of the roles and responses of these caregivers deserve and receive separate chapters.

THE SITUATION

The reactions of caregivers are, of course, not only influenced by their background but also by the variables that surround the death.

Dying children present three special disadvantages and problems. Dying patients tend to turn away from the dangerous future and toward the past for solace, but children and even most adolescents do not have this ability. They are, by their cognitive inability to master the adult's sense of time, trapped in the present. Second, ultimately, and most literally at death, everyone is alone. Because it is well known that children require parental closeness to be happy and to survive, to witness the loneliness of a dying child is especially painful for adults. Finally, the premature death represented by a fatally ill child brings home forcefully the fact that no one is guaranteed a long life, only a life time.

One general variable that affects all caregivers' responses to dying children is how close psychologically they are to the age of the patient. This closeness may be brought about by knowing another child or children who died at a similar age or by having a sibling, son, or daughter of the same age. Especially hard for young caregivers is the dying adolescent. Not only is adolescence the time for strength, beauty, and independence developmentally, and death is an especial anathema to these goals, but the proximity of the caregiver's age awakens a kinship with fatally ill adolescents that is powerful. The dread of death before fulfillment is particularly pervasive among students in the health professions, who have had to endure inordinately long periods of training and who are looking forward to now obtaining the professional and financial benefits of their study.

I have in the past suggested that one way of looking at the situation of a dying child is to divide the problems associated with care into three time periods, each having its particular difficulties.[11]

The first is the period of impact. Being the first to know the diagnosis and prognosis when life is threatened by illness, the pediatrician is the first to feel the impact of the tragedy. Telling the parents is difficult, and it is not unusual for the family's physician to rationalize having the "expert" in the hospital do this chore. In fact, most parents prefer to hear important medical news from the physician whom they know and who knows them best. When it is necessary for a specialist to explain the complexities of a condition or its treatment to the parents, the family physician should also be present, if possible. The disclosure to the parents that their child has a condition that might prove fatal usually triggers a series of reactions that include shock, disbelief in the diagnosis, disbelief in the prognosis, anger, guilt, acceptance, and anticipatory mourning. In order to clarify the communication, both parents should be told at the same time if at all possible. It is not unusual for parents to find this event more overwhelming than the actual death, depending on how much anticipatory mourning can be accomplished. Parents occasionally blame the physician as an omnipotent, malevolent person who could change the diagnosis and prognosis if he or she wished. Although parental feelings of anger and failure may be projected onto the pediatrician, most parents find it difficult to be angry with the person in whom they must put their faith for good care, and they therefore displace their hostility onto other caregivers, spouses, or other relatives, neighbors, and so on. Because a child's death is a threat to one form of parental immortality, there may also be anger toward the child; but being so unacceptable under the conditions of impending death, this anger too must be placed elsewhere. Of all the caregivers, nurses are most likely to receive the brunt of parental anger, because they are most available and most involved in day-to-day care.

It is important during the period of impact for all the caregivers involved to know what facts are told to whom, and if information is withheld, why. It is damaging to ward morale when staff members must be careful not to answer certain questions or reveal secrets when they do not understand or approve of the secrets.

Although it is generally accepted that parents should know the facts of the case, it is difficult to know how much should be told the child. Obviously, hope should never be completely withdrawn from anyone. Most fatally ill pediatric patients do not ask whether they will die, but most know that something terrible is wrong with them. In fact, once parents know the prognosis, their reactions to the child change so dramatically that is it impossible for the child not to realize that something very worrisome is occurring. What is most important is that there be an atmosphere of openness that allows the patient to ask as much or as little as he wishes. The more painful a decision is, the more we wish to establish a rule to cover it: it would be much easier if there were an age, type of diagnosis, family circumstance, or other indicator that could be relied on to determine correctly what to tell the child. The only true indicator, however, is the child, and the only measurement is the caregiver's sensitivity. Grief is not only painful for the sufferer but also for the observer, and this is one reason why we tend to believe children know less and feel less than they do. It is not unusual, for example, for dying children to tell caregivers that they are dying, but add that others should not be told, because the patient knows he or she is not supposed to know.

When a patient seems aware of what is happening but is reluctant to talk about it, there are ways to encourage communication. For example, "You must sometimes worry about dying," or even less direct, "You must sometimes wonder if you are ever going to get well." Some children who know they are dying still do not want to be told. An adolescent once explained this to me when she said, "If *you* tell me I'm dying, it's a fact; but if only I think it, I can believe it or not believe it depending on how I feel that day." It is crucial that caregivers know what questions the patient is asking whom and what the answers have been. Although all caregivers should be available to the patient and parents, it is mandatory that one person be in charge to coordinate the child's care. It is all too common that hospital care, especially of patients who are difficult to treat medically or emotionally, is diffused and confused by frequent staff changes or the lack of a single person who is responsible for the care being given in a complete and consistent way.

The second phase of care may be termed the period of battle and consists of the time of management until the child is in extremis. These periods, of course, are not as clearly demarcated in practice as on paper, and a number of emotions, such as denial, grief, guilt, and anger are common to all three periods.

Along with anger, guilt is ubiquitous when one is working with a dying child. Parents must be assured and reassured that their child's illness is not their fault. Caregivers also tend to feel guilty. This may be because one's treatment is not working, one's counseling is less than completely successful, one feels anger toward the child for not responding, one is withdrawing from the patient and the family more than is therapeutic, and so on. Guilt often leads to a variety of reactions that cause problems. The use of secrets regarding diagnosis and prognosis has already been discussed. Secrets are also sometimes kept in regard to physical tests and procedures or in regard to drug side effects. Guilt also has a tendency to cause parents and staff to become overly permissive, even though dying children respond best when there is structure and when their schedule is kept as routine as possible.

Anger is an important factor in the reactions of caregivers. A child's death is a threat to physicians' feelings of omnipotence, and working with a patient who does not respond is difficult for all the staff. Becoming angry is a common substitute for depression, and at times one senses that some caregivers look for reasons to criticize others in order to feel less bad themselves.

The reactions of caregivers are often affected by other variables. Patients who require severe dietary or fluid restrictions, who suffer remissions and exacerbations, who become progressively debilitated over a long period of time, or who are very demanding tend to bring out anger from the staff. Caregivers' reactions may include blaming the parents as overintrusive or underinvolved, treating the dying child as inferior, or allowing hospital routines to take primacy over dignity, respect, and humanity. The latter reaction is especially frequent and causes hospital personnel to be so busy taking care of routines that they learn nothing about a process that they themselves will eventually experience.

The third and final phase of care is the period of defeat. This includes the terminal phase of treatment, the death, and the period of contact with the family thereafter. Whenever there is a high census of dying children or there are multiple deaths over a short period of time, the staff is likely to become depressed. With multiple deaths, even the most experienced and competent caregivers admit to an unrealistically severe scrutiny of their own role in the children's care.

The length of time the staff members have known the child influences the emotional intensity they feel. Children who are preverbal or who die quickly tend to cause less personal anguish than adolescents or those who are cared for over a protracted period of time. Patients whose deaths are due to accidents are sometimes an exception to the finding that quick deaths have relatively little impact on caregivers. Accidents are the most common cause of death during all but the earliest part of the pediatric age range. It is striking how little has been written about the reactions of caregivers toward children who die because of accidents. This paucity is partly because many of these patients die either before arriving in the hospital, in the emergency room, or following only a brief stay on the ward. Staff contact is therefore brief. I believe there are also emotional factors that have influenced the lack of attention to accidental deaths. Compared with staff reactions to children who die from illness, reactions to children dying from accidents contain more anger than guilt. There is less a feeling of medical failure and a greater sense of blame, either at parents for not protecting the child adequately or, more often in adolescence, at the patient for causing the mishap. A focus on blame sometimes causes the staff to resent caring for the patient and affects adversely the quality of care given. This reaction is most pronounced in regard to adolescents who have made serious suicide attempts. A common reaction here is "Why is this patient bothering us with his craziness?"

During this terminal phase, the reaction of caregivers toward children that is most frequently noted in the literature is withdrawal. Although withdrawal is a natural part of anticipatory mourning, and the patient may exhibit it as well, staff withdrawal should be neither abrupt nor extensive. Staff withdrawal from the patient is often accompanied by withdrawal from the family as well at the time they need support most. It is important for all staff to follow the old adage that the fewer the treatments available to the physician the more the physician must be available.

Following a death there may be a feeling of relief as well as defeat, especially if the child has suffered for a long time. It is common for the staff to want to withdraw, but it is crucial that the family not be abandoned. Staff members' presence and willingness to listen are usually more important than what is said. In fact, much of what is said is not heard. Often parents complain that once their child has died, the staff forgets about them and their child. Contact in the following weeks or months by the physician, psychiatrist, social worker, psychologist, and/or chaplain to see how the parents and siblings are reacting to the death is seldom done but very useful.

With our ability through technology to keep patients' lungs oxygenating and their hearts pumping, the question of how long to keep patients alive has become an increasingly difficult one. In addition, especially with cancer patients, there is the problem of how long to press aggressive treatment during the terminal phase. On the one side are the possibility of a remission and the possibility of gaining important new knowledge, while on the other side are the possibilities of providing unnecessary pain and prolonging death rather than life. Again, there are no pat answers, and the patient and family should, as much as possible, be included in the decision making. In general, those closest to the physical care of the patient are the least willing to prolong the terminal phase. Staff friction sometimes occurs when attending physicians, radiologists, or oncologists continue to prescribe uncomfortable treatments to children in extremis. Unless the rationale for the treatments is well communicated, other caregivers may in various ways undermine the patient's and parents' confidence in the care they are receiving. When this sort of staff split occurs, anger and depression are the common sequelae for all involved.

A prolonged terminal phase causes individual staff members considerable emotional pain. The wish to avoid this pain is strong, but it is confounded by the realization that a wish for the pain to go away may include the wish for the child to die. For some these wishes are conscious, but for most caregivers they are not, because there is at the same time the wish that the child will not die. The usual response to such ambivalence, especially on the part of physicians, is to reject any course but keeping the child alive for as long as possible. With increasing frequency, however, and usually among caregivers who are not physicians, there is seen a very different reaction: an enthusiasm for "allowing" the patient to die or even a definite push for the use of some type of euthanasia. Carried to an extreme, both approaches get rid of a dying child whose presence is anxiety provoking. In the first approach the child, a treatment failure, is changed into an interesting medical exercise in keeping an organism alive, and in the second approach the child and the painful situation are removed through the hastening of death. There is no one formula or timetable, but the vigor applied in keeping the patient alive during the terminal phase should be based on the wishes and needs of the parents and patient rather than on those of the caregivers. By the midteens and with the appropriate information, the patient can often become a full partner in deciding what approaches should be used and for how long.

USEFUL APPROACHES

In this concluding section, I will describe the sorts of approaches and techniques that I have found helpful for caregivers in their work with dying children and their families. The first part of the section will focus on the training of staff, the middle portion on approaches to aiding the parents in ways that will allow the caregivers to work more effectively, and the final part of the section will be a discussion of various techniques that promote better communication and interaction among staff members working with a fatally ill child.

At present there is not much teaching done in thanatology in preparing one to become a medical caregiver. This is changing somewhat, and perhaps most is done in nurses' training. The greatest resistance is found in medical school education. Because death is the ultimate failure for a healer and it is natural to avoid failure, there will always be some resistance. Other reasons for resistance include the fact that many chiefs of service believe, as voiced by Vaisrub,[19] that patients' and families' feelings about death are not important and not really available for hard scientific study. Another factor in resistance is that most medical caregivers are action-oriented individuals and tend to avoid anything that smacks of passivity.

In spite of this resistance, however, some significant education can be provided students with only a modicum of curriculum change and time. The expectation of perfection and the messages that a physician's and nurse's job is to stamp out death are routinely conveyed in most schools. These are not necessarily said overtly, but are absorbed through the conspiracy of silence regarding caregivers' professional and personal mistakes and problems. The teaching of students that they and their peers *will* make mistakes and that death is something that must be faced as well as fought will, it is hoped, remove some of the pressure that is generated by unrealistic expectations. This knowledge may also help to modify the cold, ineffective routines that hospitals have traditionally used to protect staff from feelings and from patients.

Often when thanatology is taught, it is done through one or more didactic lectures. This is ineffective unless accompanied by direct interaction with dying children and/or through rounds or discussions with staff who are caring for these patients. In general, students accept teaching about the care of the dying best from members of their own discipline. Although this may be due partly to elitism, it is enhanced by identification and the knowledge that the teacher has been through what they will go through and that they will eventually experience and have to master what their teachers have. With this subject, as with others, the best teachers are often those who are not more than a few years ahead of the students. In medicine, for example, a house officer who is articulate and interested in the problems of the fatally ill can be a valuable teacher. It is interesting that the urgency transmitted from experiences of a colleague who is just senior to the student can have credibility through the experience alone, whereas the far more extensive experiences related by a much older practitioner may be dismissed as so much prattle.

A number of specific points should be stressed with students regarding working with fatally ill children and their families. None pertains exclusively to the dying, but all are especially important in these cases. The most general point concerns the maintenance of continuity of care. Many terminally ill patients require, or at least obtain, the services of a multitude of specialized caregivers. Each person has charge of a part of the child, but often no one is in charge of the whole. Every medical professional knows that such fragmentation leads inevitably to poor care, but the phenomenon can be corrected only if it is looked for. The fact of the possibility of this danger must be repeated and repeated to students. Second, it must be stressed that when one is working with the dying, listening may be more important and helpful than acting. This is especially true in the impact and terminal phases. Finally, the student must be made aware of the ubiquity and power of the feelings of guilt and anger. These affects abound in patient, family, and staff. The situation of a fatally ill child commonly causes anger in one or more of those involved. The anger may be at the wasted past, at the absent future, at the cost in time, energy, and money, at the narcissistic injury, at fate, at God, at one another, or at oneself. There is also the powerful existential anger that something so repugnant as a child's death must be somebody's fault. Anyone's fault, even one's own, may seem more acceptable than the mockery of blind fate. The realization that guilt and anger are usual rather than unusual can help remove their venom.

The response of parents to their dying child has a major effect on the reactions of caregivers, and there are ways of working with parents that direct their grief into constructive rather than destructive actions.

During the period of impact, it is useful to warn parents of a fatally ill child not to hurry to tell others of the tragedy. Until they have had a chance to begin to assimilate the news along with its meaning and demands, it is better to tell as few people as possible. When parents do seek solace by immediately informing family and friends, the result is usually counterproductive, because they are not yet able to respond to the multitude of questions, to the outpouring of sympathy, or to the covert rebuke that accompanies some peoples' tendency to "blame the victim." It is better for the parents to first have some idea of how they feel and what they are going to do before they face the additional problem of explaining the situation to others.

We have found that a good way to help parents face the diagnosis and prognosis is not only to have professionals convey the information repeatedly but also to encourage parents to meet together in groups. These groups may consist of parents of the children who are together on the ward at the same time, parents of children having the same medical condition, or parents of children who are dying. The makeup seems less important than the skill of the leader in providing an atmosphere of mutual support and comfort. A common difficulty with such groups, however, is that parents seldom remain after their child dies. Although the postdeath period is one in which they could use the continuity of care provided by the group and the group could benefit from hearing of their experience, the feeling of having been let down or of having let the group down is common and frequently strong enough to keep the parents from continuing.

Already mentioned, but worth repeating, is the helpfulness of drawing the parents into the care and planning of their child's treatment. Mothers are usually better able to do this than fathers, who tend to be more fearful of hospitals, but it is best when both are involved. When parents feel they are part of the plan, their feelings of guilt and anger are reduced. Anger and guilt are emotions that often generate one another. Strong feelings of parental anger and guilt may trigger similar reactions from the caregivers and reduce staff efficiency. There are constructive ways to channel parental anger, and one of the best is to encourage parents to join, if appropriate, a society to help raise money, lobby, change laws, educate, and aid in other ways to further the understanding of leukemia, sudden infant death syndrome, cystic fibrosis, or whatever condition their child suffers from.

There are also a variety of techniques that promote better communication and interaction among staff members. Communication with the patients can be enhanced through patient meetings.[14] Some patients would rather write their concerns than speak them, and this option should also be made available. We accomplish this through a ward newspaper.[15] It is especially important with adolescent patients to provide opportunities for them to maintain their self-esteem.[13]

Who supports the caregivers? Here, too, communication is the crucial ingredient. Besides communication of information, already mentioned, communication of personal feelings is also important. I was impressed by a type of communication used by nurses in a renal dialysis unit. The nurses and patients wore white gowns. At times nurses or patients would stick a red bandaid on the sleeve of their own gown. This was known by all to mean that the person was irritable that day, wished to be left alone, and should not be bugged. There are other techniques that are more expressive. The writing out of dreams about patients who are dying or have died can be used to evoke feelings and thoughts that were not previously realized.[12]

Although it is sometimes useful, especially with inexperienced caregivers, for a preceptor to supervise them with their work with the dying, group meetings again seem to be more effective. This is true especially when the group meets regularly and the members know each other well. Such groups can be formed from the staff of a ward or a specialty clinic. Physicians seem to have the most difficulty in these groups, because their training and status tend to encourage a suppression of feelings and a wish to give a definitive answer. It is also difficult when a member of the staff, whether or not he or she is a physician, is considered an expert in thanatology. When this occurs, the person tends in the extreme either to be looked to for answers that will alleviate staff anxiety and pain or to be avoided as an unwanted reminder of death.

This brings up the final point that must be stressed to caregivers: teaching personnel about thanatology does not make difficult problems or emotions go away. Understanding and skill allow an impossible job to be done better, but after all we say and do regarding the fatally ill patient, the child still dies, and being human, we still mourn.

REFERENCES

1. Cramond, W. A.: Anxiety in medical practice—the doctor's own anxiety, Aust. N.Z. J. Psychiatry **3:**324, 1969.
2. Fox, T.: Purposes of medicine, Lancet **2:**801, 1965.
3. Geis, D. P.: Mothers' perceptions of care given their dying children, Am. J. Nurs. **65:**105, 1965.
4. Gyulay, J.: The forgotten grievers, Am. J. Nurs. **75:**1476, 1975.
5. Hinton, J. M: Facing death, J. Psychosom. Res. **10:**22, 1966.
6. Kutscher, A. H., and Kutscher, A. H., Jr.: Medical school curriculum and anticipatory grief; faculty attitudes. In Schoenberg, B., Carr, A., Kutscher, A., Peretz, D., and Goldberg, I., editors: Anticipatory grief, New York, 1974, Columbia University Press.
7. Livingston, P. B., and Zimet, C. N.: Death anxiety, authoritarianism and choice of specialty in medical students, J. Nerv. Ment. Dis. **140:**222, 1965.
8. O'Connell, W., and Covert, C.: Death attitudes and humor appreciation among medical students, Existential Psychiatry **6:**433, 1967-1968.
9. Paykel, E. S., McGuiness, B., and Gomez, J.: An Anglo-American comparison of the scaling of life events, Br. J. Med. Psychol. **49:**237, 1976.
10. Peabody, F. W.: The care of the patient, J.A.M.A. **88:**877, 1927.
11. Schowalter, J. E.: Death and the pediatric house officer, J. Pediatr. **76:**706, 1970.
12. Schowalter, J. E.: Pediatric nurses dream of death, J. Thanatol. **3:**223, 1975.
13. Schowalter, J. E.: Psychological reactions to physical illness and hospitalization in adolescence; a survey, J. Am. Acad. Child Psychiatry **16:**500, 1977.
14. Schowalter, J. E., and Lord, R. D.: The utilization of patient meetings on an adolescent ward, Psychiatry Med. **1:**197, 1970.
15. Schowalter, J. E., and Lord, R. D.: On the writings of adolescents in a general hospital ward, Psychoanal. Study Child **27:**181, 1972.
16. Simmel, E.: The "doctor game," illness and the profession of medicine, Int. J. Psychoanal. **7:**470, 1926.
17. Solnit, A. J.: Who mourns when a child dies? In Anthony, E. J., and Koupernik, C., editors: The child in his family; the impact of disease and death, New York, 1973, John Wiley & Sons, Inc.

18. Vaillant, G. E., Sobowale, N. C., and McArthur, C.: Some psychologic vulnerabilities of physicians, N. Engl. J. Med. **287:**372, 1972.
19. Vaisrub, S.: Dying is worked to death, J.A.M.A. **229:**1909, 1974.
20. von Brauchitsch, H.: The physician's suicide revisited, J. Nerv. Ment. Dis. **162:**40, 1976.
21. Watterson, D. J.: Psychiatric illness in the medical profession; incidence in relation to sex and field of practice, Can. Med. Assoc. J. **115:**311, 1976.

CHAPTER 11

The chronic care specialist: "but who supports us?"

BRUCE H. AXELROD

The purpose of this chapter is to discuss the delivery of chronic care, primarily from the perspective of the physician, but also to explore some of the unique problems presented by patients with chronic, progressively terminal illness. I will focus on the delivery of care to patients with cystic fibrosis (CF), because this illness exemplifies in a dramatic and poignant way the issues that are common to all chronic illnesses in children and their potential for catastrophic impact on the individuals afflicted and their families.

CF is a progressively debilitating illness for which no cure presently exists. Care for children with this affliction has traditionally been provided through approximately 120 centers, mostly in university settings, throughout the United States. As is true for diabetes, there is no antenatal test to determine whether one is a carrier for CF, nor is there an intrauterine diagnostic procedure currently available. Like many chronic diseases, it is a genetic disease that follows a traditional mendelian pattern of inheritance. Until recently, children rarely survived beyond their teenage years; but, with the increasingly effective use of antibiotics and an awareness of the spectrum of the disease, patients with CF now live into young adulthood, and a number of adults in their 30s, 40s, 50s and 60s have been diagnosed.

Unlike many of the malignancies that result in a rapid downhill course over a period of several years, most patients with CF survive well into adolescence and many into young adulthood. Chronic malabsorption and repeated pulmonary infections result in progressive weakness, debilitation, cyanosis, and ultimate death. As has been pointed out by McCol-

I would like to express my appreciation to the center directors who afforded me the privilege of getting to know them during the years of my training and, most recently, during several fireside chats at the Cystic Fibrosis Spring Meeting. I hope that I have been able to portray their triumphs and disappointments in a way that gives justice to the dedication and integrity of these individuals. Their willingness to be vulnerable with me formed the basis for much of this chapter.

lum[5] and others, the impact of CF on the family is often catastrophic, resulting in an exceptionally high rate of divorce, enormous financial hardships, and often behavior problems, not only for the children who are afflicted, but for their siblings as well. The annual cost of medical care for a child with CF may range as high as $15,000 per year.[2] Few families have the financial resources to provide this care without state and local assistance, a problem that has become increasingly acute with the progressive limitation of federal funds for health care delivery. Unlike a child with diabetes, who can take his shot of insulin in the morning and then go about a relatively normal day, the child with CF coughs throughout the day and rapidly develops the stigmata of the disease: stained teeth as a result of tetracycline, clubbing of fingers and toes as a result of chronic hypoxia, and the not uncommon state of dyspnea as a result of progressive lung involvement. Delayed puberty is common, as is short stature. Thus, for many children with CF, adolescence is a particularly stormy time, during which the children face repeated humiliation and rejection from their peers. Most patients who survive into their 20s have significant difficulties in obtaining employment, maintaining financial independence, receiving appropriate care from adult physicians, and most important, in dealing with the progressive downhill course of their illness.

Because of the enormous complexity of needs that these children and their families present, once they have become established as patients of a specific CF center, they are extremely reluctant to leave. In part this is undoubtedly due to the fantasy that only their doctor has the magic to help; but there are also realistic benefits, such as financial and psychosocial support, that have often been obtained only after much struggle. These families become extremely dependent on the CF director and staff, resulting in a patient population for a given center that has a stability unique among most medical clinics. It is not at all uncommon for many CF patients to receive care throughout their lives from only the one pediatrician who has run their CF center.

DELIVERY OF CHRONIC CARE

What motivates the chronic care specialist to get into this business at all and to give care in a setting in which the rewards, on the surface, appear to be so limited? Almost without exception, center directors I have known have cited the personal contact with families, the opportunity for intimacy, and their basic admiration for the courage of the patients and their families as having led them to remain in a field that has made far less progress than many had hoped. The delivery of chronic care has not been seen as a highly desirable talent in most training institutions. Chronic disease has only been "in" for the past few years. Before this time, the directors of oncology programs, diabetes centers, CF centers, or multidisciplinary birth defects programs were, for the most part, individual practitioners who were frequently tolerated by the university medical complex as a necessary addition to the program to provide a well-rounded education; but they were rarely given either financial or institutional support to create the multidisciplinary comprehensive care program that many desired. Unlike their surgical colleagues who had the built-in support of an operating room team, a large cadre of house staff, and institutional support, many of these individuals fought a lonely battle for their patients, daily combating institutional ambivalence, apathy, antipathy, and avoidance.

What are the major issues with which the center directors must cope? Without doubt, the single, overwhelming issue is the fact that the specialist is engaged in a battle that cannot be won. If one cannot appreciably affect the duration of life, then one must be content to improve the quality of it. To do this, it is essential that the center director have the intimate contact with the child and his family that will enable him to understand the physical, psychological, intellectual, and developmental difficulties with which all children affected by CF must cope. As one center director put it, "When most people come to see a doctor, they hope they will never have to see him again. But with our patients it's different; they know that not only will they *have* to see you, but they *want* to see you again. They want the personal contact with you. It's not the social worker, the dietician, or the pulmonary therapist they want; they want that one-to-one time with *you,* and no one else will quite substitute for it." And yet the center director knows that he must ultimately lose. It is this internal struggle for closeness and intimacy with patients on the one hand and on the other the desire to distance oneself from the patient to help minimize the pain of loss when his child patients die that presents the most difficult dilemma for the chronic care specialist.

There is an enormous educative role that the center director must fulfill, not only at the time of diagnosis, but throughout the life of the child. Coping difficulties occur at all stages of development, and families are greatly in need of anticipatory guidance and crisis intervention.[5] As mentioned previously, the financial consequences of this disease can be devastating, and the center director not only must be an excellent physician but also must be aware of the political scene as well as an expert on insurance, social programs, and voluntary agencies.

Repeated pulmonary infections frequently result in unexpected and prolonged hospitalizations. It is in this setting that the CF director must not only address the needs of the patient and his family, but must deal frequently with disinterest and avoidance on the part of house staff and nursing personnel. Unfortunately, the children with CF, who are repeatedly hospitalized with pneumonia, like the diabetic recurrently hospitalized in acidosis, have traditionally been patients who have attracted little interest from the house staff. Exposure to these children evokes enormous anxiety in many house officers because of the fear that these patients will die. Although there have been numerous articles in the literature describing innovative and creative programs for teaching house staff and medical students about death and dying,[1,4,7,8] it has been my experience that for the most part they are ill-prepared to deal with the enormous demands of the dying child and his family. The chronic care specialist usually has the expertise and experience to help house staff handle these situations, but this educative process requires time and a receptive setting.

When terminal patients with CF are admitted to the hospital, the center director must deal with ethical as well as medical issues: Should a child be placed on a respirator? How heroic should one be? Should the child die at home? Should one accelerate the inevitable downhill course of the disease? All are questions that inevitably exist but may not be immediately discussed at the time of admission. As a result, nursing staff as well as house staff become increasingly anxious and may avoid the patient or displace the anger that they feel toward the CF director for not being able to cure this patient onto the family or other staff. Ideally, the family members have had anticipatory counseling and have come to accept the child's impending death. But frequently this is not the case. In an attempt to deal with their feelings of inadequacy, helplessness, and hopelessness, the family make increasing demands on the house staff. This heightens alienation and increases the anxiety and anger that the house staff feel, with a resultant increase in ward conflict and lack of mutual support. Thus, the CF director must not only care for the patient and the patient's family, but he must become the mentor for the ward staff as well.

ATTEMPTS TO INTEGRATE AND COPE WITH CONFLICTING NEEDS

How then does the CF director attempt to integrate and cope with the often mutually conflicting needs of patients, staff, and himself? The remainder of this chapter will focus on the CF director's roles in managing patients' medical care, coordinating the health care team, handling the pressures of academe, and coping with his own isolation.

Managing medical care

It has been my experience that most center directors express relatively little concern about their own medical competence. In general, the field is sufficiently delineated that mastery is possible, and the techniques of treatment have remained essentially unchanged over the past several decades, with the possible exception of the discontinuation of mist tent therapy. In addition, there are multiple opportunities each year for center directors to meet through the Cystic Fibrosis Foundation to exchange information regarding current medical practices and, as in programs dealing with other types of chronic disease, such as oncology programs, there is rapid and reasonably complete dissemination of information from center to center. Of increasing concern to some center directors is the continuing care of their patients who are now living into young adulthood, well beyond the range of normal pediatric care. Most center directors, however, continue to provide care for these patients, in part because of the scarcity of internists who are interested in and capable of handling patients with CF, but also because of the intense bond that forms between the center directors and many of the patients they have cared for over many years.

Managing the health care team

A second major area of responsibility for the director is managing the health care team. Patients with CF have significant difficulties medically, economically, and of course psychosocially. The day-to-day management issues demand a multidisciplinary approach. To effectively manage CF, one needs a pulmonary therapist, a dietician, a social worker, and ideally, some psychiatric input as well. Because of limited funding, however, it has become increasingly difficult for many center directors to establish and maintain this multidisciplinary approach. Also, although many center directors have seen the need for the development of such teams, they are often ambivalent about actually using them. Given the realities of the multiple psychosocial demands of these children and their families, it is virtually impossible for most center directors to function without a team. At the same time, many express concern that the creation of a team is a response, not to the multifactorial needs of the patients, but to the physician's desire to distance himself from patients for whom he has no cure and with whom he must spend 15 or more years of his professional life. One center director jokingly said, "If you're really successful, you'll get a group of house staff, and they'll see the patient first, and then you'll get some social workers, and then a psychologist, and if you're really lucky, you'll be able to build a large enough team so you can spend all of your time in the laboratory." Although clearly this was said in humor, it accurately reflects a dilemma that many center directors feel. Few individuals would disagree that there is a need to share the burden of this kind of care, for without the opportunity to get away, the center director would quickly burn out. But for the patient and for the physician, it is in fact the bonding, the personal contact, that seems to be crucial. Another center director told me, "When a patient is dying, he wants *you* at his bedside, not the social worker, not the psychologist, not the pulmonary therapist. Even when the family knows there is nothing more you can do, it is the personal contact with you that seems to make all the difference."

Many center directors who have had limited exposure to multidisciplinary education feel an initial reluctance to delegate responsibility to team members. Programs that are initially sufficiently limited in scope and number and can be handled by the physician himself soon increase in complexity and inevitably require additional staff members to help share the burden. There is often a period of adjustment when a team is formed. The center director frequently has not been prepared for nor has the skills to cope with interpersonal problems within the team itself. At the same time, there is always the lingering concern and guilt that somehow this team is serving, not as a facilitator of care, but as a barrier between the center director and his patients.

An additional member of the team, who by virtue of his training status is usually a transient one, is the house officer. The center director is frequently torn between providing a reasonably nonrestrictive environment that will enable the house officer to have an appropriate clinical exposure to these patients, and maintaining control over the house officer's activities so that his inexperience or anxiety will not result in inappropriate and possibly destructive approaches to the patient. As an unfortunate example of the latter, a CF director once told me of an incident in which a 22-year-old CF patient with diabetes and congestive heart failure was seen by a house officer who walked into the room and said, "Gee, I'm surprised you're alive at all—we thought you'd be dead 2 years ago." When episodes of this type occur, the family becomes understandably distrustful of and angry at the institution, the house officer, and most important, the center director, whom they hold responsible for all that transpires. It is all too easy for most physicians to accept this omnipotent image, because it fits both his patient's wish and his own latent hope. However, the ultimate death of his patient is a painful reminder of his own fallibility, and he must repeatedly experience frustration and despair, when, despite all his dedication and good intentions, his patients still die.

When a team is functioning well, it is a major source of support and also comfort for the center director, the members of the team, and the individual patients and their families. The skills that social work brings to the delivery of chronic care are sorely needed, and, although many center directors experience some initial discomfort with mental health professionals, a feeling of trust is established when the psychiatrist or the social worker provides appropriate interventions, enabling many CF directors to comfortably delegate some of the responsibility for handling the psychosocial issues of their patients to other trusted members of the team. In an era in which one out of four families moves every year, it is not surprising that frequently the composition of the team will change as well. If the team has worked well with him and has enabled him to share the burden of his position, a disruption, because of the departure of a trusted member, will be experienced as a profound loss by the center director and will compound many of the other losses that he must experience when his patients die.

From the perspective of inpatient management, the center director must cope with a number of extremely difficult issues. Patients with CF are hospitalized on general pediatric wards, unlike their counterparts with oncological illnesses, who are often hospitalized in defined units with a stable nursing and support staff. The center director must therefore deal with staff who may have had minimal exposure to the care of terminally ill children and little opportunity to discuss their own feelings and reactions as participants in that process. Thus, at the time when the center director must cope with the death of his patient, he must simultaneously establish a support system within the hospital to assure adequate care for the child and the child's family. I have found that it is extremely uncommon for most inpatient pediatric wards to have a resident social worker or access to psychiatric consultation on a regularly scheduled basis. Thus, the opportunity for the ward staff to work as a group and establish a mutually supportive network is frequently unavailable. When a dying patient is placed in an unsupported setting, the results are frequently chaotic, punitive, and destructive. House staff tend to avoid dying patients, as do many of the nursing personnel. Those who are sincerely motivated are frequently without skills or experience to be able to handle the dying patient well. As one center director put it, "When a CF child is about to die, you have to have a meeting. You have to call all the people together—the nurses, the social workers, the dieticians, the medical students, the house staff—and get them all to talk. Because if you don't do that, especially in those situations in which the family has elected not to continue heroic measures, you will find yourself spending all day and all night at the hospital. It is dreadful to see how painful it is for people who have had so little experience. It's the young nurses who so frequently are left with the responsibility for caring for these patients and who rapidly become attached to them. Without benefit of support and guidance these staff members experience the loss as a tragic and painful experience." Frequently, at those centers that have well-functioning teams, conferences are held on a weekly basis to discuss the current status of the dying patient. The team members are able to support each other and to share some of the burden of establishing a supportive network on the inpatient floors as well.

Managing the problems of academe

As mentioned before, most patients with CF receive care in centers located in university hospitals. Thus, superimposed on all the service demands of the CF director are the problems of academe. Somehow the center director must find time to publish a requisite number of articles or risk losing promotion, tenure, and ultimately his job. For most chronic care specialists, this departure from direct care is not done without certain pangs of guilt. Although many center directors are recognized as definitive bench scientists, others have a more limited bibliography. They often achieve less status within the academic community than colleagues engaged in basic research. Because few other physicians deal on a day-to-day basis with the debilitation and progressive deterioration of patients, it is often difficult for the center directors to seek support from their peers, especially those for whom a more intellectual and distant approach to patient care has been their personal style of coping.

Academic advancement is presently predicated on publications. Commitment to comprehensive care, role modeling, expertise with psychosocial issues, and serving as an ombudsman for the patient rarely have been rewarded with endowed chairs in pediatrics. Thus, the center director must fulfill both roles if he is to achieve academic success and gratify his emotional and intellectual needs. This is not to say that many center directors do not derive great benefit from their basic research efforts. More will be said about this later.

It is well known that pediatric outpatient departments rarely make much money, and those that deal with chronic illness tend to make even less. For this reason, as well as a basic lack of commitment to chronic disease, institutional support for CF programs has been meager at best. It has been difficult to obtain either training funds or financial support for individuals who would comprise an effective health care team. Frequently the size of the CF population is significantly less than some of the more ubiquitous chronic diseases, such as diabetes, epilepsy, or arthritis. Administrators are often less than willing to invest in social work support for what appears to be a poor dollars-and-cents return. But as has been illustrated in this chapter, although their numbers might not be great, the scope and depth of the problems presented by these children and their families are profound indeed.

The chronic care specialist:
the individual

One of the most significant problems for the CF director is isolation. Because few physicians in the institution are likely to have had the experience of dealing with death and dying so frequently, it is unusual for a CF director to develop an intimate relationship with a colleague with whom he can share some of these burdens. As Rothenberg[6] has pointed out, when physicians feel they cannot cure, there is often a sense of hopelessness and helplessness that is at variance with the more omnipotent stance that many doctors have been cultivated to assume. Success is cure in modern medicine, yet with chronic disease one can at best palliate. How can one feel successful, when, as one center director put it, "The toughest thing about this job is that you know you're going to lose, you can never win." When faced with these feelings of inadequacy, some physicians will often attempt to compensate by increasing activity or by developing a blind adherence to regimens that may be of marginal medical value (excessive daily testing of urine for diabetic management, religious adherence to mist tent treatment, and so on). Some physicians find the opportunity to go to the laboratory a welcome respite from the day-to-day realities of the CF patient. One can thus redirect much pain and anguish into productive research that will, it is hoped, advance the state of the art. For others, opportunities to extend the principles of care for chronically ill children to other settings by attending on a ward or in outpatient clinics provide extremely gratifying experiences; and having patients who can be *cured* is a confirmation of one's medical ability and skill.

An area about which unfortunately little is known is the impact of the CF director's professional life on his family. A number of center directors have said to me that when they return home, they are frequently upset, depressed, withdrawn, frustrated, and at times emotionally unavailable to their wives and children. A number of the children of center directors have expressed a desire to make an appointment with their parent so that they would have an opportunity to see him or her more. Still others claim to have no knowledge of what their parent does, a reflection not only of the lack of opportunity for children to observe parents at work generally, but also, I feel, a defense on the part of the children against having to deal with the fact that their parent is involved with such a serious and potentially catastrophic disease.

Given the nature of this book, there has been perhaps more emphasis on the issues of death and dying than really occupies the attention of the physician on a day-to-day basis. However, the issues are constantly pres-

ent, and when a child is in a terminal state, the center director must deal
with still another ramification of the impact of death: the *anniversary
phenomenon*. Selma Fraiberg[3] has pointed out that the behavior of parents toward children often has antecedents in their relationship with
their own parents. For many, there are ghosts from the past that lurk
within the nurseries and affect the care of the new infant until they can
be exorcised. In a somewhat similar way, when a child is dying, the
center director is haunted by the ghosts of past patients as silent testa-
ments to his fallibility. Although he may not be consciously aware of it,
the ghosts of other children are in that room with him, and unless they
can be exorcised, these feelings result in an unusual amount of guilt and
depression following succeeding deaths. It is as though there is an aggre-
gate mourning, not only for the present child, but for all those who have
preceded him. Although these physicians deal frequently with death,
there has been little systematic study of center directors' attitudes toward
death.

Despite all these difficulties, there are presently 120 CF centers in
this country, and the number is increasing. Why do center directors stay?
Why do they continue? Why do they persevere? How do they acquire the
skills that enable them to cope with the issues that have been described
above? Perhaps what is most basic to many of them is a belief in comprehensive care for their patients, the opportunity for intimate relationships with children and families, and a sense that they are doing something that very few people wish to do. There is a sense of the "last of
the frontier docs" about these individuals, who have manned a lonely
vigil, long before chronic disease was "in." It is not that they see themselves as saints or as crusaders, but as people who have accepted the challenge of a devastating illness and, through their relationships with their
patients and families, have experienced a sense of community that is so
painfully absent in most of American society today. The title for this
chapter is based on a comment by one of the center directors that, on
many occasions when he has felt himself on the verge of despair, it has
been the strength of the patient or the family that has enabled him to
carry on. While it is clearly the responsibility of the center director not to
be a burden to his patients, it is at the same time this capacity for
reciprocity, in a reasonable and supportive way, that continues to foster
their commitment to these families. Many center directors find enormous
gratification in the personal relationships they form with house staff as
well. They are frequently seen as comprehensive care physicians, often
sought out for personal problems as well as for more intimate learning
experiences. A number of center directors have found themselves giving
lectures, not about CF, but about how it feels to handle a child who is

dying. They become role models for the kind of physician that many of the medical students and house staff wished to be when they entered the field of medicine.

Clearly there have been significant gains in the treatment of cystic fibrosis: life is prolonged, and the quality of life has improved. Although it is far short of what anyone would have wished, it is improvement nevertheless. There have also been changes in the nature of the center directors themselves. In the past 5 to 10 years, interest in the delivery of comprehensive care and in chronic illness has increased tremendously. As a result, many young people are working in CF programs and are bringing fresh insights, dedication, energy, and commitment to continuing the fight. Significantly, these young physicians have attempted to deal with their personal isolation by meeting in groups to talk about common problems—not medical management issues, but what it feels like to have a child die: Do you go to the funeral? How do you allow a child to die at home? How do you use a social worker or a psychiatrist? Is it okay to go out and fish for a week? Why do I feel so guilty when I take some time off? By beginning to explore their own feelings, they are developing a sense of mastery over extremely painful problems, and in contrast to many of their predecessors who relied only on their own experience, they are learning new techniques to handle the psychosocial issues that in the past have received little support or concern. Increasingly, national meetings are providing opportunities for the acquisition of these skills, not only intellectually, but also experientially.

With the large number of individuals currently involved in the care of chronically ill children, it should come as no surprise that not all CF directors have achieved the level of competence that they would like. Many isolate themselves from patients, adopt a stance of rigidity that enables them to avoid many of the painful effects of loss, fail to see the need for a multidisciplinary team, and wish to continue their position as individual practitioners. What is most important, however, is that *there is not only one way* to cope with the delivery of chronic care. Furthermore, the specialist must recognize that it is indeed the personal contact with him that is most significant to patients. As one center director put it, "After the child has died, many families have come back to thank me, not for the medication that I gave, for they knew the disease was fatal, but for the care that I gave and the personal relationship that I had with them and their child." It is the specialist's personality that will have a great impact on the way in which the other caregivers treat the patient, as well as the scope of services that are provided by these individuals. None of us can do it all, none of us can do it in the same way, and most important, none of us can do it alone.

REFERENCES

1. Barton, D., and Crowder, M.: The use of role playing techniques as an instructional aid in teaching about dying, death and bereavement. Omega **6:**243, 1975.
2. Cystic Fibrosis Foundation Young Adult Committee: Personal communication, 1977.
3. Fraiberg, S. F., Adelson, E., and Shapiro, V.: Ghosts in the nursery, J. Am. Acad. Child Psychiatry **14:**387, 1975.
4. Gould, R. K., and Rothenberg, M. B.: The chronically ill child facing death—how can the pediatrician help? Clin. Pediatr. **12:**447, 1973.
5. McCollum, A. T.: Coping with prolonged health impairment in your child, Boston, 1975, Little Brown and Co.
6. Rothenberg, M. B.: The unholy trinity; activity, authority and magic, Clin. Pediatr. **14:**585, 1975.
7. Schowalter, J. E.: Death and the pediatric house officer, J. Pediatr. **76:**706, 1970.
8. Tietz, W., and Powars, D.: The pediatrician and the dying child. "Physician know thyself." Clin. Pediatr. **14:**585, 1975.

ADDITIONAL READING

Patterson, P., Denning C., and others: Psychosocial aspects of cystic fibrosis, New York, 1973, Columbia University Press.

CHAPTER 12

Reflections of a physician caregiver

PETER H. VILES

> We must live within the ambiguity of partial freedom, partial power, and
> partial knowledge.
> All important decisions must be made on the basis of insufficient data.
> Yet we are responsible for everything we do.
> No excuses will be accepted.
>
> *Sheldon Kopp*[11]

I have been asked to write this chapter on the reactions of a physician caregiver to the dying child from an "intensely personal yet analytic and constructively critical" perspective as both a pediatric cardiologist and a director of a pediatric intensive care unit (PICU). As a cardiologist, I seldom think of my patients as "dying," for death often follows an attempt at a palliative or corrective operation in what is viewed as a hopeful situation, regardless of the estimated surgical risks. In the intensive care unit the stresses are multiple, because illness usually comes swiftly, dramatically, and unexpectedly. Death, while not unfamiliar, occurs after a short but intense struggle by patient, parents, and caregivers. The unexpectedness and lack of preparation for the fatal outcome in both situations create special problems for all concerned. Others[3,4,18] have written on the ethical and moral dilemmas of the intensive care unit. The following, therefore, will be a personal, and admittedly anecdotal, reflection on some of my experiences in cardiology and the PICU.

It is commonly said that we learn from experience when, in fact, we learn from *reflecting* on our experience. I will, therefore, follow a format that can be understood by the mnemonic E-I-A-G; that is, the *experience* will be related, an *individual* aspect of that experience will be selected, I will try to *analyze* my thoughts and feelings about that aspect and then *generalize* to some position that seems valid, at least for me. I hope that other caregivers will find that the analyses and generalizations stimulate their own thinking, perhaps not to agree with my conclusions, but at least to prompt reflection and discussion about their own experiences.

Jason, a 16-month-old child, was transferred from another hospital because of coma. His illness started with vomiting, and he was hospitalized with stupor and dehydration. Initially the diagnosis of aspirin intoxication was made because of a high blood salicylate level. When he failed to improve despite appropriate therapy, however, transfer to the PICU was made. Despite some atypical features, the admitting diagnosis was Reye syndrome with stage III coma.[7] This quickly deteriorated to stage IV coma, and signs of intermittent uncal herniation were present. Intensive supportive care preserved his life but left him severely brain damaged in a persistent vegetative state.[8]

At the time of admission Jason was dying and, in fact, the person he was and could have been had died, despite the continuation of vital functions. For reasons not completely clear to me, Jason and his family sparked a special sense of identity in me at the time of his admission. For the first few days of his illness, when his eventual outcome was probably decided, I was as emotionally unprepared for his death as the family. Now, 3 years later, I ask myself, "Did I do enough? Did I do too much?" Intracranial pressure monitoring[15] allows better recognition and, presumably, better treatment of cerebral edema, but it was not in widespread use at the time of his illness. Nonetheless, much of my discomfort about Jason, then and now, resides in this issue of uncertainty of outcome and the guilt I feel in this situation of having helped create that outcome. I seek forgiveness, but do not know whom to ask. Perhaps it is I who cannot forgive myself.

I believe that compassion and empathy are essential to being a competent and effective caregiver. To the degree that as caregivers we identify with patients and families, we run the risk of being less effective in our care, although lack of identification probably creates the risk of ineffective care as well. Here I am not talking just of lack of objectivity, always a risk in such situations, but of becoming too emotionally vulnerable to function effectively, both in giving definitive care to the patient and in fulfilling our supportive roles to patients and families. Being a member of a team may serve to distance the individual from the situation and reduce this hazard. Ideally, a prime function of the team is to monitor the well-being of each member as they approach the difficult task of caring for the potentially dying child. In retrospect, I am not aware that any member of the PICU staff fulfilled this role for me with Jason. Either they were unaware of my need, or I would not let anyone share my pain. An awareness, however, that I do have pain in these situations creates the possibility that I will be free to share my pain or recognize the supportive team member when he or she reaches out to me.

Andrew, a 15-year-old boy, was in excellent health until 36 hours before admission to the hospital. At that time he complained of cough and fever. By the following morning he was short of breath and, when a chest x-ray film at another hospital showed extensive bilateral pulmonary infiltrates, transfer to the medical center was made. On admission he was severely dyspneic and cyanotic in 40% oxygen. Arterial blood gases showed hypoxemia without hypercapnia. He was intubated and placed on a volume-controlled respirator. Over the ensuing 24 hours, further deterioration occurred despite high levels of positive end expiratory pressure, use of 100% oxygen, and measures to optimize cardiac output and oxygen delivery. Survival seemed unlikely for more than a few hours. At this point, extracorporeal membrane oxygenator support was discussed with the family and, with their concurrence, was begun 48 hours after admission. Viability of the right leg (site of arterial inflow) was questioned, and acute renal failure subsequently occurred. Hyperkalemia was controlled with exchange resins. Decreased oxygenator efficiency required a change of membrane, during which time he developed irreversible cardiac arrest.

The seduction of technology in the intensive care unit is great[22] and often difficult to resist. Although extracorporeal membrane oxygenation in the setting of acute inflammatory pulmonary disease is not of clear benefit,[6] it seemed to offer the only chance of survival. The decision not to begin hemodialysis for renal failure may be seen as an inconsistency in treatment (as it was by several members of the nursing staff in the PICU), but by that time the course of the illness seemed irreversible, and more important, the family was prepared for their son's death. In post-death counseling, both parents spoke at length about the importance to them of the additional time they had to understand Andrew's terminal illness. They expressed gratitude to all who had cared for their son.

As a caregiver, I wish to cure all my patients. When that is not possible, I may feel inadequate and responsible for the failure of treatment. It is important for me to remember that the "caregiving" is often the most important thing I do and that benefits result even when "cure" does not happen. Andrew's family appears to be one that "rings with a clear, beautiful tone" when struck by adversity; I am grateful that I and others were able to hear it.

Emily died at 2 years of age after a lifelong struggle with congestive heart failure and repeated pulmonary infections secondary to congenital heart disease (atrioventricular canal defect). At about 5 months of age, her condition worsened with increased left AV valve (mitral) regurgitation and ECG changes that suggested myocardial infarction. Hemodynamics were marginal at rest, and she was unable to increase cardiac output to meet the needs of activity or fever. She was hospitalized repeatedly, and family stresses were great. Surgical opinion was that poor ventricular function precluded successful corrective surgery. She died one evening en route to the hospital with one of her many episodes of fever and collapse.

Because of the chronic nature of Emily's illness, all members of the cardiology group came to know Emily and her family well. The night she died, the mother drove her to the hospital alone. She stated, "I knew she was going to die sometime, but I thought this episode was just like all the others." Her husband arrived later in the night, and both parents were able to express and share their grief. I went home about 2 o'clock in the morning. The house was empty, for my wife was away at the time. For several weeks thereafter I was unusually depressed. Although I recognized this as grief for Emily, my affect did not improve. It was not until I was able to work out my grief and express my love for Emily in a Gestalt group some months later that closure occured.

Physicians grieve for the loss of patients close to them as surely as parents and other family members do. Closure must occur and resolution of ambivalent feelings of guilt, anger, and despair take place. For most of us, such understanding has come slowly or not at all, because it has not been part of our formal medical school teaching or residency training. To show emotion is to lose objectivity and to be "unprofessional." Nonetheless, I am human, and as a compassionate physician I need to do my own grief work regularly and to keep the "accounts balanced" so that I can continue to be effective. The importance of this understanding has not been stressed in teaching or training. Each of us has been left to our own devices to see that it is (or is not) accomplished.

Janice, an 11-year-old girl with known cystic fibrosis but with excellent pulmonary status, was hospitalized for the first time with pneumonia. Four days after admission, abdominal distension and diarrhea with dehydration resulted in transfer to the PICU. She was alert, in moderate respiratory distress with adequate blood gases, dehydrated, and mildly hypotensive. Her clinical condition rapidly deteriorated, with worsening pulmonary function, the appearance of generalized edema, and increasing abdominal distension. A pulmonary artery catheter was placed in order to help guide fluid replacement therapy and monitor cardiopulmonary function. Free air in the abdominal cavity prompted surgical exploration, which revealed peritoneal fluid, edematous bowel, and cecal perforation. Despite efforts to maintain circulating blood volume, the use of a volume-controlled respirator, antibiotics, and steroids, Janice died. The duration of the acute phase of her terminal illness was 36 hours. In addition to the expected findings of cystic fibrosis, the autopsy showed pneumonia and membranous enterocolitis.

Nellie, an 8-year-old girl, was visiting the zoo with her classmates when a thunderstorm struck. Nellie and others were unable to find appropriate shelter and took cover under a large tree. Lightning struck among the group of children, knocking several to the ground and rendering Nellie and a companion unconscious. When she arrived at a nearby hospital, ventricular fibrillation was present. Cardiac action was restored with cardiopulmonary resuscitation, appropriate drugs, and electrical defibrillation. A burn was present on her abdomen and the sole of her left foot. She required ventilator support and bilateral lower extremity fasciectomies in the next few days. Renal failure did not occur. A tracheostomy was eventually performed to facilitate tracheal toilet, and she was weaned from the respirator. About 3 weeks after the injury, respiratory distress again appeared, an infiltrate was present on chest roentgenogram, and arterial blood gases deteriorated. At that point she was transferred from the receiving hospital to the PICU. A pulmonary scan was consistent with multiple pulmonary emboli. Blood gases stabilized and improved, and respiratory failure did not occur. Her neurologic evaluation was consistent with the persistent vegetative state. A decision not to use anticoagulants or to place an inferior vena caval sieve was made. Efforts were directed at removing the tracheostomy tube, which was accomplished 10 days after transfer, and she was discharged from the PICU. Eventually a chronic care facility was located where Nellie remains, still unresponsive to her environment, but in a stable condition.

There are similarities in my reactions to Janice and Nellie. In neither case did I perceive myself as the primary physician, and I was separated from their initial care by some time and distance. With Janice, my role was to bring my expertise to her acute, devastating illness and to support her primary care physician and family, both of whom had dealt with her chronic illness in an atmosphere of hope and encouragement based on her excellent clinical course. With Nellie, I had not participated in her initial resuscitation and stabilization. I saw my role as improving her medical status so she could be moved to a chronic care environment and as counseling the family and nursing staff about a realistic expectation for her future. In both situations I felt this was accomplished: Janice's physician and family expressed gratitude for the supportive care given them and their daughter, who died apparently unafraid; in Nellie's case, while death appeared to be the desired outcome, there was no "plug to pull," but the staff's and family's feelings of anger, ambivalence, and helplessness were recognized and allowed expression.

In cases where I am aware of some distance from the family, child, and other caregivers, my role seems clearer and my skills can be applied more specifically, ideally with positive results. The tension of closeness and distance is one that exists in all patient-physician relationships; its importance seems magnified in dealing with the acutely ill and dying child. Distance may be intentional (Janice) or occur by circumstance (Nellie). Lack of a prior relationship with the patient and family may sometimes work to advantage. In these two situations, at least, it appeared beneficial.

George, a 4-month-old infant with a large ventricular septal defect and congestive heart failure, was admitted to the PICU with probable bacterial pneumonia. Blood cultures were initially positive for *Streptococcus pneumoniae* (pneumococcus) and later for gram-negative organisms. Respiratory failure required long-term ventilator support. With the appearance of gram-negative sepsis, renal insufficiency and jaundice were noted. Although his basic lesion (congenital heart disease) was correctable, George's medical condition never stabilized enough to allow consideration for surgery, nor was it clear that surgical correction of his heart defect would allow resolution of his other medical problems. The final decision not to prolong intensive supportive care and treatment to maintain his life (or prolong his dying) was made after many discussions with family, nurses, consultants, and the primary physician.

George was with us in the PICU for several weeks. The nursing staff, who spent many hours with him, expressed their wishes that he improve and their anger and frustration when he did not, despite all their efforts. I was one of the first to realize our efforts were prolonging his dying rather than preserving his life. At that point, while I had sadness, of course, there was also a sense of renewed purpose in that my efforts with George, his family, and the nursing staff could be channeled more effectively as we helped him with his dying and prepared ourselves for it.

"A dying man needs to die, as a sleepy man needs to sleep, and there comes a time when it is wrong, as well as useless, to resist."[1] The decision to let death come is never easy, but must be faced many times in the intensive care unit.[2] Our fear seems to be that we might give up too soon, so that guidelines for decision making have been suggested,[19] although evidence exists that in many cases we persist in our efforts too long.[4] With George it seemed appropriate to admit our limitations and not prolong his dying.

Kari, a 1-day-old infant, was transferred to the medical center with congestive heart failure. The clinical picture was that of a hypoplastic left ventricle, confirmed by echocardiography. Supportive care, including digitalis, diuretics, and oxygen, was given until her death on the fourth day of life. Autopsy showed mitral and aortic valve atresia. During her life, Kari's parents were continually at her bedside, showing grief as would be expected, but also being very supportive of their child and each other.

If there is such a thing as a good death, Kari experienced it. The newborn can no longer be viewed as a passive recipient of care,[12] and maternal-infant bonding plays an important role in the experience of grief following the death of a newborn infant.[10] Mother, father, and Kari used the time available to them to express their concern and love for each other. The resolution of the parents' grief was to see Kari's life as "4 happy days on earth."

Watching the process, I agree. In later conversations with the nursing staff, however, I found those who did not view the process in the same light. They were left bitter and angry at this "wasted" life. Because neither parent felt that way and had expressed that to the staff at a visit to the unit several weeks after Kari's death, I conclude that, for some, death can never be seen as an opportunity for growth and even perhaps for rejoicing. To the contrary, death is the enemy to be resisted with all one's strength and abhorred with all one's energy. It may be that such persons are particularly drawn to intensive care settings. Each must resolve his own feelings about death. I have found great comfort and solace in Tillich's words, "Nothing can prevent us from fulfilling the ultimate meaning of our existence. There is a creative and saving possibility implied in every situation, which cannot be destroyed by any event. The daemonic and destructive forces within ourselves and our world can never have an unbreakable grasp upon us, and the bond that connects us with the fulfilling love can never be disrupted."[20]

There are two themes common to the vignettes presented here. The first concerns the tension between intimacy and distance, emotional involvement and objectivity. I would submit that these are not exclusive positions and that it is the job of the caregivers to the dying child to try to synthesize these positions into a stance that allows caring in the context of dying. I would not claim universal, or even frequent, success in achieving such a stance (for example, Jason) and am bothered at times when the distance seems too great (Nellie). Likewise, I have no answer to the tension between technology in the ICU (Andrew) and the need for the patient to die (George). At the moment, to be aware of the polarities and to struggle with the process of synthesis in each case seem adequate.

The second theme concerns the vulnerability of the caregiver—specifically the physician. Most intensive care units I have been associated with have paid little, if any, attention to the psychologic well-being of the staff.[9] Approaches to the psychiatric problems of patients in the ICU, both adults[13] and children[16] have been suggested, and, of the staff, nurses have been the subject of the most investigation and intervention.[5,14] Documentation of the reactions of resident physicians in the ICU have been few[21] and attention to senior physician staff essentially nonexistent. I would suggest a model of a team approach in which the members of the team have as one of their prime values and goals an awareness of the psychic well-being of each member. Such a goal could be achieved through team meetings with this as a specific agenda item,[17] in the context of patient-oriented conferences, or by frequent informal "checking out" of the emotional status of team members. As caregivers in crisis situations, we need to make ourselves vulnerable to one another, share our doubts and fears, and gain strength to continue the struggle. This will not be any easy task for most physicians I suspect, because it requires surrender of authority and claims to infallibility and admission of our own finiteness.

> We must learn the power of living with our helplessness.
> We have only ourselves, and one another. That may not be much but
>   that's all there is.
>
> *Sheldon Kopp*[11]

I would like to gratefully acknowledge the care and love for me shown by the nursing staff of the Neonatal Intensive Care Unit and the Pediatric Intensive Care Unit of Strong Memorial Hospital, my wife and family, and the Community of Genesis II during the period of time I helped care for the patients described above.

REFERENCES

1. Alsop, Stewart: Stay of execution, Philadelphia, 1973, J. B. Lippincott Co., p. 299.
2. Cassem, N. H.: Confronting the decision to let death come, Crit. Care Med. **2:**113, 1974.
3. Curran, W. J.: The proper and improper concerns of medical law and ethics, N. Engl. J. Med. **295:**1057, 1976.
4. Duff, R. S., and Campbell, M. B.: Moral and ethical dilemmas in the special care nursery, N. Engl. J. Med. **289:**890, 1973.
5. Hay, D., and Oken, D.: The psychological stresses of intensive care unit nursing, Psychosom. Med. **34:**109, 1972.
6. Hill, J. D., Ratliff, J. L., Fallat, R. J., and others: Prognostic factors in the treatment of acute respiratory failure with long-term extracorporeal oxygenation, J. Thorac. Cardiovasc. Surg. **68:**905, 1974.
7. Huttenlocher, P. R.: Reye's syndrome; relation of outcome to therapy, J. Pediatr. **80:**845, 1972.
8. Jennett, B., and Plum, F.: Persistent vegetative state after brain damage, Lancet **1:**734, 1972.

9. Kachoris, P. J.: Psychodynamic considerations in the neonatal ICU, Crit. Care Med. **5:**62, 1977.
10. Kennell, J. H., and Klaus, M. H.: The mourning response of parents to the death of a newborn infant, N. Engl. J. Med. **283:**344, 1970.
11. Kopp, Sheldon B.: If you meet the Buddha on the road, kill him! Ben Lomond, California, 1972, Science & Behavior Books, Inc., p. 166.
12. Lozoff, B., Brittenham, G. M., Tause, M. A., and others: The mother-newborn relationship; limits of adaptability. J. Pediatr. **91:**1, 1977.
13. Maron, L., Bryan-Brown, C. W., and Shoemaker, W. C.: Toward a unified approach to psychological factors in the ICU, Crit. Care Med. **1:**81, 1973.
14. May, J. G.: A psychiatric study of a pediatric intensive therapy unit, Clin. Pediatr. **11:**76, 1972.
15. Mickell, J. J., Cook, D. R., Reigel, D. H., and others: Intracranial pressure monitoring in Reye-Johnson syndrome, Crit. Care Med. **4:**1, 1976.
16. Reinhart, J. B. Kampschulte, S., and Nuffield, E. J.: Psychiatric rounds on a pediatric intensive care unit, Crit. Care Med. **1:**269, 1973.
17. Rosini, L. A., Howell, M. D., Todres, I. D., and Shannon, D. C.: Group meetings in a pediatric intensive care unit, Pediatrics **53:**371, 1974.
18. Skillman, J. J.: Ethical dilemmas in the care of the critically ill. Lancet **2:**634, 1974.
19. Tagge, G. F., Adler, D., Bryan-Brown, C. W., and Shoemaker, W. C.: Relationship of therapy to prognosis in critically ill patients, Crit. Care Med. **2:**61, 1974.
20. Tillich, P.: The meaning of providence. In The shaking of the foundations, New York, 1948, Charles Scribner's Sons, p. 106.
21. Todres, I. D., Howell, M. D., and Shannon, D. C.: Physicians' reactions to training in a pediatric intensive care unit, Pediatrics **53:**375, 1974.
22. Waisbren, B. A.: Simultaneous and sequential use of multiple organ support systems, presented at Third Annual Meeting of the Society of Critical Care Medicine, Anaheim, Calif. February 18 to 20, 1974.

CHAPTER 13

A staff nurse's view

PATRICIA A. BALON

The role of the staff nurse in caring for the terminally ill child and his or her family can be as superficial or as involved as each individual wants it to be, and thus will vary from nurse to nurse and family to family. Some nurses cannot give of themselves as much as others for a variety of reasons: past experiences, role perception, personal style. In addition, I believe that, difficult as it is, one must confront one's own thoughts about dying and death before one can effectively help other people deal with this part of life.

To promote the kind of mutual sharing and commitment that the care of any child requires, a primary nursing program has been instituted on the pediatric units at the University of Rochester Medical Center. By definition, a primary nurse assumes 24-hour responsibility for planning the care of the patient, beginning with the first admission and continuing throughout all subsequent admissions. When the primary nurse is not on duty, an associate nurse assumes responsibility for care for an 8-hour period in accordance with the overall management plan for the patient. This system lends itself well to the development of long-term relationships with patients.

The primary nurse is also responsible for communication between the staff and all other health disciplines about the treatment and needs of the patient and his family during the hospital admission and upon discharge. Thus this system also helps to facilitate communication among the patient, the family, and the caregivers.

As a safeguard to both the patient and the professional, the option of changing a primary assignment if a conflict arises between the patient and nurse is always available. If there is a problem, it is important to recognize it and resolve it if possible. If not, seeking the help of another staff member whose personality may mesh better with that of the child and the family is an alternative.

Although I will base most of my remarks on my experiences with hematology/oncology patients, other services and children and families facing crises with other kinds of illnesses have helped to shape my thoughts about my role as a primary nurse. I urge the reader to consider some of the broader applications possible with chronically ill children as well as with those who have fatal illnesses.

At the time of diagnosis and later, the hematology/oncology team of our hospital routinely asks the primary nurse, or if she is not on duty, the associate nurse, to be present at all major conferences with the family so that whatever information is given or feelings are expressed will be known to all the involved health care givers firsthand. I have found, as others have noted before me, that when a family is initially told of a fatal diagnosis, they are overwhelmed, and many questions are either not asked or the answers only partially heard. It is, instead, during the weeks and months that might follow that the staff nurse must support and reinforce the answers already given to many of the patient's and family's questions and help to foster the family's inherent strengths. The staff nurse may be asked by the family to help them deal with the guilt they often feel and also to help them continue to hope without encouraging false hope. I have found that most families maintain hope to the very end; it is a strong emotion that seems essential in helping them to cope both with a fatal diagnosis and with the problems and stresses of daily living that such a diagnosis often carries with it.

The terminally ill child is usually a frequent visitor to the outpatient clinic or the inpatient service, or both. Our hematology/oncology staff always offers to notify the primary nurse when his or her patient has a clinic appointment. I have found it extremely helpful to stop by the clinic to say "Hello" and keep in touch with the child and parents. The few minutes spent in the clinic refreshes the child's memory of me, thus making me a more familiar figure when he is rehospitalized. This brief visit can also be an excellent time to assess how the family is coping.

Periodically I encourage parents to bring their child to the unit before or after an outpatient visit in order to see me in that setting as well. It seems to help build up the child's trust in me if he does not always see me on the ward only in a threatening situation.

In addition to these in-hospital meetings, I feel that picking up the telephone and checking on a patient at home is a natural, human, caring response that can provide an excellent opportunity to talk at some length, if necessary, about the functioning of other family members. Siblings, especially, are at risk, because parents tend to become involved with their ill child sometimes to the extent of conscious or unconscious neglect of their other children. Yet siblings, because of their unique relationship, are particularly susceptible to fantasies about personal responsibility for the catastrophe that has befallen their brother or sister. Brief contacts can help families maintain an awareness of each other's feelings and their various needs for information or reassurance.

Impending death unites some families and divides others. I have frequently given my phone number to parents with the invitation to call me any time they need to talk. A husband or wife, even though fairly open in their discussions with each other, may still need other sounding boards outside the family unit. Neighbors sometimes provide this outlet, but even they shy away during this time because of their own perceived inadequacies in dealing with the emotionally charged feelings that come with a fatal diagnosis and progressive illness. Because I am usually comfortable with direct personal contact or service between hospitalizations, I occasionally make home visits and suggest to the mother that she take an hour for errands or other personal business while I babysit. I have found this to be especially helpful for a mother because, unlike a father, who may be able to use work as an escape from the burden of daily care or constant preoccupation with a sick child, she may be literally confined to her home. Aggravating this feeling of confinement are fear of leaving the child with someone who may not be experienced in intricate medical care and potential guilt if anything should happen while she is away. If, on the other hand, the mother has confidence in me as a nurse, she will sometimes let me assume this caregiving role, thus allowing herself a respite from constant responsibility. These natural responses are appreciated at the time and are long remembered.

When a child is actually hospitalized, it is important to him and to the parents to keep admission procedures as smooth and short as possible. Because the primary nurse keeps nursing records from one hospitalization to the next, many routine admission questions need never be repeated.

Hospital stays can be emotionally draining times for both the family and the staff. I attempt to maintain as much normalcy as possible in my contacts with the child and family. To accomplish this, I try to visit the room often, even if only briefly, and to intersperse pure conversation, some of it lighthearted when appropriate, into my talk with the patient and the parents. However, I have also found that parents at times need to be alone with their child in the hospital. If the patient is not in a private room, providing an unused office where the family can go and just be together without being disturbed by other visitors and medical staff can be an invaluable service.

When a unit is extremely busy and has one or more terminally ill children on it, frustrations mount and tempers become short. Often I feel as if I am being pulled in many directions at once and have no idea which way to turn first. I may be aware that a parent needs to talk, but I have no time at that moment. Parents feel my frustrations. I have had parents say to me "I needed to talk, but I saw how busy you were."

Personally, when I find myself being drained emotionally, I tend to become more subdued in my relationships at work. I find myself wanting to spend more time with the fatally ill child at the expense of my other patients. Such involvement or overinvolvement, can, very subtly, become unhealthy. At the other extreme, some staff members tend to avoid the patient's room because their feelings have become so intertwined with the family's that they can no longer separate and be supportive. Other nurses eventually become unable to talk with families at all. Instead, they become caught up with the technical aspects of patient care: monitoring, counting, and measuring become all-important and time-consuming. When the family is present, they appear constantly busy and so avoid more personal contact. I have found that although a nurse may be able, on an intellectual level, to come to terms with the fact that a child is terminally ill, he or she may have tremendous difficulty in attempting to handle both personal mourning and that of the family at the same time.

When the atmosphere of the unit becomes tense and parents and staff alike are responding with short gruff answers to innocent questions, the time has arrived for the staff to stop and ask for help. Sometimes the change takes place almost imperceptibly. Working out the tension that develops on a ward when a fatally ill child is admitted is often a whole staff problem best dealt with by someone trained in group dynamics who is known, but peripheral, to the staff. Occasionally the problem is truly an individual one best handled privately with the help of senior nursing or medical personnel.

If disagreements arise between the nursing staff and the medical staff about the way a terminally ill patient is being managed, muttered grumbling is unproductive; sitting down as a team with the physicians and discussing the matter, including both management and feelings, is almost always feasible and much more constructive. It is close to impossible to support a child and family if the staff is concurrently struggling with opposing feelings and thoughts.

When one of my primary patients is actually dying, I try to be there. If I am not on duty, I leave word to be called for any significant change for the worse. I might not be able to say or do anything, but an arm around the shoulder, a hand to hold, or even a tear shed can have tremendous meaning to the family then and later.

Over the past few years, I have also come to realize that as the primary nurse my commitment is not over when the child dies. After the death, the family seems to be expected to leave the hospital and pick up their lives as before. It should come as no surprise that they cannot do this: they are unable to sever so quickly all the relationships that they have developed over days, weeks, and months.

Hospital staff attendance at the funeral service is much appreciated by the family. But even after the death and funeral, parents need to talk about what happened with someone who experienced it with them. Often this individual needs to be a person outside the family yet not a stranger. Keeping in touch with the family can be invaluable, even if it is merely by phone. Although the first few attempts to make contact may be rebuffed because the family is not ready, occasional repeated contacts help to remind them that if and when outside support is needed, it is available from someone whom they know.

The following three case histories help to illustrate some of my experiences.

Case 1

TL was 1 year old when he was hospitalized with an abdominal mass later found to be a Wilms tumor. Today, 18 months after his death, his parents can say that although their pediatrician tried to prepare them for the diagnosis, neither heard the warning. When they were actually told the diagnosis in the hospital, they reacted with shock and disbelief. T had a stormy 7-month course before he died. During that period the family had great confidence in the oncologist, feeling that he never offered more than they could hope for, yet he helped them maintain hope throughout the illness. One of their major frustrations was that they had to put their son's fate in the hands of someone who was merely human. They found themselves thinking of the doctor as God, even though, at some level, they realized otherwise.

During T's illness, Mr. and Mrs. L appreciated the continuity of care that we were able to provide their son. They also appreciated the fact that neither he nor they were ever avoided. Breaks in conversation when people talked about lighthearted subjects and some bending of the rules to accommodate them were also remembered positively. Interestingly, despite their preoccupation with their son, the parents were aware of nursing frustrations and felt our pressures. As might be expected in any long illness, especially one with a poor prognosis, they also experienced personality conflicts with certain hospital staff members.

Mr. L feels that it was probably easier for him to cope during and after T's illness because of his work, whereas his wife was almost constantly at home. T was extremely difficult to care for during his illness. After his second hospitalization, he would never sleep in a crib again. His parents took turns holding and rocking him 24 hours a day. He would eat very little, and then when his mother did insist, he would vomit, causing her to first become angry with him and then feel tremendous guilt. Toward the end of T's illness, his mother found it difficult to take him to the hospital for his treatments. His father then took over this responsibility. Mrs. L eventually reached the point where she wanted T to die, because she felt she could no longer cope with his illness and its demands.

Mr. and Mrs. L found that their lives revolved around T, to the exclusion of their other two sons. Yet T's brothers were also experiencing tremendous upheaval coupled with separation from their parents, because they were cared for by out-of-town relatives during much of the time just before T's death. The parents feel that they attempted to explain T's illness as much as possible to the boys. The 6-year-old understood that T was seriously ill and often asked if he were going to die. The $2^{1}/_{2}$-year-old did not really understand what was happening except that his parents were away frequently and that he himself eventually was sent to his grandparents' home. Although relatives helped the family greatly, they were also a burden at times. Mr. and Mrs. L. found it necessary to emphasize and reemphasize that they wished to remain in control of their family despite the need for prolonged absences from home.

I was T's primary nurse. He was hospitalized only twice during his illness, because he received most of his therapy as an outpatient. I asked the hematology clinic to notify me each time T came in for treatment, and I tried to see him then if I was on duty. After T's death, at which I was present, I tried to contact the family on several occasions, but received no answer on the phone. Weeks and months afterward I met the father several times in the hospital halls when he was working on a project for an oncology parent group. I saw the mother once, more than a year after T's death, when she was in the hospital to work at a seminar on the dying child. But it was not until 16 months after T's death, when I was writing a term paper for a course I was taking, that I sat down and talked with these parents for an evening. The discussion was beneficial for us all, and I learned much, including the fact that T's mother's grief reaction had been and still was severe. She had found that after her son's death she could not dismantle his room—it remained intact in hope that he might return home. In addition to preserving many rituals that had been important while T was alive, picture albums containing snapshots of the child were taken to neighbors for safekeeping when the family was going to be away from their home for a few days.

Mr. and Mrs. L feel that they were eventually brought closer together by their experience, although the style and pace of their individual grieving brought them into some initial conflict. Whereas shortly after T's death, Mr. L became very active in a hospital group for bereaved parents, fulfilling the need to do positive things in T's name, for many months Mrs. L could not face close contact with other families and children going through a fatal illness. However, after an automobile accident involving Mr. L and one son in which the boy had to be hospitalized, Mrs. L again began to appreciate how much her remaining family meant to her. This incident marked the beginning of her reemergence into her family and, finally, the community.

Today, the parents talk about the difficulty they have looking at later pictures of T because of the physical changes associated with his illness, which they are now really seeing for the first time. They both still find it difficult to look at any child with cancer.

One of T's brothers, now 8, appears to be having some psychologic problems. He is an intense child who voices many fears of the uncontrollable: floods, tornadoes, and poisonous snakes. He cries easily and has a need to win at all he does.

T's other brother, now 4, is much less serious and more sociable. Although he may not have really understood T's death, last summer when he was hospitalized, he needed much reassurance that he would go home. His hospitalization and its successful termination became positive experiences for him.

In retrospect, what would I have done differently? I regret that I did not make more home contacts during T's illness. But it is for the events after T's death that I feel the most regret: I wish that I had been more persistent in trying to contact the family so that possibly I could have made their grieving a little easier. It is interesting that T's parents do not feel as I do. Although I realize there are limitations to what I can do, nevertheless I feel I could have given them more support during the time when they were expected by others to resume their normal lives but were not able to do so.

Case 2

JA is a charming 3-year-old today, who over 2 years ago had surgery for a rhabdomyosarcoma followed by a full course of chemotherapy. Presently, she is disease-free without medication. I have followed J since her first admission. It has become a routine (and a beneficial one for both J and me) that her mother almost always brings her to the ward to visit either before or after clinic appointments. J has thus had the opportunity to build up a trusting relationship with me at times when she was not threatened with hospitalization. As a result of these extra few minutes, during admissions Mrs. A can leave her daughter at night, without difficulty, whether I am present the first day or not, by telling J that in the morning I will be there to care for her. In the morning J is sitting up waiting for rounds! She even enjoys accompanying me while I care for other children. Procedures have always been explained to J and, at 3, she knows exactly what to expect and uses the terms brain scan, bone scan, and x-ray appropriately and without fear.

Case 3

CR was 1½ years old when he was admitted for chemotherapy for a yolk sac tumor. As with T, I had visited him in the clinic, and as with J, his mother often brought him to the ward to visit. C learned to trust me through many conversations about his favorite things—ducks, fire trucks, and his dog. Even when he was home he would mention things we had talked about. When caring for C in the hospital, many small efforts, such as carrying him, complete with IV tubes, to the window to see the fire trucks, meant a tremendous amount to his mother then and still do now, 8 months after his death.

I maintained close contact with this family after C's death. I was able to help his mother, especially, during this period when she needed to talk about C. In giving support to this family, I have also become a close friend.

In retrospect here, I would have made some home visits during C's illness to enable his mother to get out of the house more. I would also have been there when he died. Unfortunately, after much contemplation that weekend, I went out of town and was not near enough to return when the staff called me about his death. The parents were told I would be in contact with them the next day—a promise I kept.

In summary, I do feel strongly that one can become involved and yet remain supportive when caring for a terminally ill child. I have learned not to be afraid of natural responses such as a touch, a smile, or a tear. Something that I admit I am still learning is that some caregivers will be able to give more than others, but that no one individual can be all things to all people.

There is an enormous challenge in the fact that the staff nurse can be a cohesive force that brings and holds together the health team and the child and his family. Throughout life we are raised on the premise that the young bury the old. It is contrary to our society's thinking for the old to bury the young. We seem to come to terms more easily with the death of a grandparent than we do with the illness and death of a young child. Thus, caring for the dying child is emotionally draining for all of us, but it is also a fulfilling experience, as expressed in the saying on a plaque given to me by the parents of a terminally ill child: "The heart that gives gathers."

ADDITIONAL READINGS

Elfert, H.: The nurse and the grieving parent, Can. Nurse **71**:30, 1975.
Jackson, P. L. : The child's developing concept of death; implications for nursing care of the terminally ill child, Nurs. Forum **14**:204, 1975.
Kastenbaum, R.: Is death a life crisis? On the confrontation with death in theory and practice. In Datan, N., and Ginsberg, L., editors: Life span developmental psychology; normative life crises, New York, 1975, Academic Press, Inc.
Lindemann, E.: Symptomatology and management of acute grief, Am. Psychiatry **101**:7, 1944.
Mann, S. A.: Coping with a child's fatal illness; a parent's dilemma, Nurs. Clin. North Am. **9**:81, 1974.

CHAPTER 14

A nurse specialist's view

PATRICIA E. GREENE

A typical reaction to the knowledge that one has chosen a career in pediatric oncology is admiration and sympathy: "I don't know how you do it; you must feel depressed often." Others imply suspicion of freakish callousness: "I could never do that; I love children too much."

Several years of encountering such reactions led me to examine closely my philosophy of nursing and my motivation for my career choice. Early in my preparation for a professional nursing role, Virginia Henderson's definition of nursing was offered as a sound foundation for a practice broad in scope:

> Nursing is primarily assisting the individual (sick or well) in the performance of those activities contributing to health, or to its recovery (or to a peaceful death) that he would perform unaided if he had the necessary strength, will, or knowledge. It is likewise the unique contribution of nursing to help the individual to be independent of such assistance as soon as possible.[2]

Implicit in this definition is the active role the patient and his family play in giving care and their partnership with health professionals. It speaks not of cure but of a spectrum of outcomes ranging from maintenance of health to a peaceful death. It encompasses prevention, rehabilitation, and death with dignity. The emphasis is not on arresting, reversing, or controlling a disease process, but on caring for a patient who may or may not be affected by illness.

It has been my impression that this is the major difference in the orientation of nursing and medicine. The tremendous yield of medical technology and the nature of specialization force the physician to focus on treatment of disease. Cure, not care, is the measure of success.

In recent years the nursing process has received considerable attention. It is a systematic series of steps the nurse takes in planning and evaluating nursing care. It involves the ability to make an assessment, identify nursing care problems based on patient needs, decide how to manage or solve these problems, and then evaluate whether the prescribed methods did indeed effect a satisfactory resolution.[1]

Just as Henderson's definition of nursing was firmly implanted in my mind, so was the concept of nursing practice. And, like so many graduate professional nurses, I arrived on the clinical scene eager to engage in a partnership with patients and work to achieve mutually agreed-on goals of care.

My setting, general pediatric nursing in an acute care unit, offered varied opportunity for this experience. For many children, hospitalizations were brief and problems were self-limited. I found I preferred to care for chronically ill children. The duration and repetition of their hospitalizations provided an opportunity for a long-term relationship, which was more satisfying for me.

The children with cancer seemed particularly resilient and motivated to fight to overcome the implications of their diagnosis. When I questioned the appropriateness of therapy, their strength and determination provided the impetus I needed to continue in the struggle.

For many laymen and health professionals, the thought of a child with cancer evokes a mental picture of a heavily sedated child in a dark room surrounded by grief-stricken loved ones awaiting the long-anticipated moment of death. Though this may have been the case 20 years ago, recent advancements in therapy have totally changed the picture, as shown by the following description of a typical course of illness and the inherent opportunities for coping.

The diagnosis of childhood cancer has an amazing impact on the child, his family and friends, and health professionals. The process of grief and grieving is set into motion instantaneously. An elaborate treatment plan, encompassing both physical and emotional considerations, must be devised and implemented. What is created is a fertile environment for a clear-cut and gratifying nursing role. The problems become apparent precipitously, and individuals involved agree on the necessity of dealing with them. Suggestions for interventions are appreciated and faithfully carried out by patients and staff (whose anxiety is often as great as the patient's). Generally, response to therapy is prompt, and side effects are temporary. Progress is made in a reasonable period of time, and all feel a sense of accomplishment.

Initially, the goal of treatment is cure. The truly cured child must be free of cancer, mentally and physically healthy, and able to function at an age-appropriate level in society.[5] For an increasing number of children this goal becomes a reality; for almost all children a period of remission is attainable. The benefits of a difficult therapeutic regimen are realized and appreciated. Patient, family, and staff are euphoric. The child and his family live life to the fullest with an intensity and meaning seldom experienced by well children and their families.

The nurse specialist participates in the administration and management of the ongoing therapy that "makes it all possible." Continuing involvement with the patient and family earns the right to share in the joy of wellness. This phase of illness is the cornerstone of my coping system. I can always leave the bedside of a dying child and find a "well" child with cancer who is full of life, love, and appreciation. If I need to, I can suppress the unpleasant feelings evoked by the dying child and focus on the satisfying experiences of caring for well children.

There is evidence that many specialists from a variety of disciplines use this mechanism. Articles about the treatment of childhood cancer are prefaced with statements about promising cure rates. Conferences and books are devoted to the needs of the cured child. Indeed, it is reassuring to see this possibility realized and have the option of occasionally stealing away from the distressing circumstances of impending death.

Unfortunately, for many children the hope for cure is lost with recurrence of disease. The grief felt by all at this time is often greater than that felt at the time of diagnosis. Some diseases, such as leukemia, offer several reprieves through subsequent remissions. Generally, however, therapy is progressively more intensive and demanding and less effective. Efforts are focused on getting through the next phase of therapy, and the hope is that therapy will be of some benefit. In spite of increasing adversity, life and living continue, and the child and family carry on with amazing, inspiring strength. Small milestones and victories are enthusiastically and genuinely celebrated.

In the terminal phase, the goal is death with dignity and optimal functioning of surviving family members. Complications may develop that are painful, debilitating, and deforming. Caring for the child becomes difficult, and team members may withdraw. The most commonly expressed feeling is overwhelming frustration and impotence aroused by the sight of a dying child and a grieving family.

In managing care, the nursing process provides a starting point that otherwise might be difficult to find: anticipation and planning may prevent many complications, such as pain and skin breakdown; fractionating the overwhelming, complex situation into discrete, manageable problems decreases feelings of helplessness. By setting goals that are both acceptable and realistic, the nurse can feel successful when the child dies, if the best possible physical and emotional care has been provided. This is not always true for the physician, whose evidence of success is a cured child.

The choice to specialize creates a number of changes in the nurse's relationship with the patients and other health professionals. Most nurse specialists agree that formal preparation and experience build a body of knowledge that can be translated into more effective care. In turn, effective care decreases frustration and anxiety and enhances satisfaction.

For example, patient education is a vital nursing function. This entails teaching about the physical and emotional effects of the illness and treatment and providing anticipatory guidance. I have found that staff nurses are reluctant to become involved in patient education. Although they may feel comfortable discussing some aspects of care, such as control of symptoms, they are uncertain about other issues, such as response to therapy and prognosis. This hesitancy is entirely appropriate and based on the fact that therapy is complex, rapidly changing, and only barely comprehended by most staff nurses. With specialty experience and knowledge, the nurse can offer explanations and advice that are more accurate and more consistent with information offered by other team members. For the family under stress, this confident and consistent approach is essential, because even the slightest contradiction in information is confusing and alarming.

There are, however, many aspects of care, such as activities of daily living, coordinating activities on the unit, and controlling symptoms of disease and treatment, that are clearly better managed by the staff nurse. When nurses are planning care, it is essential that they realize their areas of expertise as well as their limitations and capitalize on the varied experience represented in the total nursing team.

Typically, chronically ill children are treated in referral or research centers. Many parents fear that their child will be used for experimentation and learning. The predominance of students and young, inexperienced caregivers accentuates their fear. It is not at all surprising that they readily trust and rely on a nurse, doctor, or social worker billed as a "specialist" who appears to be speaking from experience. They quickly learn the nature of the chain of authority and decision making. Quite naturally, if they are articulate, assertive, and accustomed to controlling their child's environment, they become demanding of expertise and even hostile if they feel this is denied. Obviously this is comfortable for the specialist and shattering for the rejected student, intern, or graduate nurse. When caregivers are inexperienced and insecure, it may be difficult for them to appreciate and accept this attitude. The potential for conflict between patient and staff and among staff is great. When conflicts do arise, they generally concern the day-to-day aspects of management of therapy, such as the performance of technical procedures.

Herein lies another important part of my coping system. I find myself responding with disproportionate anger when I encounter situations I should have learned to expect: an intern who unsuccessfully needles a child repeatedly before calling for help, a nurse who fails to medicate a child in pain for fear of addiction, a student who tells a child not to cry, "it won't hurt," when it will. No doubt some of this is displaced anger at the senselessness of a suffering child. I have to struggle to control my emotions and consider the needs of the staff as well as the patient. Sometimes I fail, and I rant and rave and feel much better.

In my experience, the reaction of staff nurses to a nurse specialist has been varied. Apparently there are several contributing factors. Morale on the unit is the most significant. When nurses are overworked and inadequately supported by their supervisors, they are threatened by a consultant or specialist. They may feel the specialist is rewarded by patients while staff nurses do all the work. However, if a unit is well staffed, and nurses have the time and energy to deliver good nursing care, and the quality of their care is recognized and appreciated, they are likely to be more receptive. Rather than viewing the specialist as a threat to their relationship with the patient, they view him or her as a resource and a collaborator in the delivery of quality care.

The volume of patients is also important. There must be enough patients to "go around." If the specialist is the primary nurse for all patients, staff nurses will feel excluded. A wise specialist will encourage staff nurses to establish a primary relationship with patients and then foster the relationship by helping the staff nurse obtain the necessary information for teaching and planning care. In discussions with patients, he or she can maximize the value of the staff nurse's input. This approach can only enhance job satisfaction for the nurse, quality of care for the patient, and acceptance of the specialist.

I learned this lesson slowly. Initially, when I was insecure in my role as specialist, I needed to be all things for all patients. Later, as I became more comfortable, I was better able to use my own personal resources helping others expand their roles by sharing the burden of these difficult patients.

The attitude of the supervisory personnel (nursing supervisors and head nurses) toward the specialist is reflected in the attitudes of the staff. If supervisors are accepting and supportive, the staff will follow their lead. If they are not, the specialist will find that recommendations for care are not followed, prompt notification of patient admissions or crises is not made, or attendance at rounds, conferences, or lectures is poor. The manifestations of rejection of the role are numerous, but the end result is always a compromise in patient care and the feeling of failure for both staff nurses and the specialist.

A difference exists in the roles of the nurse specialist and the staff nurse in regard to the nursing process. Generally the specialist acts as a consultant, assisting in planning and evaluating care and interpreting the plans to the patient. The staff nurse's role is the implementation of the plans. As a result, the staff nurse may feel a greater sense of entrapment when problems seem overwhelming. It is the staff nurse who must wait at the patient's bedside to evaluate the results of pain control measures, dress a malodorous wound every 4 hours, or support a parent who is afraid to stay in the child's room alone. For the specialist, it is tempting and convenient to retreat to a less threatening position of intellectualization or theoretical postulation. This situation may exist in the medical team as well. The attending physician must be able to provide rationale for the use of an antibiotic or antineoplastic regimen, but it is the house officer who spends hours at night starting an IV line. As a result of this common sense of entrapment shared by the patient and primary care providers, they may form an intense and meaningful relationship that may equal or surpass those established between the patient and specialists over the duration of the illness.

Unfortunately, the events that surround the death of a child may minimize the benefits of that relationship. While the nurse is preparing the body for viewing and the intern is completing the necessary forms, a host of people may arrive. The group may include off-duty doctors, nurses, or secretarial staff who have become close to the child and family throughout the illness, or the members of the specialty team. Often their notification of the child's death is in response to their written request left on the chart or Kardex or with the nurse or doctor on duty. Their purpose in coming is to console the family. A chaplain (who may or may not be known to the family) is frequently called. What often happens is that the nurse and doctor who cared for the child at the time of death, when free to talk with the family, find it logistically impossible to do so.

Some professionals believe that others should step in and relieve the staff at the time of death. They claim that the staff must be exhausted and distraught by the events leading to death and are not able to support the family adequately. I agree that they are exhausted and distraught, but I do not feel this necessarily detracts from their ability to support the family. Indeed, they may be best able to support the family, who are also exhausted and distraught. At times, because of other responsibilities or feelings of inadequacy, the staff may choose to be less involved after the child's death. In this situation, others must assume primary responsibility. I feel that it is appropriate for the other professionals who have become close to the child to participate in support of the family at the time of death, but they should be sensitive to the ward staff's wishes to be involved and supportive of their ability to do so.

Perhaps the greatest advantage of specialization is geographic assignment. The inpatient staff nurse's responsibility is only to hospitalized children. Contacts are limited to children who are newly diagnosed or those who are admitted for complications or terminal care. The nurses in the outpatient clinic lose touch at the most difficult period and may never experience closure of a longstanding relationship.

The specialist is responsible to both hospitalized children and those being treated as outpatients. Children are seen at clinic visits and at home when possible. With this arrangement, the specialist is able to share their joy and gratification during periods of wellness, and grieve with them when setbacks are encountered or when aggravating complications further burden their difficult lives. It is thus possible to obtain a more accurate understanding of the quality of their lives: to know what successful therapy has afforded and what is lost when treatment fails. Nurses who are not able to have this continuity in their relationship with patients develop a biased view of the value of treatment. Seeing only the bad times, they ask why the children should endure the hardship of therapy to no avail.

By maintaining an ongoing relationship with the child, the nurse specialist can begin grief work earlier, at the time of recurrence. She may be more aware of the long downhill struggle that often ensues. When the time for death comes, it may be easier to be accepting.

Having realized the advantages of this continuity, I have attempted to make the opportunity available to other nurses. Outpatients are encouraged to visit the inpatient units to demonstrate the benefits of therapy. Often they bring souvenirs of their well lives, such as school papers, music recital programs, or softball team photos. On a rotating schedule, inpatient unit nurses spend a day in the outpatient clinic. Weekly conferences are held with the nursing staff, and a progress report on outpatients is given. Good news about well children and bad news about recurrences or complications are shared. This offers a more realistic picture of the quality of life for the patients and gives the staff warning when hard times are ahead.

In discussing my experiences with children with potentially fatal illnesses, I have referred to children with cancer. I am certain, however, that the lessons I have learned from these children are applicable to other nurses and to children with other illnesses.

Perhaps the most important lesson is that the diagnosis of a fatal illness does not make a child a "dying child." For me it has worked well to concentrate on helping children live until their death.

Another fact has become clear. Just as there are many styles of living, there are many styles of dying. To return to Henderson's definition, we are "assisting the individual . . . in the performance of those activities . . . that he would perform unaided if he had the necessary strength, will, or knowledge," *not* those that *we* would have him perform.

I remember one situation that demonstrates this clearly. Charles, a lovable 15-year-old boy with acute leukemia, was in the midst of a long and stormy hospital course. He had been patient and tolerant of numerous traumatic episodes. His family was supportive and capable of participating in his care. Since the time of his diagnosis, the entire family had been open in their discussion of his diagnosis and treatment. The probability of his death and the family's feelings about it were not, however, open for discussion. As his death became more imminent, the staff became increasingly concerned that someone should talk with him and allow him to express and share his feelings. He declined numerous opportunities to discuss this with staff members who made themselves available. At one point another adolescent with leukemia died. Charles chose to discuss this with me, and we had a lengthy and open discussion about his awareness of his death, his feelings about it, and his wishes regarding our behavior at the time of his death.

This encounter was a "good" experience in the staff's value system. We hoped that, "having broken the ice," Charles would continue to share his feelings. He did not. One day he asked to talk with me and seemed impatient that I was not available. Everyone was sure he wanted to talk about death, and they were relieved. When I arrived, I learned that his concern was not his death, but very much about living. He had been secretly smoking in the bathroom for 2 months. He was out of cigarettes and had no idea where he could get his next supply. He hoped I would get them for him.

The lesson Charles taught was learned in time. We scolded him for smoking in the bathroom. We agreed to allow him to continue, but we established with his parents very strict rules about where and when. In addition to enjoying the cigarettes, he appreciated being disciplined and having limits set, two normal experiences of adolescence frequently denied the dying child. One week later he died.

I am concerned that our tendency to plan Charles' ideal approach to dying and guide him in that direction is not unique. I have observed this pattern in several different settings.

Kübler-Ross's stage theory, when misinterpreted by well-meaning health professionals, predisposes to an approach of pushing the dying person through stages until the ultimate acceptance occurs; many have come to rely on this orderly progression as part of their own coping mechanism.[4]

Indeed, it is attractive to believe that most, if not all, patients will die accepting their fate. This attractiveness combined with the fame and popularity of Kübler-Ross's work has played an important part in the thanatology revolution. It is timely to operate from a theoretical framework and apply planned interventions.

Kalish[3] aptly described the situation: "Health professionals have the delicate task of sailing a safe course between the Scylla of being stamped by the impact of Kübler-Ross's work and personal charisma and the Charybdis of refuting a concept that has gained a wide following and that appears to have substantial heuristic value, at least to some medical personnel."

Middle ground has proved to be a safe and comfortable course for me. I care for children and their families with the awareness that their behavior in response to dying may or may not fall into a described stage, that it may cross stages, fluctuate, or remain unchanged. I use this knowledge in interpreting behavior for myself, students, staff, and patients. I strive for consistency in demonstrating my acceptance of patients' feelings and behavior and in supporting their hope.

I recognize that there are times when I am able to do this and times when I am not. Therefore, I am constantly aware of individuals who serve as resources either to facilitate my coping mechanism so that I can continue to work effectively or to relieve me when I must have a reprieve. It is this combination of knowledge to understand the process and resources to make it work that has made my career both challenging and rewarding.

REFERENCES

1. Becknell, E. P., and Smith D. M.: System of nursing practice, Philadelphia, 1975, F. A. Davis Co.
2. Henderson, V.: Harmer's textbook of principles of nursing, ed. 5, New York, 1955, Macmillan, Inc., p. 4.
3. Kalish, R. A.: A little myth is a dangerous thing; research in the service of the dying. In Garfield, C., editor: Psychosocial care of the dying patient, New York, 1978, McGraw-Hill Book Co., p. 221.
4. Kübler-Ross, E.: On death and dying, New York, 1969, Macmillan, Inc.
5. Van Eys, J., editor: The truly cured child; the new challenge in pediatric cancer care, Baltimore, 1977, University Park Press.

SECTION III

SURVIVORSHIP

CHAPTER 15

The rites of death: thoughts of a funeral director

J. ALBIN JACKMAN

It is only natural that all of us want to deny death, particularly our own. It seems that all we have to do is ignore it and it will go away. This oversimplification is passed on to our children by unintentional, or intentional, remarks and actions.

When dealing with the unknown, children are often bewildered by the fact that their parents do not know all the answers. Parents, in turn, compound this uncertainty by ignoring their children's questions or by giving long, complex explanations that do not satisfy their children's wishes to know and understand.

Children are people with needs, emotions, and individual personalities. Unfortunately, this fact is often forgotten when the crisis of loss arises. Adults, wanting to "spare" the child, tend to minimize any loss for a child or ignore it. The loss of a possession, for example, no matter what its value, is frequently treated lightly, without really allowing the child to express himself. What should happen, instead, is that anyone concerned with the well-being of a child should take a step back and assume the child's eye level to see what the child is seeing. His perspective is different from that of an adult.

When a child asks a question, it is usually about an event that has occured or that he has observed. When the questions are about death, they deserve honest and simple answers given promptly with love and understanding. These are natural and innocent questionings by the child and should not cause the adult any undue apprehension.

When adults are answering these questions, it is important that they not give explanations that they do not accept or believe. The child will eventually discover discrepancies that can destroy an entire relationship through distrust. Honest discussions on all topics provide for a strong relationship built on confidence.

It is a common belief that a child in our society should not suffer disappointment or grief. When a disappointment or loss occurs, a replacement is quickly offered, denying the child the opportunity to appreciate the fulfillment that he had received from the lost possession. Thus, the child is never allowed to experience, express, or manage his grief. In reality, children do encounter a variety of situations in their daily lives in which they experience emotions of loss that lead to diverse forms of grief. They also go through the various steps of resolving the loss. Much, of course, will depend on the magnitude of that loss and the attitudes that they have acquired through the observation of their parents, other elders, and their peers. However, a child should never be ignored or belittled during these periods of resolving loss, no matter how trivial the matter may seem to others.

When a death occurs in the immediate family, the children or grandchildren are frequently pushed aside and ignored while the other members of the family experience their own grief and are not able to provide support to the children. At this time, there should be an understanding and familiar person who is able to relate to the children, offering them comfort and a readiness to answer their questions honestly. The children should be encouraged to express their emotions and, if they feel like crying, be reassured that this is a normal feeling. In a family where experiences are shared regularly, the children should be invited, but never forced, to participate in the activities surrounding the funeral. Through these activities they will be able to express their grief more freely.

As a funeral director, I welcome children and try to make them feel that they, as part of the family, can share in the funeral itself. If the children are not present during the funeral arrangement interview, it should be determined what their relationships have been to the deceased person. For example, there can be a distant blood relationship but a very close personal relationship or vice versa. Many observations must be made in a short period of time during the arrangement conference. We are all aware that the age of the person who has died, the manner of death, the duration of the final illness, and previous expectations for recovery all have a great deal to do with the emotional state of the survivors. A sudden or accidental death, for example, has enormous impact upon a family, because no anticipatory grieving has been done.

During the interval between the death and the funeral service or for some period of time after the service, the family usually receives the relatives and friends who gather to offer consolation. It is during this time that the children can be present to experience the warm feeling of mutual support and see that the deceased member had worth and meaning, not only to themselves but to many other people, and that they themselves have worth and meaning to others. It should not be expected that younger children remain perfectly behaved. They may become restless. There should be arrangements for them to spend some time with someone who can, if necessary, comfort them. Also the very young should be allowed time with their toys and friends.

The strength of the family unit rests within the members of the family when they are joined together in a common experience. For this reason, it is often recommended that children from the age of 5 or 6 be present at least for the funeral service. Sometimes the parents want and need to have even their infants with them, to provide a realization that life will continue: there is hope of survival when we gather with our children.

The children should always be encouraged to share in the decisions about how they will participate in the rituals surrounding death. As children grow older, they are able to express themselves more readily. Here again the individual child helps decide what will provide the comfort and peace of mind that he needs to close his relationship with the person who has died. At times, funerals have become so organized and structured that they have not met the needs of the survivors, especially the young survivors. Teenagers particularly are expected to act like adults, but they are often treated like outsiders.

If a child elects to participate in the funeral service, there are many ways that his participation can be structured. With the cooperation of the officiating clergy, various members of the family may take part by reading passages from Scripture or literature. In some cultural backgrounds, acknowledgments are spoken in relation to the deceased's life and accomplishments. Placing a written note or letter or a gift or an article of special significance in the casket can help a child express his sentiments.

The funeral service is most frequently concluded in the cemetery. The children should be invited to go to the cemetery on the day of the funeral. Attending this part of the ceremony can alleviate a child's feeling of suspicion or mystery about burial. If this is a first visit for the youngster, a simple but adequate explanation of the function of the cemetery should be given.

Information is frequently sought before a death, and many funerals are arranged before there is an immediate need. One observation must be made: funerals should not be so tightly prearranged that the survivors have no decisions to make. Only general plans should be discussed, because what is pertinent today may not be so later. Some preferences, if followed to the letter, could actually be detrimental to the survivors. The prearrangement conference is also a unique opportunity for the funeral director to provide information to the family on explaining death to children.

A delicate time for both families and funeral directors occurs following the death of a newborn or stillborn baby. Many times the funerals, or non-funerals, for these children have been unduly rushed in an effort to spare the mother any "unnecessary" grief. The wisest decisions are made by taking the mother's needs into consideration, and those needs may include her very strong desire to be part of the funeral, both as a planner and a participant. Denial of these desires may cause difficulties later with unresolved grief and feelings of unfulfillment.

Friends should be encouraged to respond to the mother's needs by telephoning or sending cards or flowers to the hospital. The fact that the baby lived, either in utero or for a few hours or days, cannot and should not be denied or ignored; to do so prevents the kind of closure necessary for effective mourning to take place.

Unresolved grief can take many forms, and some parents are reluctant to discuss their feelings with anyone, including their spouses. Support is necessary for all the members of these families following the death of a child. Much help can be obtained through the various volunteer groups of parents who have had similar experiences. The Society of Compassionate Friends and the Sudden Infant Death Syndrome Foundation are examples of groups of parents who have gone through the death of a child. They can readily identify with the family and offer help during this period. Other sources of support include, of course, members of the health profession and the clergy.

The funeral service profession, through various international and national organizations, has published and distributed many pamphlets and publications dealing with the subjects of dying, death, and bereavement. These organizations provide information and resources either directly or through their members to those who request it. The National Funeral Directors Association, whose headquarters are in Milwaukee, represents almost all the funeral directors in the United States. This national organization is the federation of the individual state associations, which generally have their headquarters in the state capitals.

There are additional funeral director associations that have provided research and assistance for their members' service to families. Special programs have been developed for community presentations and individual counseling. Among the most prominent are the International Order of Golden Rule Funeral Directors in Springfield, Illinois and the National Selected Morticians of Evanston, Illinois. The members obligate themselves to follow the code of ethics established by these service organizations. The Order of the Golden Rule provides audiovisual programs through its members to serve their communities and other professions. The Order has a continuing commitment to the development of new programs and publications to provide needed information to the public. The National Selected Morticians has supported research in grief therapy and counseling through relationships with university and medical school counseling services.

The role of the funeral director in the community should be one of service to all, providing comfort and understanding. He should also be available to offer facts, information, and counsel. The funeral director should be skilled in human relations and assistance to families at the time of death and during the succeeding weeks.

If all the caregiving groups provide support in harmony and remain available to those who are in need of their services, then most of the families will resolve their grief and reenter the mainstream of life with positive feelings of relationship to the person who has died and those survivors with whom they continue to share their lives.

The children who have experienced the death of a close member of the family can best be guided by true love and affection. If they have been included in the funeral and have been given adequate opportunities to express their grief and ask their questions, they will have a more comfortable adjustment. In no way should there be any unresolved grief or any unresolved guilt feelings for them. They should never be made to feel that they are being punished for a death that has occurred. This can, however, be close to impossible at times when the adults around them have these same feelings and are having difficulty resolving many of these issues for themselves. Understanding that children do mourn and helping them to express their feelings in constructive and meaningful ways, beginning immediately after a death, help to form the basis for a mutually shared and, ideally, mutually resolved grieving process.

Children are people with emotions, needs, and individual personalities. They are a vital part of the family unit and should be treated and cared for as such.

Funeral director organizations that can provide assistance:

National Funeral Directors Association
Howard C. Raether, Executive Director
135 West Wells St.
Milwaukee, Wis. 52303

International Order of Golden Rule Funeral Directors
Dale W. Rollins, Executive Director
929 South Second St.
Springfield, Ill. 62704

National Selected Morticians
Frank B. Miller, Executive Director
2121 Sheridan St.
Evanston, Ill. 60201

State funeral director associations
Usually located in the state capitals

Audiovisual aids that are immediately available:

"With His Play Clothes On" (Film strip/cassette)
International Order of the Golden Rule
929 South Second St.
Springfield, Ill. 62704

"Death of a Wished-for Child" (16-mm film with sound)
International Order of the Golden Rule
929 South Second St.
Springfield, Ill. 62704

"Understanding Death—Series" (Film strip/cassette/record)
Educational Perspectives, Inc.
P.O. Box 213
DeKalb, Ill. 60115

"Children in Crises Series" (Film strip/cassette/record)
Parents Magazine Enterprises, Inc.
52 Vanderbilt Ave.
New York, N. Y. 10017

"Death and Dying: Closing Circle" (Film strip/cassette/record)
Guidance Associates
757 Third Ave.
New York, N. Y. 10017

The reactions of children and adolescents to the death of a parent or sibling

MARION J. BARNES

A death in the family, especially the death of a parent, is a trauma for a child. How he will adapt and react to such a tragedy depends on many factors: the age of the child when the death occurred, the sex of the parent who died, the child's special relationship to the deceased, the nature of the death (sudden, prolonged, or violent) and the sensitivity and assistance of the surviving family members in attending to the emotional needs of the child.

Special attention should be given to children under 5, because so often it is felt that they are too young to understand about death, that they have an incapacity to mourn, or that they should be shielded as much as possible from such a harsh reality.

REACTIONS OF CHILDREN

In her book *A Child's Parent Dies,* Furman states:

> Mastery of the experiences of the first stressful days is often important in its own right and also sets the stage for all aspects of the mourning — the understanding and acceptance of the concreteness of death, the attitude to stressful feelings, and the need for the surviving parent's physical presence and emotional closeness. As long as these goals are kept in mind, different families find their own ways of achieving them.[7]

How old does a child have to be before he understands what it means to be dead? It helps when a child already has had some concrete experi-

---

Editor's note: The case history vignettes that the author includes in her text are gleaned from her own and others' experiences in the settings of both a therapeutic nursery school and individual practice. In this context, the severity of the children's responses to death that are illustrated generally fall into the more disturbed range of a whole continuum that spans all the psychologic permutations, from no detectable effect through situational adjustment reactions to frank psychosis. What is of special benefit in this chapter is the inclusion of specific therapeutic interpretations of particular behaviors that help us gain valuable insight into the conscious and unconscious workings of the minds of children.

ence with death. Some children of 2 can already name something as dead, such as a goldfish, turtle, bird, or insect. They do not comprehend death in an abstract way, but they do use the word and understand that the animal, bird, or fish will never live again. If they have had no such experience, the surviving parent can at least introduce the child to what it means to be dead. Bodily death and a life hereafter, if that is the belief of the family, should be kept separate. So often families whose religious beliefs do not embrace immortality will leap to this explanation to avoid their own pain and to shield the child from an even greater pain. A child under 5 thinks concretely, and his first thoughts will be about the burial.

Four-year-old Wendy and 2½-year-old Winnie had been told about their mother's death and burial.[1] The father explained that she had stopped breathing, that she was not alive any more, that she could not feel anything, that she was gone forever and would never come back. She would be buried in the ground, protected in a box with a cover on it, and nothing would hurt her—not the rain or the snow or the cold. Wendy asked, "How will she breathe and who will feed her?" The father explained that when one is dead, one does not breathe any more and does not need food.

On the evening of the mother's death, even after a visit to the cemetery, the children seemed relatively unaffected. They were both "happily" playing "London Bridge Is Falling Down." In this game, what is down is built up again.

A second game that Wendy played concurrently was a twirling game in which she became dizzy, fell down on the floor, and then quickly demonstrated how she could get up. She laughed in getting up and commented "You thought I was dead, didn't you?"

I encouraged the relatives to tolerate these games, in spite of the anxiety that this play aroused in them, because it meant that Wendy was trying to master her fear and the painfulness of death by actively reversing the process.

A week after the death, Wendy went to visit two little cousins, who, in an effort to be comforting, told her that her mother was an angel in heaven with their grandfather. Then they showed Wendy her mother's picture, indicating that she really was not dead. Wendy cried hysterically and said her mother was in the ground.

In the third week after the death, as Wendy was being dressed by the maid to come to nursery school, she had what the maid felt was an unreasonable temper tantrum about the clothes she was to wear that morning. Not only did she refuse to get dressed but was adamant about not coming to nursery school. The maid, feeling that Wendy was acting like a spoiled child, slapped her. As we talked over this incident, the family recalled what was no doubt behind the expression of this anxiety. At Christmastime the mother had taken both little girls shopping and to look at the toy window display. In one decorative scheme, along with Santa Claus, were angels dressed in black leotards with little white overdresses. These were commercially known as angel costumes. The mother had bought one of these dresses for each of the girls, and they were delighted with them. Their pictures in these outfits had even appeared in the Christmas holiday supplement of the newspaper. It was this dress that Wendy objected to wearing. She was unable to verbalize the reason why. I suggested the family talk with her about the associations that this evoked—an older memory of a pleasant shopping trip with the mother and its new association with the anxiety aroused by an angel's synonymity with death.

A child's almost immediate reaction to hearing about a death where the relationship is close is, Could this happen to me? Could this happen to the surviving parent? It therefore is essential to give the child some facts about the illness so that he can differentiate himself from the deceased. All illnesses can be explained in simple terms that a child can comprehend—not that a single explanation settles once and for all the question as to the cause of death, because it will reemerge for months and years as he grows in maturity and develops intellectually. However, once the subject has been introduced and an open communication has been established, the child feels that it is all right to ask questions, and this will stand him in good stead as he corrects fantasies and misconceptions with an explanation of reality.

Almost all caregivers have had experience with the child who has a misconception about illness and carries the burden of his anxiety for years. I have in mind a boy of 9 who was referred because of a learning disability. He also had a limp, which his pediatrician had determined was of psychologic origin. In the course of his treatment, he brought up his confusion between a limp and a lymphoma. He was consumed with an anxiety lest the fate of his father, who had died of a lymphoma, befall him.

Many children equate the sex of the parent with vulnerability to death. If the child is of the same sex, he especially needs help in differentiating himself from the deceased. Many children will express the feeling that they do not want to grow up and be like Mommy or Daddy. Sometimes this is misunderstood as a negative and unfeeling reaction on the part of the child. Often children will regress to wanting to forever be a baby—their way of expressing the danger of growing up and dying. Even when such a feeling is righted with time, a family can become disenchanted and sometimes react punitively, thereby compounding the problem. Caregiving adults have a more constructive attitude when they learn that this is a child's anxiety related to the death.

In helping a child with his feelings about death, one needs to evaluate burial service, the cemetery, the grave, and the gravestone using a child's perspective. A child should not be excluded from the mourning process, a meaningful involvement with the family of which he is a member. On the other hand, he should not be overwhelmed. A crucial issue is whether the adults in bereavement can attend to their own sorrow but have sufficient affect available to support the child. Furman states:

> These concrete evidences and reminders of the bodily death are an important part of the acceptance of death and of the child's ability to differentiate himself appropriately from the dead. The parent who is able to be in tune with his child can best gauge when and how much his child can integrate.[7]

If a young child remains at home with a family friend, he should be told what is happening while the relatives are gone. If he is taken to the zoo or an entertainment program is arranged instead, he will usually find it more difficult to grasp the reality of death. Children can bear the sadness and grief of family members better than silence, avoidance of the feelings of bereavement, or deception.

A boy of 8 was hospitalized with his brother as a result of carbon monoxide poisoning. The older brother died. The younger boy's expression of loss was mild. For the most part, he acted as though nothing had happened. However, several weeks later when he visited the family mausoleum where his brother was interred, he was grief-stricken. He cried again when the brother's bicycle was given away.

Painful as it is, there must be an expression of grief over an important loss, and sometimes this does not occur until the finality of death becomes a reality.

In many children with whom I have worked, the tasks of mourning and adapting to the loss were delayed because of the necessity of coping with other external realities. There was a change in homes, often a change in the city, thereby adding to the loss through death the loss of friends and familiar surroundings. When it was the mother who had died, there were sometimes, unavoidably, a variety of baby-sitting arrangements. This only added to the psychologic complexities of loss. It is only when there is stability in the environment and when the child feels his reality needs are provided for by a principal caregiver that the child is able to attend fully to the important tasks of mourning and coping with his feelings about death.

In the young child, there is often not an immediate acute reaction to the loss, even though there has been an appropriate sadness. Several months may elapse before the child reveals his many-faceted anxieties. If the child's distressed behavior persists the surviving parent may need to seek some counseling for his own understanding in an effort to help the child.

A reaction to death shown through a change in behavior

Stevie, a 3-year-old boy, was described as suddenly developing very "naughty" behavior 3 months after his father's death from acute coronary thrombosis. He displayed a new defiance and took fiendish delight in breaking every home and family rule. The mother, who was very sensitive and understanding, said she found herself becoming enraged. Was Stevie spoiled by all the special considerations the family had received since the death? He gave up naps completely and fought about going to bed at night until he literally dropped from fatigue. Separations from his mother when she went out in the evening were characterized by crying spells and a need to control. When she returned, he kicked her. Many mornings he could not tolerate her leaving him at school, but when she became firm and left he would yell, "Go and never come back!" One day at school he and another boy accidentally collided, and he was unconsolable over the possibility of some injury. On another occasion he deliberately tripped a little girl (uncharacteristic behavior for Stevie), and when the teacher asked why, he replied, "I'm so angry—because I'm so full of fear." A remarkable answer for one so young.

In subsequent work with the mother, she listened very carefully for expressions of affect. One day Stevie was taking a Popsicle from the icebox and out of the blue blurted out, "You know our daddy died—he died." To a neighbor he commented, "Did you know my daddy died? When I'm sleeping in my bed I cry for him."

He asked many adults if they had a father. Whenever the answer was no, he asked about the cause of death. The usual answer was that death occurred because of old age. This didn't satisfy him, for his father had been young. Finally he made a more pointed remark to his mother: "Before my daddy died, I forgot to ask him how he got sick."

One evening at bedtime he talked about trying to help people and not being able to. He said he had wanted to help his older cousin hammer nails but could not. He then shifted into a very sad mood and said that he just had not been able to help his dad. When his mother tried to discuss this further, he dug his nails into her arm and would not answer.

This case clearly brings out how Stevie confused sleep with death, and how brief separations from his mother and trips to nursery school had become associated with the forever separation of death. Also, the quietness of bedtime and the relinquishment of waking control caused him anxiety that he, too, might die. He had many unanswered questions about heart attacks, and implicit in this was his anxiety that he, too, would suffer the same fate.

Painstakingly a parent will have to clarify over and over for the child these confusions that exist because of an immature ego. A simple explanation of the specific cause of death is indicated. The question usually comes up innumerable times in various contexts as the child continually seeks to grasp the full meaning. Much parental support is necessary to clarify misconceptions satisfactorily.

One might ask why these reactions were so long in expressing themselves. One explanation might be the many outside distractions in family life concurrent with a death. More important is that psychologically it takes a period of time before the full impact of the terrible loss through death becomes a reality.

A reaction to death with the development of a symptom

Four months after his young father's death from a short terminal illness, 3½-year-old Seth was referred to Hanna Perkins Nursery School.* The father had been hospitalized during most of the illness, with certain medical procedures being visible, such as occasional IV equipment, nasal tubes, bandages, and so on. Seth observed some bodily and facial changes, although he was shielded from most traumatic situations. There was always a member of the family who went to the hospital solely to support Seth.

Three weeks before this untimely death, a baby brother was born.

After the father's death, the mother was in deep mourning and continued the grieving process well into the second year.

Seth was the first-born child in his family on both sides, and he was greatly cherished. His development was normal, and he enjoyed excellent relationships with both parents. He was a verbal child and in close touch with his feelings. He had just recently successfully completed an important developmental task, that of becoming toilet trained, when his father first became ill.

After the father's death, Seth shared in the mother's profound grief and was indeed a sad little boy. Three months after the death, a severe conflict developed. He was unable to use the toilet for bowel movements, withheld

---

*A therapist gives weekly mother guidance or parent guidance to the family of each child in the nursery school. She also meets weekly with the teachers so that the work and observations of school and home may be integrated into a meaningful whole.

feces, and when he did have a bowel movement it was either in his pants or on a newspaper. This conflict over the toilet followed a visit from friends, with their two young children, from the family's previous city. There was much reminiscing about the deceased father and much sorrow expressed. In retrospect about this event, we postulated that Seth had a fantasy that his father would return with these former friends. He was sad and cried a lot that weekend and asked where his daddy was. When told that his father was buried in the ground and could not feel anything, Seth was horrified. "They can't put my daddy in the dirt!" His mother and he talked a lot about this, but it was after the friends left that Seth developed a problem with his bowel movements. It seemed he had "dirt" and "buried" mixed up and thought that giving up bowel movements meant giving up daddy.

At a time when he did not want the toilet flushed, the mother reassured him that no parts of little boys go down with the flush. Seth added, "And you can't flush a daddy away." Then he modified this to, "When I was little, I used to think you could flush a boy away, but . . ."

Adding further energy to this conflict was the presence of a baby brother very much in diapers.

This regression was not completely worked through until Seth one day described his bowel movements as monsters. When his mother talked to him about his angry feelings, he described the destructiveness of his feelings— how they could blow up the whole room. He was angry with his baby brother and angry about his father dying and being unable to return. The prominent affect of the mother at this time was one of anger—the unfairness to her husband that he should have died at the beginning of a promising career. Another feeling that emerged was that Seth had once in a while been angry with his father during the illness, because his mother did not have the usual time to spend with him and much of her affect was diverted to a preoccupation with the illness.

Seth was entered in our therapeutic nursery as a preventive measure to assist the family educationally in integrating the many facets of his response to his father's traumatic illness and death.

It became clear that the constellation of affects that was embodied in the encopresis involved a little boy's omnipotent thinking about the power of angry feelings having the potential of making a person disappear forever and the necessity of his inhibiting these feelings, particularly toward his little brother. Then there was the anxiety of equating feces as very much a part of the self and the fear that he, too, could die—just disappear forever.

When these feelings were put into perspective through sensitive interpretations by the mother, the conflict expressed in soiling and inability to use the toilet was resolved.

Another anxiety that he occasionally revealed was a preoccupation about small hurts. He was covered with Band-aids for the slightest little cut. Any illness that he or other children acquired immediately raised anxiety about the possibility of death. A popular toy at Christmas that had a pliable face that could be distorted (not particularly constructive for any child) caused him excessive anxiety until he could understand why this was especially anxiety-provoking for him. There were constant explanations by teachers and mother correcting his infantile fantasies with reality interpretations. During another period, there was excessive preoccupation with skeletons and dinosaurs that prompted him to ask innumerable questions about the disintegration of the body. He talked about his visits to the grave and eventually came to emphasize many memories of the living father.

Until these anxieties about death and dying were worked through, Seth's ability to identify with his father in a positive way was not possible. He did not want to be tall, to follow in his father's profession, or to have wavy hair. As soon as these anxieties were placed in their proper perspective, the happy and tender memories could also emerge. At school he wore an engineer's cap, a gift from his father, and his dad's neckties, and he recounted many incidents he had shared with his dad. He said to the children one day, "You know my dad didn't want to leave us."

Although the soiling and inability to use the toilet had long since disappeared, the inhibition of aggression showed itself in the form of never being angry, for he was working very hard at being in control and being a perfect child. He did not play in the block corner, he never asserted his rights, and he was exceedingly cautious in outdoor play. That anger and death were closely linked with worries about bodily injury was vividly illustrated when Seth was looking at a picture of an x-ray in an alphabet book. He became flooded with thoughts of his dad and of how his dad did not get better. Then he complained of a headache, a stomachache, and a backache, and held on to all parts in turn. After Seth had expressed many times his fear that anger can make you dead, the teachers began pointing out little things in play situations that he might be having angry feelings about and supporting him in the fact that it was safe and constructive to have such feelings. A quote from the nursery school record states: "As Seth became freer to express anger, he became less inhibited. This child who could not participate in music can now sing with enthusiasm. Now he can climb with free and agile movements. He does not need to watch as though looking for danger."

A reaction to death that is bound in a psychosomatic symptom and completely repressed

When a child is unable to master the traumatic experience of death, he may become partially fixated at the developmental level where he was when the trauma occurred; that is, his development becomes uneven. There is an incapacity to move fully forward, because childish fantasies are not able to be modified by experiences in reality. When this occurs, professional intervention is necessary.

Sophie, 6½ years old, was referred to the child psychiatry clinic from pediatrics. She was the oldest child in the family. A younger brother had died when she was 2. He was grossly defective and never came home from the hospital. The family were in deep mourning over the loss of this son, the father's namesake. They made frequent visits to the grave, and there were periodic masses for him in the church.

Sophie had had repeated hospitalizations for dehydration as a result of continuous vomiting. After intravenous feedings, she would recover and function ably until the next crisis, which was triggered by a mild physical condition such as a cold or some undefined psychologic source. She was a bright student, a model of good behavior, and adequate in her social functioning.

In her play sessions she was shy, polite, and well behaved. Only through symbolic play did another side of her affectual life emerge. In her drawings there were innumerable volcanoes destroying whole families. Belief in magic also dominated her play: if one wished for ten dolls, the dolls would appear.

From the first session, a small plastic horse became important. This toy horse was unhappy because he had a stubby tail. He was magically to acquire a more proper and beautiful tail by stealing tails from other animals and eating them. At times this horse ate babies with the greatest pleasure. Another piece of repetitive play was the enactment of the story of Noah's Ark. She brought all her own equipment from home to ensure a full stage production. The message she communicated through this story was that evil and bad people are punished by God through death.

This was a little girl who had inhibited most outward manifestations of aggression but was consumed by aggressive fantasies. At the time of her brother's death, magical and omnipotent thinking was appropriate for her age. She had deeply resented her brother's arrival and wished him gone. When he died, she interpreted this as the result of her angry wishes. With the arrival of a second brother, these feelings of aggression and resentment continued. Her wish to be a boy and her infantile fantasies of acquiring a penis were also evident in the play. The real cause of the brother's death had remained a complete mystery to her, so that she was left with her own inner fantasies about the cause of his death. Because of her enormous guilt, as seen in the Noah's Ark play, the slightest illness or emotional breakthrough triggered a fear of death.

It was only through psychologic work closely coordinated with pediatric management that this symptom began to subside.

A child's reaction to a violent death: suicide

In the first two examples that I have given, the children had reached adequate age-appropriate development in all areas of their personality functioning. It was the trauma of death itself that the immature ego could not assimilate. However, when there is a disturbed family environment for whatever reason, a child may already be showing disturbances himself. The addition of the death of a parent only complicates the stress and makes it virtually impossible for the child to master this trauma.

When Peter was 3 1/2, he was already showing serious signs of disturbance. He was not toilet trained and had a severe eating problem—just hovering at acceptable weight—constantly sucking his thumb, and evidencing the symptom of echolalia. The mother had been depressed for two years, and there had been a period of hospitalization for her. Different housekeepers had substituted for her during her periods of unavailability, so that Peter already was reacting to separations through regression in toilet training and hyperactive behavior. His mother had been working with me for several months specifically around toilet training and his feeding disturbance. (She saw a psychiatrist for her own depression.) She had achieved a constructive relationship with Peter through reading stories and providing ample educational toys and records. Just at the time when things seemed to be significantly improved, she locked herself in the bathroom and shot herself through the head. Peter and a baby brother were home with her. For several hours Peter cried and tried to kick open the door. When the father returned from work, he put the children in a room and broke down the door. The scene was unpleasant; blood was everywhere. The father tried to lift the body and in the effort dislocated his shoulder. He turned around to telephone for help, only to find Peter standing outside the door taking in the whole scene. The police and an ambulance arrived. Not only was the mother taken away, but the father, too, had to go to the hospital.

These confusing and terrifying circumstances complicated Peter's ability to cope with the facts of death, to mourn, and to progress in his development.

The first responsibility was to find a reliable caregiver who could act the role of a substitute mother. There were, unfortunately, several changes before a suitable housekeeper was found. This sad but frequent reality of finding a housekeeper to take the place of a mother occurs in a great many cases. Fortunately, by the time Peter entered Hanna Perkins Nursery at the age of 4, there was the stability of good emotional and physical care by a motherly housekeeper. This is an essential prerequisite before one can address oneself effectively to the psychologic issues disturbing the child with some hope of resolution.

Peter showed the effects of this trauma in the nursery school by frequently lying on the floor, overcome with anguish, stating that his mother was dead and had jelly all over her face. On one occasion he told a visitor that his father had killed his mother. The child was so anxious and so overwhelmed that direct treatment was necessary.

His reactions to the death, his bereavement, and all the defenses utilized in coping with the loss were unfolded in his treatment. He re-created the relationship with his mother by sitting very close to me and having me read stories, just as he and his mother had enjoyed doing. A book that he requested repeatedly was one entitled "I Can Fly," a fanciful story about a little boy pilot. This story expressed a boy's ambivalence about going to heaven to join his mother or focusing on interesting earthly objects. The story made a point about the little pilot dropping messages to his grandparents.

Another story he wanted repeated over and over was about a fire fighter who successfully rescues a mother and dog from the flames. Peter also played out that he was a fire fighter successfully rescuing all kinds of people. He acted out a character known as Mr. Fix-It over and over—there was no wreck so demolished that he could not fix it.

I talked with Peter over a period of time about how much he would have wanted to prevent his mother's death. He chanted television commercials that expressed his feelings, such as "All my troubles will be over when I get Head and Shoulders." His sadness was expressed in the Maxwell House Coffee advertisement "That first day in the new house was the loneliest day of my life. Dad was at work and I was alone with the baby." Then enters Jean, a neighbor, with a cup of coffee and companionship.

Peter's denial of the death was expressed in many ways by a Sears commercial he chanted: "Through wind and snow and rain and sleet Die Hard batteries never die."

In a neighborhood play group, he never tired of playing a game called "Briar Rosebud," the story of Snow White. He liked to be chosen to be the prince and eagerly waited his turn to wake Briar Rosebud, who had been asleep so long, with his touch.

Separations were exceedingly difficult. When the school secretary went out to lunch, Peter repeated over and over the times when she left and when she would return. An absence of a teacher from school filled him with dismay. For months there was always great concern that his housekeeper would not pick him up exactly on time. For a year he could not go on little school field trips away from a familiar setting unless his housekeeper accompanied him. Each illness of his own or another child's caused him much anxiety that it might result in death.

Peter showed the positive side of the relationship with his mother through his interest in being read stories and in telling stories. Some children thought he could read, because he could repeat verbatim about 20 stories. This was a way he had of remembering his mother. He also showed the negative aspects of his interaction with his mother by being teasing and provocative with food retaining, a pathologic reaction in his effort to retain the memory of his mother. In this area around food, he revealed a fantasy that he was responsible for her death through his bad behavior.

His anger toward his mother for leaving him by dying was also revealed through his anguish over broken promises. His mother had promised him that when they moved into their new home she would take him often to the library and the fire station nearby.

Mention has been made in previous examples about the importance of giving children simple, factual information about the circumstances of death. The appropriate time to tell a child under 5 about suicide is difficult to determine and depends on the child's ego strength. This is a hard concept to comprehend. Children understand about murder more readily, because they are in touch with their own aggressive feelings. Difficult as suicide is for the young child to understand, it is necessary to talk about it. There is always the possibility that other children will mention it. When the surviving parent chooses to keep it a secret, the child always knows that some important forbidden information is being withheld. This creates a barrier to open communication between parent and child.

There was a lapse of several months before Peter was given the exact details of his mother's suicide. He showed his readiness by a preoccupation with a story called "Blue River." This is a story of pollution that raises the question, How did it happen? Could they save Blue River? Radio and television stations told everyone that the river was dying. Great factories dumped their waste into the river, and the river was full of dead fish. The plants were killed, and the fish had nothing to eat. Peter commented, "I don't understand. How did they all die?" I thought that he probably was wondering about another death—his mother's.

"Yes," he said, "I'd like to know how did she die." I asked if he had any ideas. "Yes, she died from pollution in the toilet."

He pressed on in the book, which traced the life of the river from colonial times. He focused on an Indian log cabin and asked me to draw it. An Indian woman was sitting on the floor engaged in work. A warrior was standing in the door looking on. Peter distorted what was in the picture and said, "See that Indian mother lying on the floor. She's dead." I asked how she died. "She died of high blood pressure and heart disease." I asked just what high blood pressure was. He answered, "That's blood all over you." I wondered how that could happen, and he explained that the Indian man had thrown the mother on the floor, and she died. I told Peter it was time for him to know how his own mother died and that his dad would tell him that very day.

The father told Peter that his mother had died of a special kind of sickness that made her want to die and she had shot herself with a gun. The doctors in the hospital tried to help her in every way, but they just could not. There was nothing that the father or Peter could have done to save her. She had died as soon as Peter had heard that noise.

A week after this explanation Peter was pretending to be the captain of a tugboat. He was accompanying the Queen Elizabeth. The Queen Elizabeth struck an iceberg and went down. Peter commented, "The wreck was too big. I just couldn't save her."

Hearing the real facts prompted another spurt in this little boy's growth. It relieved him of the burden of guilt and dissipated the anxiety that his father had had some part in the death—a natural conclusion considering what Peter had seen.

Young children do not ask painful questions directly. They do, however, try to cope with a resolution through symbolic play or through the use of stories. It is not my purpose to discuss therapeutic techniques in dealing with defenses or methods of slowly strengthening the ego but to illustrate the constant and painful struggle a young child engages in to work through the multiplicity of feelings that emerge. It takes a long time to integrate and cope with such a trauma.

A prominent defense mechanism intermittently used by children of all ages is denial, even though intellectually there is a comprehension of death. The pain of coming to grips with a loss understandably extends over a long period of time. With young children, their magical thinking and their powerful fantasies and wishes work toward undoing the loss. For a variable length of time there is always the hope and expectation that the loved one will return. This is a normal reaction for a child with an immature ego. The adult is constantly correcting a child's inner misconceptions in all areas of his development. With the pain of a death, adult support is even more necessary. In the case of Peter, I thought that after 2 years of treatment he had accepted the finality of death fairly well. However, one day he informed me that his neighbor had told him about a plant that seemed dead but came alive again—it was called a rose. One has constantly to empathize with a child who wishes so much that death were not permanent.

In contrast to these younger children is the case of a 13-year-old girl who, although she understood the finality of the death of her 15-year-old sister, returned from a trip to California 2 months after the death and, upon entering her home, had an overwhelming grief reaction, crying, "When will I see her, when will I see her?" This was only temporary, but there are occasions when the pain is too great. Her 17-year-old sister, in writing her autobiography during the same period, wrote, "I have two sisters, one 13 and one who will forever remain 15." The mother, writing her autobiographical background for an organization, wrote, "I have two children."

I have placed great emphasis on the special necessity for preventive work with children under 5 when a parent dies, because this is the most vulnerable age group. Such children depend completely on parental support for their ego development and mastery of their instinctual drives. Their reality testing is limited, and they are easily overwhelmed with anxiety. Their capacity to verbalize affects is not fully developed, and they need adult help in identifying feelings.[8] Anxiety or inner stress is prone to take the form of physical activity. Deutsch has pointed out the effect of parent loss in childhood on adult pathology. Paul also has based a school of family therapy on early unresolved grief reactions.[10]

The time to offer counseling is at the time when a death occurs, before conflicts and anxieties have resulted in behavior difficulties or symptom formation. Important areas involve helping the bereaved around burial services, clarifying with the parent the importance of discussing the nature of the illness so that the child can achieve his own differentiation, and supporting the bereaved in their grief so that they in turn can allow the expression of grief in their children.

REACTIONS OF ADOLESCENTS

Because of greater ego maturity, the normal adolescent is better able to cope with the finality of death. Unlike the younger child, he does not depend as completely on parental figures for his progressive development. He is loosening libidinal ties to parents, and emotional attachments are invested in the peer group and adult figures outside of the family. However, we are all too aware that generalizations about adolescence cannot be made, because this is often a period of transient turmoil. In particular, it would be a mistake to think solely in terms of chronologic age of the adolescent in predicting behavior.

Deutsch has pointed out that, in the ongoing struggles for identity, "many more or less severe symptoms may arise. General confusion of identity and the feeling of a lack of coherence in his ego culminates in the adolescent's painful question 'who am I?'"[5]

Also during this phase there is a recapitulation of one's earlier life, and unresolved conflicts and arrests in development are renewed.[6]

Adolescent reactions and resolutions are extremely variable and unique to an individual, and it is often only at a time of crisis that we are able to observe his adaptability and assess how well the ego can deal with anxiety. The loss of a parent or sibling through death does not automatically lead to pathology. The impact of a loss on the adolescent's psychologic development will be determined by the level of drive development, the quality of his object relationships, and the degree of ego maturity attained before the loss. Object loss, while itself not pathogenic, can become the nucleus around which earlier conflicts and latent pathogenic elements are organized.[9]

The potential for suicide often arises in the adolescent group.

A 15-year-old girl was hospitalized after taking a large overdose of aspirin 4 months after the death of her father. She was his favorite child, and an overly close relationship had been maintained between father and daughter since early childhood. The father had been delinquent, in conflict with the law, and held in disrepute by other family members. This attitude only strengthened the tie between father and daughter. It was clear that she had never properly relinquished the earlier oedipal attachment, and as an adolescent she had never gained satisfactions from her peer group. Although devoted to her father, she was also ambivalent about his delinquencies, because they paralled a conflict she was going through—cutting classes in school. She longed intensely for her father and wished to rejoin him in death. Another causative factor in her attempted suicide was aggression toward the father because she identified with his delinquent behavior and was punishing herself by death. Just before her suicide attempt, she expressed a strong belief in immortality, which had previously not been a part of her personal belief or consistent with the philosophy of her particular religious group.

We are all familiar with a number of adolescents who develop a renewed interest in immortality or a preoccupation with immortality for the first time. Deutsch has made the point that as the adolescent struggles with intense anxieties, he is confronted with one of life's sharpest paradoxes—namely, that on the threshold of a new life he also feels the threat of death.[5] She feels there are various ways of conquering this specific anxiety: at one extreme, real achievements; at the other, flight into fantasies—either fame and immortality of an earthly character or eternal life.

The normal interest in immortality as part of the adolescent growth process can sometimes be employed defensively to deny the horror of death, avoid sadness, and perpetuate the fantasy of a reunion in the physical sense. Any spiritual connotations are usually missing. A meaningful death in the life of an adolescent can result in suicidal thoughts, using a negative approach to thoughts of an eternal life.

Another normal adolescent process, working through the stages of achieving a solid identity, can be interfered with if the adolescent cannot differentiate himself from the one who has died.[3] During this period the group and peer members have assumed the greatest importance. Whether he will identify with the healthy, more mature members or temporarily overidentify with pathology is always a risk and depends on a myriad of factors—his reality testing, the strength of his ego, and the level of his anxiety. It is not uncommon for adolescents to imitate and identify with persons in their environment. It is particularly crucial when this identification is with one who has died. If carried to an extreme, this process can lead to suicidal attempts or suicide. Blos[2] has noted that in early adolescence the group serves as a support for some of one's own deficiencies, especially in the area of body image. To cope with this anxiety, adolescents often place themselves in dangerous positions and activities as if to test out the very bodies about which they are anxious.

The adolescent needs much emotional support and the opportunity to verbalize his concerns so that misconceptions about death can be clarified. This often comes from the peers and/or adults associated with adolescent groups—teachers, clergymen, and youth leaders. From the constructive side, most adolescents have a greater capacity to deal with death than the younger child. They are more able to cope with the immediate impact of the circumstances, to mourn, and to resume and continue their emotional life in harmony with their level of maturity. They take a more active role in funerals and participate in memorials to the dead, such as raising money for research and eradication of certain illnesses. They remember and mourn through constructive acts for the living as well as remember the loss through death.

REFERENCES

1. Barnes, J.: Reactions to the death of a mother, Psychoanal. Study Child **19:**334, 1964.
2. Blos, P.: The second individuation process of adolescence, Psychoanal. Study Child **22:**162, 1967.
3. Caplan, L. M.: Identification; a complicating factor in the inpatient treatment of adolescent girls, Am. J. Orthopsychiatry **36:**720, 1966.
4. Deutsch, H.: Absence of grief, Psychoanal. **6:**12, 1937.

5. Deutsch, H.: Selected problems of adolescence, Monogr. Ser. Psychoanal. Study Child No. 3, 1967, International University Press.
6. Freud, A.: Adolescence, Psychoanal. Study Child **13:**42, 1958.
7. Furman, E.: A child's parent dies; New Haven, 1974. Yale University Press.
8. Katan, A.: Some thoughts about the role of verbalization in early childhood, Psychoanal. Study Child **16:**184, 1961.
9. Laufer, M.: Object loss and mourning during adolescence, Psychoanal. Study Child **21:**269, 1966.
10. Paul, N. L.: Psychiatry; its role in the resolution of grief. In Kutscher, A., editor: Death and bereavement, Springfield, Ill., 1969, Charles C Thomas, Publisher.

CHAPTER 17

The impact of parent suicide on children

ALBERT C. CAIN

Although the topic of suicide is still surrounded by taboos, stigma, and wide-ranging social discomfort, recent decades have witnessed sharply increased scientific studies of and professional attention to suicide. Massive formal suicide bibliographies,[7] an outpouring of book-length studies and collections of papers, the brief but catalytic appearance of a center within the National Institute of Mental Health, special training programs and curricula, specialty journals (*Bulletin of Suicidology, Suicide and Life-threatening Behavior*), and a growing list of local suicide prevention centers all attest to the vigorous development of concern for the special anguish, despair, and tragedy inherent in the act of suicide. The preponderance of both clinical and formal systematic investigations has focused primarily on the *suicidal individual:* psychodynamics, personality, diagnostic status, ego state, precipitating events, early background, current family constellation, interpersonal relations, age, race, sex, occupation, socioeconomic status, religion, "predictability," inpatient or outpatient management, method employed, and so on.

By contrast, stunningly little study or clinical attention has been directed to those individuals profoundly affected by a suicide. The understandably intense focus on the individual who contemplates or commits suicide has almost completely overshadowed the unique immediate stress and longer-term vulnerabilities of those "survivors" of suicide: family members and others outside the family genuinely involved as well. The conservative formal data on annual incidence of suicide in the United States, based on death certificates, indicate approximately 25,000 deaths by suicide each year. Given the shame and stigma attached, it is widely recognized that suicide as a cause of death is often concealed by underreporting both socially and on death certificates. Conservative extrapolations to more realistic figures suggest approximately 50,000 suicides in the United States each year. Shneidman[18,19] thus estimates some 200,000

---

*Such data have led many observers to suggest, paradoxically, that perhaps the most effective locus for suicide prevention will be "postvention" with surviving family members following a suicide!

"survivor-victims" of suicide *per year.** If serious suicide attempts and effects on individuals outside the family are included, the numbers swell enormously.

A few autobiographical and biographical studies poignantly translate such statistics into compelling depictions of the destructive effects suicides may have on surviving family members.[15,24] So too do a small but growing number of intensive clinical case reports.[2] As convincing as those documents are, several large sample studies are perhaps more persuasive about the general pathogenic potential for the bereaved family members: these studies consistently demonstrate the grossly higher incidence of a family background of suicidal behavior in the histories of adolescents and adults who attempt or commit suicide than occurs in the backgrounds of nonsuicidal control groups.[8,11,14,20]

The presentation here will be limited specifically to the impact of parent suicide on children, recognizing of course that a suicide's impact on a surviving spouse is a significant component of the postsuicide constellation with which the child must contend. The utter neglect of the children of parents who have committed suicide is symbolized by two basic facts. First, in the numerous detailed demographic studies on suicides, virtually none include data on whether the individuals had any children, much less the number or ages of those children. Second, of the approximately 200 suicide prevention centers across the country, containing many devoted and informed professionals and volunteers committed to working with problems of suicide, only a bare handful have programs, projects, or even mechanisms for working with bereaved family members following a suicide.

Obviously, the information base is a narrow one.* There has been a scattering of instructive individual case studies[1,6,12,16,21-23] atop some earlier, truly awesome if tantalizingly sketchy references to "anniversary" suicides and suicides repeated across generations of families.[9,13,25] Also relevant are those studies previously cited that indicate a high incidence of suicidal behavior in the parents of individuals who attempt or commit suicide. A series of clinical studies of significant samples of children whose parents committed suicide contains data that not only confirm particular pathogenic elements and family vulnerabilities in this context but also suggest a markedly elevated incidence of developmental disturbance in "children of suicide."[3-5]

What follows, then, is an attempt, using these sources and additional

---

*It is essential to expand the study of the impact of suicide on survivors in nonpsychiatric survivor samples, that is, samples derived from the general suicide survivor population, as in the pioneering studies of Henslin[10] and Rudestam.[17]

case material, to delineate briefly some major dimensions of the impact of parent suicide as a uniquely tragic variant of childhood bereavement.*

DIMENSIONS OF THE IMPACT OF PARENT SUICIDE

In order to discuss some common, widely shared dimensions of children's reactions to parent suicide, a massive caveat is necessary.

1. Each act of parent suicide is unique in its nature, timing, and locale.
2. Each family context is unique: for example, an "only child" family; a family amid custody determinations; a family utterly controlled by an aging grandmother; a multiparent, third marriage, "merged" family, and so on.
3. The parent suicide is superimposed on a preexisting personality structure and state of development in the child; thus the child's reactions inevitably are highly individualized.
4. In many instances there exist, long before the suicidal act, substantial developmental disturbances in the children, some that are clearly related to the nexus from which the suicide evolved, some that are separate in nature and origin.

Despite frequent denials by parents and many professionals who encounter these children, the child is frequently directly involved in or immediately presented with some facet of the parent's suicidal act. Here are some case illustrations:

- A 7-year-old watched as her father first shot three holes in her mother's picture, then pumped the next bullet into his own brain.
- A girl found her mother's body hanging in the girl's closet on her thirteenth birthday.
- An 11-year-old boy had been sent to the drug store to pick up the medication (another "open prescription") that his mother used to kill herself.
- A 7-year-old boy saw his father attaching a tube to the car exhaust pipe, had some awareness of its implications from prior suicide attempts, but was unable to summon help.
- A girl, in a family meeting during divorce proceedings, asked to live with her father, then watched as her mother declared that she was no longer of any use to anyone and then threw herself to her death from the balcony of their high-rise apartment.

These are vivid, overt examples; it is hoped that they will not obscure to clinicians many children's quieter but perhaps more pervasive involve-

---

*The clinical data come not only from continuing studies of families who have sought child psychotherapy for various conditions some years after the suicide but also from families seen on a different, *preventive* basis within a few days or weeks after the suicide.

ment in parent suicides: suicides immediately following blowups over a child's misbehavior, suicides occurring amid parental battles focused on (or displaced onto) a child, or suicides in which a child had been told to "keep an eye on" the suicidal parent.

If such case material leaves any doubt as to the pathogenic potential of parent suicide for children, a few fragmentary case vignettes may briefly illustrate some eventual outcomes of the forces unleashed.

- George, a 23-year-old music student kills himself with the same gun his father had used to commit suicide 15 years earlier. George's brief, gentle suicide note states that he forgives his father and realizes that his father too "must have known it was the only solution for people like us."
- Billy, a 12-year-old whose father committed suicide 3 years earlier, is referred because of behavioral difficulties and deteriorating school performance, with special concern about recent threats of suicide when he is disappointed, disciplined, or falling short of his mother's expectations. In initial contacts he speaks with relief of the office being at a ground floor level: "No way I could jump or fall out the window and be hurt." At a later point in treatment, he tells in a halting, depressed manner how he decided a year earlier that he will have to kill himself "before it does it to me." The "it" he describes as an inner urge (occasionally experienced as an inner voice) that he fights off, a force that "will kill me unless I do it first."
- Mike, age 8, has a peculiar symptom of semichoking, gasping, and struggling for breath, which remains without explanation after repeated pediatric workups and is resistive to a variety of attempts at symptom management. He is seen in outpatient psychotherapy for completely separate reasons (increasing passivity, inhibition, constriction, and phobias); the "gasping" symptoms emerge as stemming from an identification with what he fantasied to be his mother's struggle to breathe during her suicide by carbon monoxide in the garage. The symptom disappears after a number of sessions in which he plays out various versions of her death amid interpretations of his guilt and fright over her death and his identification with her fantasied choking.

Guilt

Generally the child's guilt stemming from his parent's suicide is so intense and suffocating that its effects are plainly visible in the child's disturbance: insistent direct statements of guilt and self-recrimination; depression; provocative and self-punitive behavior; obsessive, guilt-laden ideas; self-destructive behavior; or desperately driven efforts by the child to prove defensively that he is utterly good and in no way damaging, dangerous, or bad.

In many instances, the previously depressed patient had long made family members feel guilty about and partially responsible for his despair; they feel even guiltier then about the subsequent suicide. Similarly, in cases with severely disturbed parents, the children had often been repeatedly warned about upsetting or worrying that parent, which placed a large implicit responsibility for the parent's psychologic well-being on the child's fragile shoulders. Furthermore, because children typically exhibit concreteness, distorted concepts of causality, egocentrism, and naiveté regarding psychic realities, many children perceive specific incidents immediately preceding the suicide, especially parental argument over or anger at the child's misbehavior, as having *caused* the suicide. Single, partially precipitating events are confused with causes. In addition, the child's guilt often centers about the actual suicidal act—how he could have, *should* have stopped it; reality considerations rarely reduce or undo the child's guilty sense of responsibility in this respect.

Denial, distorted communication, and reality distortion

As noted earlier, significant numbers of these children have to some degree witnessed the suicidal act or its immediate aftermath. Nevertheless, in a fashion difficult to imagine, most surviving parents and adult relatives avoid communicating honestly and openly with their children about the suicide. In many instances in which the children have directly witnessed some aspect of the suicide, the surviving parent tells the children that the death was due to an accident or illness, not suicide. Children who had watched their father threaten suicide and immediately shoot himself were told it was a gun-cleaning accident; children who found and read a parent's suicide note were told they misread or misunderstood what they read; children who found their father hanging from a rafter in the house were later told he died in a car accident, and so on. When children insist on what they have seen, they often are shamed or variously censured and quieted. Often they are told that they have confused everything with a bad dream, or that they have been watching too much television.

In many instances of parent suicide not witnessed by the children, communication is completely blocked or distorted. Flagrant, transparent lies are told; evasive statements are constant. Some parents simply refuse to discuss the matter with their children. Many mothers report that they pray their children will never ask them about the death. Upon seeking treatment, numerous parents insist that the therapists not reveal to their children the truth of the suicide.

Suffering amid the suicide-precipitated stigma, shame, and social embarrassment, as well as their own guilts and tumultuous affects,[4] the surviving parents' profound reluctance to communicate openly with their children is understandable. But it leaves the children no opportunity for catharsis, for relieving guilt, or for clarification and reality correction of fantasies surrounding the death. Instead, they are left to deal with marked confusion, a doubt of their own sense of reality, a wedge of distrust between them and their surviving parent, and often a frightening message that they must not tell, must not even *know* of the suicide—this latter often evolving into disturbances of communication and learning.

A further complication: these children often hear contradictory versions of the death from the surviving parent at different points and also are exposed to additional conflicting accounts from other relatives, ministers, neighbors, or peers at school. The degree of sheer cognitive confusion, as well as the complex demands of simultaneously knowing and not knowing about the suicide, is a harsh burden for these children.

Identification

It is clear from some of the previously presented case material that one major pathologic sequela of parent suicide is a tendency to identify with the parent who committed suicide. Suicides by the children of suicide, a few days to 2 or 3 decades after parent suicide, illustrate all too painfully this identificatory undertow. Suicide on the anniversary of a parent suicide, or suicide at the same age or by the same method or at the same location as the parent's suicide, demonstrates unequivocally the strength of the identification involved. Although we frequently see, at a straightforward behavioral level, suicidal threats by such children, more complex internal processes are often equally at play: fears of one's own suicidal impulses; panicky avoidance of materials, activities, or places related to the suicide; inner urges to kill oneself; frantic efforts to "identify away" from the parent (that is, children struggling against such fatal identification desperately attempt to define themselves and behave in a manner totally different from the parent who committed suicide). In all these ways, blatant and subtle, direct and complex, overt and internal, the forces of identification with the parent who committed suicide often live on in the children of suicide.

Long-term impact

It is vital to underline as well the pathogenic import of continuing postsuicide interactions within the family. A few clinical examples will suffice.

- A father, identifying his daughter with her mother who had committed suicide, becomes incapable of imposing discipline or setting reasonable limits on her. His remarriage fails when he cannot accept his second wife's gentle, gradual efforts to reestablish sensible controls over the daughter's increasingly wild behavior.

- A father lives out, over a decade, a hate-laden vendetta against his son, openly blaming the boy since he was 3 months old for his mother's postpartum depression and suicide.

- A mother, whose overriding need to derogate and humiliate is temporarily thwarted by her masochistic spouse's suicide, fully redirects those needs toward their youngest daughter. Within a short time, this bright, competent girl, under her mother's new-found savage contempt, derision, and constant criticism, is feeling that she is "like Dad," someone who "can't even walk through a room without tripping."

- A father, who has never come to terms with his wife's barbiturate suicide, repeatedly explodes into uncontrollable tirades when he finds his adolescent daughter taking a few aspirin for headaches or menstrual cramps. He smashes any pill bottles in her medicine cabinet while wildly predicting she will end up "just like her mother."

In these and far more complex ways, the effects of parent suicide live on not only "inside" the children of suicide but also within the ongoing patterns of interaction between surviving family members.

CONCLUSION

It is widely agreed that the death of a parent, beyond the obvious human tragedy involved, contains multiple threats to normal child development. If bereaved children are a "high risk" group for developmental disturbance and later psychopathology, and there are both obvious developmental grounds and empirical data to indicate precisely that, then surely the bereaved children of parents who commit suicide are an even more vulnerable group. Added to the variety of potential developmental interferences inherent in parent loss and the intrinsic obstacles to adequate mourning in our society are the typical post-suicide effects of stigma, ambivalent avoidance, flurries of gossip, social embarrassment, and related concealment, denial, evasion, and "conspiracies of silence." Each of these factors further burdens the surviving family members and otherwise distorts the normal processes of mourning.

I have sought here to sensitize professionals to the virtually unique tragedy and developmental vulnerabilities of the children of suicide, seeking to reverse the general trend of scientific and professional neglect—even avoidance—of these children. Ideally, clinicians will be alerted to concealed parent suicides in patients' family backgrounds; more cognizant of the possible direct involvement of children in the actual suicidal events or events surrounding the suicide; more attentive to the pathogenic potential of parent suicide and some of its specific dimensions; and, most of all, more prepared to make early, quasi-preventive interventions rather than see such children 3—or 23—years later (if at all) when the distortions of the mourning process have frozen into major, deeply ingrained symptomatology and disorders of personality.

REFERENCES

 1. Arthur, B.: Parent suicide; a family affair. In Cain, A. C., editor: Survivors of suicide, Springfield, Ill., 1972, Charles C Thomas, Publisher.
 2. Cain, A. C., editor: Survivors of suicide, Springfield, Ill., 1972, Charles C Thomas, Publisher.
 3. Cain, A. C., and Fast, I.: Children's disturbed reactions to parent suicide, Am. J. Orthopsychiatry **36:**873, 1966.
 4. Cain, A. C., and Fast, I.: The legacy of suicide; observations on the pathogenic impact of suicide upon marital partners, Psychiatry **29:**406, 1966.
 5. Cain, A. C., and Fast, I.: Parent suicide and suicide prevention. In Fox, R., editor: Proceedings of the Fifth International Conference for Suicide Prevention, Vienna, 1970, International Association for Suicide Prevention.
 6. Dorpat, T. L.: Psychological effects of parental suicide on surviving children. In Cain, A. C., editor: Survivors of suicide; Springfield, Ill., 1972, Charles C Thomas, Publisher.
 7. Farberow, N. L.: Bibliography on suicide and suicide prevention 1897-1967, Chevy Chase, Md., 1969, National Institute of Mental Health.
 8. Farberow, N. L., and Simon, M. D.: Suicide in Los Angeles and Vienna, Public Health Rep. **84:**389, 1969.
 9. Farrar, C. B.: Suicide, J. Clin. Exp. Psychopathol. **12:**79, 1951.
10. Henslin, J. H.: Guilt and guilt neutralization; response and adjustment to suicide. In Douglas, J. D., editor: Deviance and respectability; the social reconstruction of moral meanings, New York, 1970, Basic Books, Inc., Publishers.
11. Jameison, G. R.: Suicide and mental disease; a clinical analysis of 100 cases, Arch. Neurol. Psychiatry **36:**1, 1936.
12. Lindemann, E., and others: Preventive intervention in a four-year-old child whose father committed suicide. In Caplan, G., editor: Emotional problems of early childhood, New York, 1955, Basic Books, Inc., Publishers.
13. Mudge, G. P.: The mendelian collection of human pedigrees; inheritance of suicidal mania. Mendel J. **1:**11, 1909.
14. Murphy, G. E., Wetzel, R. A., Swallow, C. S., and others: Who calls the suicide prevention center; a study of 55 persons calling on their own behalf, Am. J. Psychiatry **126:**314, 1969.
15. Pike, J. A.: The other side, New York, 1969, Dell Publishing Co., Inc.
16. Rosen, V. H. The reconstruction of a traumatic childhood event in a case of derealization, J. Am. Psychoanal. Assoc. **3:**211, 1955.
17. Rudestam, K. E.: Physical and psychological responses to suicide in the family, J. Consult. Clin. Psychol. **45:**162, 1977.
18. Shneidman, E. S., editor: On the nature of suicide, San Francisco, 1969, Jossey-Bass, Inc., Publishers.

19. Shneidman, E. S.: Foreword. In Cain, A. C., editor: Survivors of suicide, Springfield, Ill., 1972, Charles C Thomas, Publisher.
20. Teicher, J. D., and Jacobs, J.: The physician and the adolescent suicide attempter, J. Sch. Health **36:**406, 1966.
21. Tooley, K.: The meaning of maternal suicide as reflected in the treatment of a late adolescent girl. In Cain, A. C., editor: Survivors of suicide, Springfield, Ill., 1972, Charles C Thomas, Publisher.
22. Wallerstein, R. S.: Reconstruction and mastery in the transference psychosis, J. Am. Psychoanal. Assoc. **15:**556, 1967.
23. Warren, M.: Some psychological sequelae of parental suicide in surviving children. In Cain, A. C., editor: Survivors of suicide, Springfield, Ill., 1972, Charles C Thomas, Publisher.
24. Wechsler, J. A.: In a darkness, New York, 1972, W. W. Norton & Co., Inc.
25. Wood, J. M. S., and Urquhart, A. R.: A family tree illustrative of insanity and suicide, J. Ment. Science **47:**764, 1901.

CHAPTER 18

Parent groups as an aid in mourning and grief work

BETTY B. SATTERWHITE
JoANN BELLE-ISLE
BARBARA CONRADT

> For everything there is a season . . . a time to weep . . . a time to
> mourn . . . a time to break down, and a time to build up . . .
>
> *Ecclesiastes*

Grief or mourning has been described by Hodge[3] as "the normal emotional response to the loss of a loved one. It is the feeling of a personal loss and is experienced only by the survivor, by 'they that mourn.' " The intensity of grief and mourning over a deceased child is increased by the fact that a child's death is not in the natural order of events. One expects to lose a parent, one knows that one mate will predecease the other, but one does not expect to lose a child—that logical extension of one's own self into the future. The feeling that the child "hasn't had a chance at life, has done nothing to deserve" an early death adds to the anger, frustration, and bewilderment experienced by the mourner for a deceased child.

Our medical care system has been slow to respond to the needs of the dying child and the family; it has been even more remiss in its sense of obligation to assist the family after the death of the child. For the most part, the plethora of literature of the last few years on the child, death, and the family ends with the child's death.

No matter how prepared the family may deem itself, the days, weeks, months, and years subsequent to a child's actual death are devastatingly difficult. This is the time of mourning and grief work.

For the family who has lost a child suddenly, the disbelief, anger, and guilt occur and reoccur in rapid succession. There has been no time for anticipatory grief or the accrual of health care providers for support. For those who have been involved in a long terminal illness, the sense of loss and all the other emotions already experienced in the period of anticipatory grief are exacerbated by the total involvement of the family with the

211

child before death and the resulting physical weariness. When death actually occurs, the family members may be emotionally and physically at their weakest and may be ill prepared to begin the tasks of mourning and rebuilding their lives.

In this chapter we will discuss the following: (1) the use of parent support groups to lessen the sense of abandonment for parents after the death of a child, (2) the group as an aid to parents in their task of rebuilding the family, and (3) the evolution of a hospital-initiated parent group from a therapeutic to an action-oriented role.

Many factors make the present-day American family particularly at risk after the death of a child:

1. Our medical advances have resulted in a lowered death rate in children. Society therefore has little experience in helping grieving family members and so has few formal or informal vehicles to support them.
2. Technologic advances have led to the development of uniquely trained specialists. The care of children may become fractionated as the primary care physician refers patients to specialists. Children with chronic illness who require constant care by a specialized health care team often lose continuity with the primary physician. Because of this separation in the delivery of health care, the primary physician often does not see himself, nor does the family see him, as a source of support during the grieving process.
3. The Church as a supportive institution has become a less important influence in the coping process of many American families.
4. Our society has become so mobile that the family of a deceased child may be separated geographically from relatives who might be helpful. This isolation is compounded by the anonymity of our society where neighbors scarcely know one another and may be honestly unaware of the plight of others.

How and where, then, do families find help to do the grief work described by Lindemann as "emancipating themselves from the bondage to the deceased, readjusting to the environment in which the deceased is missing, and forming new relationships"?[5] Some have friends, extended family, or clergy on whom they can rely; others have found such people unable to console them or unresponsive to their needs and so have felt abandoned.

Along with, or perhaps because of, this sense of abandonment, some authors have suggested that those who have "walked the road" as parents are at least a partial answer to providing a support system to other parents attempting to do their grief work. Benoliel posits that other parents may be a far better source of comfort to grieving parents than heroic efforts to prolong the life of the child. "It may well be that effective crisis counseling for individuals and families whose lives have been changed by the constant threat of impending death will come from a system of services whereby the special talents and experiences of lay people rather than professionals will provide the help that these difficult human transitions seem to require."[1]

It is in this fashion that The Candlelighters' Society was born. Says Nancy Roach in "The Last Day of April":

> We found our greatest friend-support came from other parents going through or having gone through the same or similar illnesses with their children. We became involved in the founding of an organization called The Candlelighters' Society. . . . We met parents who had already lost children and took strength from them. . . . We are amazed to find that our most frightening thoughts and fears were common to them as well. We shared our grief, pain, love and joy. I always felt more comfortable with "another mother" because I knew she really understood.[8]

Candlelighters (whose name derives from the saying "It is better to light a candle than to curse the darkness") started as a legislative action in response to a crisis in funding a federal cancer research project.[7] Affiliate groups of this organization are now legion across the United States. Legion also are local chapters of the National Sudden Infant Death Syndrome Foundation, which offer emotional support to bereaved parents of children who have died from this puzzling and catastrophic syndrome.

In a poignant article, Fischoff and O'Brien describe the inception of a self-help group founded in 1974 by a couple who, not finding support in their experience of losing a child, called the chaplain of the hospital where their daughter had died. They were given the names of other couples who had lost children, and they began a group that has "grown via word of mouth, other couples, various media, and hospital communications. From the inquiries it is apparent that others see the group as being helpful to parents whose child has died."[2]

Others have recognized the effectiveness of the group in assisting the grieving family.[4] The group efficiently reduces the problem of which individuals will receive the counseling efforts of the therapist and enables the airing of shared experiences in an atmosphere of commonality and acceptance. McCollum[6] suggests that the group offers an especially effective environment for grieving parents, because the emotions and concerns experienced by parents after the death of a child are often confusing and frightening to them. Sharing these mutually experienced thoughts in a group diminishes their frightfulness and reassures the individual parent of his or her sanity.

It is difficult to predict the personality characteristics of parents who might attend such groups. Some prerequisites are that members share in common the fact that they have all lost children, verbalize their personal experiences, and are able to acknowledge emotionally painful situations surrounding the treatment and death of their child. Members must also desire to have their feelings and experiences confirmed and be able to listen empathically to others in the group. It must be emphasized, however, that this process of sharing and empathic listening is emotionally difficult for parents and generates ambivalence about returning to future meetings.

Many parents who have lost children and are invited to participate in such groups decline to do so. Again, we can only speculate about the reasons for this. They may include the fact that some parents have no desire to share their emotions with others and prefer to cope independently within the confines of their own family. Other parents may become too upset when reflecting on the circumstances of their child's death and are unable to maintain emotional control. Another influential factor is the situation where one parent desires to attend the group but does not receive endorsement from his or her spouse and therefore decides not to attend. When parents find it impossible to benefit from groups, health professionals must implement a plan of care to meet individual needs.

Aware that many grieving parents find solace most readily from the empathy of other grieving parents, two of us organized a therapeutic group for parent support in January 1976. The group began with 13 parents whose children had died 7 months to 5 years before from an oncologic or hematologic disease and had been treated by the pediatric hematology/oncology staff of the University of Rochester Medical Center. Members contracted for eight biweekly 90-minute sessions to discuss how each had coped after the death of the child. For many of the members this was their first opportunity to express powerful emotions, and the scheduled 90-minute sessions consistently expanded to 2- and 3-hour meetings.

Because many parents had indicated that a return to the medical center where their child had died was too painful, a nearby nonmedical facility was chosen.

Schematically, the eight sessions can be demarcated into three grief-resolving periods (tasks), which are defined as:

1. The period of *review* of the illness and death of the child with all its concomitant feelings of sadness, anger, and guilt.
2. The period of *reconstruction,* during which parents were able to

see their lives within the perspective of other members in the
group.

3. The period of *resolution,* during which parents channeled their
energies into the formation of an action-oriented group called
CURE.

The period of review was by far the most painful for most group members. The emotions of anger, frustration, powerlessness, and guilt often
seen in grieving parents were constant themes during this phase as parents relived the torment they experienced after their child died.

Mothers in particular cited an intense feeling of emptiness as they
suddenly found themselves with hours to fill that were previously spent
on management of the child's disease. One mother stated, "I was just
numb and tired. It didn't seem real." Another said, "I wondered if I'd ever
be capable of any emotion or love. It was just such an emptiness—the
very worst of human conditions."

Fathers felt a heightened sense of powerlessness as they acknowledged their inability to protect their child from death. Several found their
grief postponed because, in their father-husband role, they felt it their responsibility to "re-create the family." Another stated, "Because the man is
thrust back into his goal-oriented endeavors at work, he has an opportunity to get lost in his job." A father's grief was apt to be solitary and prolonged because, as one father said, "I felt that as the man I had to offer
support to my wife and son—the 'stiff upper lip' kind of thing—and so I'd
cry a lot driving to work. I'm not sure I'm through it, because I still cry 3
years later."

The knowledge that no one was alone in the feelings he or she experienced was a consolation. Discussions dealing with attitudes toward surviving siblings and the need to help them work out their grief were helpful at this time.

After the verbalization of these feelings, most parents were able to
undertake the task of reconstruction, putting perspective back in their
lives. The lapse in time since their child's death seemed to facilitate this
task. Parents whose child had died 5 years earlier were able to reassure
more recent mourners that the acute grief they were experiencing would
eventually dull. But also consoling was the fact that the passage of time
would not erase the memories of the child they wished to cherish. In addition, parents who became overly vigilant about the health of their other
children after the death of a child were reassured by those who had
reacted similarly, years before, that this need would also pass.

Reconstruction through these supportive interactions enabled parents whose grief had overshadowed all facets of their self-image to again
see themselves as parents of living children, as spouses, as members of

the community, as individuals with many talents to offer to those still experiencing the sadness of a child with a terminal illness. As the reconstruction phase drew to a close, members of the group sought to channel their energies into projects through which they could constructively improve conditions for families whose children were still fighting the disease that had taken theirs.

It was in the resolution phase that the CURE Childhood Cancer Association was born. CURE was founded in Rochester, New York in the fall of 1976 by the group of parents just described, others whose children were alive but afflicted by the disease, and concerned health professionals at the University of Rochester. Members and contributors also included friends, relatives, and others in the community interested in the goals of CURE. These goals encompass the four major areas of counseling, understanding, research, and education.

The evolutionary process of CURE as a self-help group parallels the development of similar groups across the nation that have emerged for a variety of reasons and have structured themselves with equal diversity.[4] The scope of CURE's interests broadened considerably after the organization became incorporated and the process of task identification was initiated. A core group of members pioneered efforts to solicit funds from the community, publish a parent-child handbook, initiate a monthly speaker series, purchase cots for parents for the hospital pediatric units, fund a laboratory assistant, and explore other areas where the goals of CURE could be realized.

A close working relationship between parents and health professionals continued as the organization tackled new projects. The local community has become aware of the collective concerns of CURE members to improve the quality of care delivered to children with malignant diseases and has been increasingly responsive to CURE's endeavors. Social events have provided an opportunity for families and professionals to share continuing concerns and to welcome new members into the group.

In essence, the resolution phase for members of this group has been a positive reaching-out process. Working hand in hand with hospital staff has made parents realize "how much hospital staff really cares" and "what problems they really have." CURE "has given us something positive to do that somehow gives our child's death more meaning. It gives us something to do for others now that we can't do for our own child." The group has gone beyond self-help and has dealt positively with grief by being a vehicle for resolution through self-involvement.

Not to be underestimated is the satisfaction CURE has given care providers, who are pleased to see parents moving through the resolution phase of their grief. As one subspecialist put it:

It's hard to break off with a family after the death of the child. There is emotional feedback between family and doctor. Though there is no need medically beyond this point, it is helpful for us to be able to follow through to see how they are managing. It is sometimes awkward to contact them. They may have problems, and we are not physically available. However, parent meetings provide us with a way to see a negative event turning into a positive, constructive force. Although the parent group was not planned with the professional in mind, it has turned out to be a source of emotional support in the above sense. The fact that they are trying to help is rewarding.

Partly because of its young age, CURE has not yet experienced the attrition that one might expect in a group as members find the group no longer meeting their needs. However, as with the original therapy group from which CURE grew, it is expected that, in time, those parents instrumental in the founding of CURE will leave the organization. As newer members join, the focus of CURE may change to meet the different needs of the new parents. The charter and bylaws of the organization will lend consistency and stability to the group at this time without precluding the flexibility necessary for a change in direction warranted by changing needs.

What are some directions that parent groups such as CURE may take in the future? Because such groups form when members share a common bond of personal experiences, one major emphasis will probably continue to be mutual support during or after crisis situations. Parent organizations may also become task oriented and may engage themselves in fund-raising projects, directing monies for the improvement of health care facilities, and continued research. Other efforts may be in the areas of consumer advocacy and involvement in group action to effect legislative changes relevant to areas of concern to them as parents.

In summary, the use of the group as a means of helping parents in their grief work is, from a practical standpoint, an efficient and effective way of meeting the needs of many people. It affords the added dimension of stimulating a climate of mutual understanding and support among parents at a time when recognition and acceptance of one's feelings are most critical.

Furthermore, groups that evolve into the type of organization that the CURE Childhood Cancer Association and the Candlelighters represent provide a vehicle for parents to deal constructively with feelings of anger, guilt, and powerlessness. No less important, such groups enable the medical staff not only to witness the despair and intense sadness that grieving families experience at the time of a child's death but also, in time, to see the families reemerge with new strength.

We have seen many descriptions of the problems of mourning and grief work, but few prescriptions for its alleviation. We offer the hospital-initiated parent group as one prescription for assistance during the time to weep, the time to mourn, the time to break down, and the time to build up.

REFERENCES

1. Benoliel, J.: The dying patient and the family. In Troup, S., and Greene, W. editors: The patient, death and the family, New York, 1974, Charles Scribner's Sons.
2. Fischoff, J., and O'Brien, N.: After the child dies, J. Pediatr. **88:**140, 1976.
3. Hodge, J.: Help your patients to mourn better, People Helping People **11:**1975.
4. Levy, L. H.: Self-help groups; types and psychological processes, J. Behav. Sci. **12:**310, 1976.
5. Lindemann, E.: Symptomatology and management of acute grief, Am. J. Psychiatry **101:**141, 1944.
6. McCollum, A.: Counseling the grieving parent. In Burton, A. L., editor: Care of the child facing death, Boston, 1974, Routledge & Kegan Paul.
7. Monaco, G. P., President, Candlelighters Foundation: Personal communication, 1977.
8. Roach, N.: The last day of April, American Cancer Society, 1974, pp. 27-28.

CHAPTER 19

Grandparents as grievers

JULIA HAMILTON

Death is the cessation of all vital functions. Dying is the process of life drawing to a close. Dying involves the possibility of avoidance or delay, whereas death is final and inevitable.

Death is an event we associate with old age: the culmination of a long, full lifetime. It is difficult to comprehend and justify the loss of a child who has not yet "lived." In our culture probably no experience is more devastating in the life of a family than the fatal illness of a child. The shock extends from parents and siblings to involve grandparents, other family members, and friends.

Former generations of parents expected, and were prepared to some extent, to lose at least one child during his early years. Today, with changing social conditions and medical advances, infant and child fatalities are no longer considered inevitable. Partly because such deaths have become exceptional, society has been forced to focus on and delineate the difficulties families face when a child dies.

Greater geographic and social mobility makes relatives less available when such a crisis does occur. Traditional sources of religious support, as well as the ceremonial aspects of death, are no longer widely valued and have declined in our increasingly secular society. As a result, when a child dies, a family is often left alone to struggle with its problems. Thus, today, more than ever, alternative support systems to help both the dying child and his family must be provided.

Although medical advances have prevented death and extended life, they have also made it harder to die, so that children with a potentially fatal illness may live for months or even years in a limbo of expected death.[3] Both the child and family can become overwhelmed with the stresses of such a situation. It has become necessary to pinpoint the problems that exist for such children and families as well as to identify strengths and effective methods of coping that can be helpful to them.

In psychoanalytic theory, man's preoccupation with death has been characterized by fear. In his later writings, Freud attributed much of the cohesiveness and structure of modern society to repression of the death

219

instinct. It is common in analytic practice to regard the fear of death that appears consciously or in dreams as a disguised castration fear.[7] Otto Rank, regarding separation fear as the primal human problem, equated it with death fear and treated castration fear as a subvariant. These theorists and others view fear of death as natural and universal: it is the basic fear that influences all others. There are other theorists, according to Ernest Becker, who support the healthy-minded argument that an individual is not born with a fear of death, and if he has a good maternal experience and develops a sense of security, he will not be subject to fears of loss of support and annihilation.[1] Anxiety about death comes from bad experiences—from nurture, not nature.

Becker puts forth a theory that is a combination of the two. He maintains that the fear of death is universal and innate and that it disappears through the mechanism of repression. Fears are absolved naturally by expansive organismic striving.[1] Man works against his fragility by seeking to expand and perpetuate himself in living experiences. Thus, the ever-present fear of death is absolved by our instinct for self-preservation, and there is an obliviousness to this fear in our conscious life. It is man's basic narcissism, which is increased by a secure environment and good childhood experiences, that gives him a sense of magical omnipotence, of imagining himself eternal. The fear of death varies in intensity according to the developmental process. So man goes along, cutting out for himself a manageable world, with his fears tucked away beneath the surface. At times, when there is a break in his world of activity, the awareness dawns, the repression does not work, and the fear of death emerges. The diagnosis of a fatal illness or the death of a child is one of these times.

Much of the literature on terminally ill children centers on the grief of the child and his mother. Yet many lives are affected; how many may never be fully realized. Generally, there are four other groups of persons who need special attention in such a situation: fathers, siblings, grandparents, and friends and extended family members.

A few comments follow about fathers. The main emphasis of the chapter, of course, is directed at grandparents. Siblings are discussed elsewhere in this book. However, there will also be others who will have difficulties and needs related to their own developmental levels and closeness to the dying child. I mention them to remind the reader of their existence and the need to be sensitive to their possible distresses.

American society places quite a load on a man's shoulders. From the time he is very young, he hears repeatedly, "Be big, be brave, be strong." Pain, physical demands, and emotional stresses are endured or deliberately induced to prove his strengths. When he marries, his responsibilities increase. He is almost never allowed to fail without feeling guilt and shame.

With this foundation, he faces tremendous stress when slapped with the reality that his child has a terminal illness. He has usually depended only on himself for strength and emotional solace. Perhaps the most accepted stages of grief allowed fathers are anger or acceptance (because of the strength both display).

Many fathers are pushed out of participation in care. In our society, mother is mother, and when the child becomes ill, she becomes super-mother. Some of this role taking is realistic. The father, usually the bread winner, continues his "normal" way of life. The mother's life frequently ends its normal routine and becomes geared entirely to her sick child.

Grandparents are certainly affected by the fatal illness of the child. Their grief is threefold as they grieve for their beloved grandchild, their son or daughter, and themselves. Often they think they should cope better, be an example through the ordeal.[5] They express guilt over not recognizing the symptoms themselves and anger that their child did not recognize them. When, after what they have offered (advice, financial aid, care, babysitting, experience, help) is neither asked for nor accepted, they feel guilt, frustration, and anger. They are usually frightened about caring for their grandchild in the context of illness. And they often have many questions: What would they do in a crisis? What could happen? What is happening daily to the child? What happens when the child comes to the clinic for treatment? How long will the child live? They have always felt in control when caring for their grandchild. Not now.

Sometimes the grandparents are not in good physical or emotional health and, therefore, are unable to help their child with the physical care and emotional strain of the illness. They may feel intense failure as parents as well as grandparents. Grandparents are more often alone than any other group in the grief process—especially grandfathers, both because of their role expectation as men and their triple-layered grief.

Grandparents display more denial than parents and tend to be less accepting of the diagnosis. More distant relatives and friends challenge reality even more frequently, because the tendency for reality distortion increases with remoteness from the immediate family. The parents appear to be surrounded by concentric circles of disbelief,[5] the most immediate circle being that of their own parents, the child's grandparents. The parents see that well-intentioned statements are meant to cheer them up, but they are put in the uncomfortable position of having to defend their child's diagnosis. As a result, they feel that others think they are condemning their own child. However, although friends and relatives can aggravate parents' distress, they can also be sympathetic listeners and provide support.

A surprising absence of emotional support from the extended family, particularly the maternal grandmother, was noted by Bozeman and associates.[2] They suggest that this may reflect a reactivation of earlier conflict between the mother and the maternal grandmother. My experience confirms the frequency of transient alienation between parents and extended family members as well as friends. However, in addition to unconscious determinants, intense overt expressions of grief and anxiety by relatives and friends may threaten the parents' initial warding-off defenses. Conversely, denial invoked by relatives may challenge the parents' struggles to assimilate the reality of the illness. The latter phenomenon is frequently observed when genetically transmitted diseases are involved; members of the older generation may be unable to acknowledge the presence of the "bad seed" in their own lineage. In some instances, initial feelings of alienation are resolved, and parents are well supported by the extended family. When this does not occur, professional persons and parents of similarly afflicted children may be needed to play a substitutive role.

Several authors describe a process corresponding to Kübler-Ross's five stages of denial and isolation, anger, bargaining, depression, and acceptance. Knapp delineates such a framework for those who learn their grandchild has a fatal illness.[4] Our experiences are similar to hers. Sometimes grandparents state that several days passed before their child called them to tell them the diagnosis. The first stage, after hearing the diagnosis, is denial. Shocked, grandparents cannot find words to comfort their child as a parent or to comfort themselves. The second stage, occurring after the grandparents realize the diagnosis is not a mistake, is that of anger and resentment. The third stage is that of bargaining, which can take many forms. Some grandparents attend church more often or overindulge the child, although buying the child everything he or she wants creates problems among siblings. The fourth stage is depression, which occurs as the illness progresses and the child's physical condition worsens. This is the stage at which the grandparents begin to feel that they do not know the whole truth about the illness yet are unable to get all the information and answers from the parents.

After observing and talking with grandparents, a group was formed for those individuals with grandchildren who had leukemia. This group met at Yale–New Haven Medical Center, where the pediatric hematology/oncology clinic provides comprehensive care for many children with oncologic illnesses. The grandparent group was formed as an extension of the parent group to provide grandparents with a place to discuss openly their fears, questions, and concerns about their child, who was experiencing pain, and about their grandchild, who had the fatal illness.

The group met bimonthly for an hour and a half. The coleaders included the pediatric social worker and a hematologist, although other physicians, nurses, and medical students participated at various times.

The format of the meetings was informal and flexible. The character of each meeting was dictated by the needs of the group on that day. The time was spent answering questions of a purely medical nature, enjoying lighthearted discussion, or sharing deep and personal feelings. Attendance was variable. In general, it tended to be up when one or more children were in relapse and down when all children were in remission.

In the group, grandparents asked about the diagnosis, questioned the medications, questioned what the parents should do with the child: Should the child be allowed to swing? Can the child go to school with other children? What will happen if he or she falls and gets hurt? They often felt that the parents were allowing the child to do too many things.

Adaptive behavior refers to those processes that help the person assimilate reality, master affective states (discharge through nondestructive channels and acknowledgment), and resolve issues. Information seeking, invoking emotional support, partialization, and rehearsal of death are examples of such processes.

Information seeking[6] is especially relevant to the group process, because grandparents seek much information and explanation, three types in particular. First, they try to comprehend the nature of the disease with respect to etiology, symptomatology, and expected course. Second, they are concerned about the status of the child, the severity and the degree of advancement of the illness. This information can be supplied only by the physician, who did attend the group. However, a social worker, for example, may help the grandparents clarify their questions. The third type of information has been designated "the search for meaning." Unable to accept the illness as a chance event, grandparents blame themselves for something that has happened in the past between them and their child. If the relationship has been poor, grandparents feel guilty and consider themselves worthy of blame.

The grandparents used the group to learn how to cope with both their own and their son's or daughter's feelings and reactions to the child's illness. The sessions provided a structure for expression of displaced feelings of guilt, anger, hostility, fears, and depression. By sharing feelings and interacting with each other, grandparents gained some understanding of their feelings and attitudes and the effects on themselves and their families. For many of the grandparents, this was their first experience in a group. They struggled with trying to decide how to express their feelings not only within the context of the group but also as part of a family.

Many benefits accrued from the group sessions:

1. The cathartic effect gained from the informal sharing of informa-

tion, problems, and experiences resulted in increased understanding between parents, grandparents, and staff.

2. Grandparents, parents, and staff recognized the need to lend extra emotional support during crises.
3. The staff members learned that didactic education of grandparents was best undertaken when stresses were minimal.
4. The problem of tactless comments about the child's condition was identified, and grandparents learned to cope more adequately with these situations.
5. The subjects of dying and death were aired, giving grandparents an opportunity to understand their own feelings and thus to prepare themselves to discuss death with the sick child.
6. Grandparents shared solutions with one another about how they and their grandchild could cope with problems related to therapy, pain, fear, procedures, and disfigurement.
7. The greatest benefit reported by grandparents was the opportunity to share and identify with one another at a level that was impossible with any other group of people.

The most meaningful help we, as professionals, can give to the family of the dying child is to provide them with an opportunity to share their feelings before the event of death and to allow them to work through these feelings regardless of how irrational they appear to be. Grandparents usually feel that they want to help more but that there is no role for them. They feel alone during the grief process. Because the grandparents are so vulnerable, the parents often feel they have to give them emotional support as well, although at times this is difficult to do. In turn, the grandparents express anger with the parents for leaving them out of their grief process. Quite frankly, however, many parents feel that they cannot put the burden of their fears and feelings on the grandparents, who may not be physically or mentally well.

Grandparents cannot assimilate the reality of their grandchild's illness unless they develop effective ways of gathering information. The health caregiver can review with grandparents their understanding of the disease and encourage them to view information gathering as a stepwise process. The caregiver can also offer grandparents significant help in gradually acknowledging and enduring their emotions and in discharging them through nondestructive channels. Ideally, by easing the guilt, tapping the rage, and involving ourselves with the grief, we can bolster the grandparents' strength to remain available and yet to let go.[8]

By offering the grandparents a predictable time and place to meet and by conveying through sympathetic listening that they are understood, the caregiver can help grandparents to begin to contain and endure their sorrow. The grandparents can be helped with guilt by reviewing with them their fantasies of omission or commission and by allowing the expression of ambivalent feelings toward the parent and the child. Family members need to ventilate their feelings by talking, crying, and mourning. Grandparents can be helped to contain their anger by exploring and ventilating it in group sessions. Apprehension and anxiety can often be ameliorated if the grandparents can explore and verbalize their feelings and fears. Grandparents can be helped to be freer not only to mourn their loss, but also to reinvest in other relationships.

One must become aware of the needs of grandparents when a child is dying. They, too, along with the mother, father, and siblings, need people who care, who allow them opportunities to participate in care, and who grieve with them.

REFERENCES

1. Becker, E.: The denial of death, New York, 1973, The Free Press.
2. Bozeman, M. F., Orbach, C. E., and Sutherland, A. M.: The psychological impact of cancer and its treatment, Cancer **8:**1, 1955.
3. Burton, A. L., editor: Care of the child facing death, Boston, 1974, Routledge & Kegan Paul.
4. Friedman, S. B., Chodoff, P., Mason, J. W., and Hamburg, D.: Behavioral observations on parents anticipating the death of a child, Pediatrics **32:**610, 1963.
5. Gyulay, J. E.: The forgotten grievers, Am. J. Nurs. **75:**1476, 1975.
6. McCollum, A. T., and Schwartz, A. H.: Social work and the mourning parent, Soc. Work J. **17:**33, 1972.
7. Natterson, J., and Knudson, A.: Observation concerning fear of death in fatally ill children and their mothers, Psychosom. Med. **22:**456, 1960.
8. Tihtinsky, J.: Working with dying children and their families, part 1, San Francisco, 1975, Mt. Zion Hospital, unpublished manuscript.

ETHICAL AND EDUCATIONAL CONSIDERATIONS

CHAPTER 20

Where is God?

JOAN E. HEMENWAY

There is no greater affront to our human experience than the critical illness and impending death of a child. Perhaps it is the disarming innocence of a child that so arouses our feelings of helplessness and rage. Perhaps it is the cruelly foreshortened life of a child that so stirs our cries of injustice. Perhaps it is the tenderness of a child that so evokes our feelings of love and sympathy, hurt and horror as death approaches, overtakes, and eventually has its way.

Feelings of relief and even peacefulness may temporarily ease the grief of those family members and staff who have seen it through to the end and are now exhausted. Special memories and a sense of gratitude for life, no matter how short, may lighten the lifelong burden of loss. But at deeper levels the experience of a child's illness and death profoundly disrupts and disturbs our inner as well as our outer equilibrium. Because of this experience, the universe is no longer as safe or as friendly as it once was. In fact, the universe may be experienced as downright unfriendly, uncertain, untrustworthy, frightening, and even malevolent. After such a traumatic event, we are shaken and we tremble. So does the universe. As a result, for the religious as well as the nonreligious, there is a spoken, or perhaps largely unspoken question: Where is God? Which is to say, what sense, if any, can this painful event have in the broader and deeper order of things?

DIFFERENT RELIGIOUS RESPONSES TO DEATH AND DYING

How parents and siblings and even the dying child himself answer this question depends on their religious background and current expression of belief (or nonbelief) as well as on each individual's personality structure and accustomed interaction in the family. These elements usually become apparent during the initial time of crisis, and those who enter into a helping relationship with the family are able to observe and use them.

For some people it is the stable presence of one or two family members (or health care givers) that gives focus and direction and meaning to it all. With no explicitly religious orientation but with a great deal of inner confidence in the naturalness and acceptability of life *and* death, such a focal person brings comfort and steadiness to an otherwise deeply troubling situation. The child as well as the family and staff senses this inner strength, and if they are open to it (but not solely dependent on it), they may be able to use it to get in touch with their own inner resources and power—power not viewed in any way as specifically "religious" but certainly experienced as deeply personal and significant.

For others it is the regular use of specific religious structures (daily prayers, the Sacraments, community worship, regular visits by a member of the clergy) that give meaning and focus to what is happening. Through these ordered expressions of faith, opportunities present themselves for a wide range of expression of feelings, from anger and depression and fear to gratitude and joy. The extent to which this sharing happens depends on the needs of the family, the realities of the ongoing medical situation, the responsiveness of the faith community, the sensitivity and training of the clergyperson, and the willingness of all involved to trust and help each other be together and express feelings, especially those that are negative. New understanding and even acceptance can eventually come when this process of sharing is an ongoing and long-term one. Although parents are sometimes resistant to this open process of communication (usually projecting their own fears onto each other or the child), with time and the accumulation of positive experiences, full participation begins to grow—to the surprise and joy of everyone.

For still others, it is the hope for cure, rather than the participation in care, that becomes the focus for religious expression. For such families and their children there is a strong need for assurance that they do indeed have the ability to endure this tragedy. One major source of this assurance can be religious in nature. Faith healers, specially blessed oils, prayers to certain saints, anointed medals and medallions, carefully performed rituals, and oft-repeated words (litanies) become the vehicles not only to keep hope (and the child) alive but also to express ongoing emotions. Although viewed skeptically by some as a rigid or fanatic religious system, these detailed, forthright, and concentrated religious practices provide the means by which a reality too harsh for anyone to bear is, in fact, borne.

Unfortunately there are families that close themselves off from all resources, those specifically religious as well as those more broadly secular. The lethal mixtures of fear and anger, guilt and helplessness, pride and self-pity can combine to isolate and poison all attempts to communicate meaningfully within the family, with the child, and among the staff, as well as with whatever might be perceived as more powerful and omniscient (and forgiving) than that which is bounded by the limits of our human experience. In such families there is much loneliness and suffering, and often for the sick child there is the very real fear of isolation and abandonment.

The child's response

It is important to realize that no matter what developmental stage the child is in, he will usually take his cues, whether positive or negative, from his parents in terms of what, if any, religious expression is appropriate, acceptable, or expected during the crisis.

- If mother feels better when 8-year-old Johnny wears his Saint Christopher's medal, usually Johnny feels better when he is wearing it, too.
- If Dad has made it clear that he dislikes "preachers," then 12-year-old Sally will relate cautiously, uneasily, and only partially to a minister when he visits her at home.
- If Mr. and Mrs. Dougherty have a warm relationship with Father Burke and have regularly taken 5-year-old Peggy to church with them, then the arrival and blessing by a priest at the hospital will be appreciated as a source of strength and affirmation for the parents and the child.
- Because 3-year-old Aaron has always participated in the weekly celebration of Shabbos (Sabbath), his continued presence at this family faith event will give him a sense of belonging and stability, which may not only ease his anxiety about more needles and pain but also impart a sense of well-being at deeper levels.
- If 16-year-old Dennis is turned off by his mother's overly fervent and somewhat oppressive religious faith, when the minister or chaplain arrives he will quickly turn his face to the wall and sink into silence.

ROLE OF THE CLERGYPERSON

One major difference between a hospital chaplain and a local clergyperson is that the chaplain knows the staff and hospital "system," whereas the local clergyperson knows the family and the community from which they come. Second, the hospital chaplain's ministry is focused on crises at the time of hospitalization, whereas the local clergyperson deals with long-term ministry to the family and child within their faith community. Third, the hospital chaplain has developed skills to respond to a wide variety of religious needs expressed by all kinds of people of differing denominations and faith backgrounds, whereas the local clergyperson is more closely oriented to his or her particular faith or denominational tradition and equipped to meet specific needs within this tradition. Because of these differences, it is helpful for a hospital chaplain and a local clergyperson to coordinate their efforts regarding a particular situation, so that the strengths of each can enhance and complement the work of both, to the benefit of all.

Whether the clergyperson is part of the hospital staff or from a local church or synagogue, he or she will seek to be responsive to the religious needs of the child and the family as these needs are being experienced and expressed, both in immediate crisis situations (initial diagnosis, the beginning of treatment, rehospitalization, before and after surgery, and so on) and during times of stability. By careful listening, by availability, by personal accessibility, by knowledge of human development and the behavioral sciences, by the observation and sensitive use of key dynamics within the family, and by quiet presence and gentle playfulness with the child, the clergyperson conveys a sense of warmth and caring, stability and competence in the midst of fearful disease, actual pain, and possible loss.

Most centrally, the clergyperson is a person of faith, whose theological training, vocational commitment, and ability to be personally present proclaims for the child and the family, perhaps more often subtly than explicitly, that beyond the exigencies of our brief lifetime there does in fact exist something profoundly greater and more powerful than ourselves. This faith, which is brought alive as the clergyperson relates in caring ways with the family, does not deny the hurt and pain and anger and anxiety, but rather like a lightning rod draws these feelings onto itself, receiving them all without question or judgment or surprise, incorporating them into the solid ground of all being.

Limits of the clergyperson's role

It is not unusual for families as well as hospital staff to have high expectations of clergy and then to become disappointed and cynical when these expectations are not met. Sometimes such feelings are well justified when emotion-laden situations are handled insensitively by the clergyperson who has been called. In such cases families and staff may go away angry and hurt and hesitant to reach out again. On the other hand, there are realistic limits, both professional and personal, that clergypersons need to make clear to the families and children to whom they are ministering as well as to the staff with whom they are working. The extent and clarity with which each clergyperson is able to explicate these limits in any given situation is an important measure of his or her own sense of professional identity and ego strength. However, a few basic general limitations pertain to all.

First, clergypersons are not miracle workers. They cannot undo lifelong family patterns of unproductive behavior; they cannot bring instant healing with a wave of the hand or an offering of prayer; they cannot make 4-year-old Johnny smiling and happy and cooperative when he feels depressed and angry and contrary. Second, clergypersons can neither take responsibility for, nor make significant changes in, the religious faith systems of those with whom they relate. This is sometimes disappointing to doctors and staff especially when the particular faith system either overtly or covertly undermines their methods of treatment. It can also be disappointing to the clergyperson, who may have had some unrealistic hopes about his or her own power in this regard. Third, clergypersons are people—they hurt, have doubts and fears, get tired, feel alone, need support and affirmation. Unfortunately they often find it difficult to ask for anything, especially caring, from others. As a result they too often communicate their own needs indirectly or not at all.

In this regard, it is important to realize that the clergy, like other people, need friends, people to whom they can express their own frustrations, anger, disappointments, and hurt. These supportive relationships can develop for the clergyperson among personnel at many levels in the hospital: physicians, nurses, aides, maintenance people, and so on. Ideally chaplains or ministers who regularly visit the hospital will encourage such friendship networks not only among themselves but also among the hospital staff. In addition, clergypeople need to have close supporting networks of their own, either their families and spouses or friends who are willing to hear the whole story at almost any time of day or night. Clergypeople also need professional networks for sharing and support, although like other professionals, elements of competition and criticism can sometimes break down trust and caring. But such professional networks are essential to one's perspective and continued competence, as well as to one's nourishment and faith. Without these various networks of support and friendship, a clergyperson can become isolated and alone and, as a result, find his or her effectiveness in ministry greatly diminished.

Finally, the presence of a clergyperson in the midst of a family crisis, whether it is in the home or in the hospital, depends on the initial request and continued consent of those directly involved in the situation. There is no obvious contract or exchange of money for services rendered. Rather, ministry depends on availability, sensitivity, receptivity, and need. It is an act that is freely given. Whether it is accepted, and how, is never certain. This situation presents the greatest liability as well as the greatest asset for those who have chosen the ministry as their profession.

CONTRASTING RELIGIOUS NEEDS

The degree to which people make explicit their religious needs varies. Specific requests for Bible reading, prayer, the Sacraments, and pastoral conversation about faith issues remain central to the clergyperson's work and ministry. But increasingly people today come into crises with little or no religious background or ongoing interest in a faith orientation or religious community. As a result, more often than not, it is the hospital chaplain who must learn to listen for the deeper concerns of such people. A new religious language is emerging today that is persistently secular in content, relational in nature, and indirect in tone. Instead of words like sin and salvation, creation and judgment, grace and redemption, modern "religious talk" is about relationships and feelings: guilt, rage, fear, anxiety, love, distrust, anger. Instead of proscriptions for behavior, there is emerging greater freedom to simply tell one's story and affirm all the defeats and triumphs, ugliness and beauty within that story. Instead of a set of rules for proper religious thought and behavior, there is participation by the clergyperson with the family and the child in the ongoing, here-and-now events of their lives. In sum, instead of universal truths and distant generalities, there is emerging a specific, personal mode of communication that is, at its deepest level, profoundly religious.

Through the creation of a milieu of openness and sharing, support and mutual respect, the clergyperson can enable the family to endure and prepare for what lies ahead. In the process, both the family and the clergyperson will be changed in direct proportion to the significance of their relationship. Even if no specific religious interpretation or observation about their experience together is ever made, the validity of what has happened will stand on its own merit.

CONTRASTING RELIGIOUS TRADITIONS

There are significant differences among the Protestant, Roman Catholic, and Jewish traditions that affect how people respond to illness and hospitalization. Most Jewish families, whether Orthodox, Conservative, Reformed, or nonpracticing, are used to living in an alien (Christian) culture. As a result, they come to the hospital equipped with whatever they need to practice their faith. They do not generally expect kosher food nor any special sensitivity or knowledge of their religious observances and holidays. Nor do they necessarily expect a visit from the rabbi or from members of their synagogue. Illness is primarily a family affair among Jews, and often few know about it other than family or close friends. If possible, members of each generation gather or, at least, stay in touch by phone or cards. And when the child returns home, the family comes together for a meal, a celebration, an ingathering. If they are practicing Jews, they go to the synagogue for Sabbath services where the rabbi welcomes them and reaffirms their identity as part of the worshipping community in which is embodied the chosen people of Israel.

In contrast, the Roman Catholic church extends itself immediately and actively into the hospital context. Catholic patients expect the nearby priest assigned to the hospital to visit, perhaps even daily, and to be prepared to offer a blessing, Holy Communion, or the Sacrament of the Sick, (formerly called Last Rites). For a devout Catholic, the church and its faith, based on the assurance of eternal life, are constant sources of consolation and hope. However, for some, the experience of illness may evoke confirmation of punishment for past sins, the need for absolution, and the promise (bargain) to return to more active participation in the rites of the church upon leaving the hospital. The priest, as absolver, is a powerful and important figure in the faith framework of a Catholic family. His importance transcends any personal relationship he might or might not have with the people to whom he ministers.

The Protestant tradition, though ranging from high-church Episcopalian to low-church Baptist, from nonchurch Quaker to new-church Seventh-Day Adventist, is generally marked by a high degree of individualism and personal initiative. As a result, an active Protestant family, when crisis occurs, call their minister. They then expect him or her to visit the home and the hospital, inform the congregation of what has happened, and offer prayers during Sunday worship services. In addition, other church members may become actively involved in the crisis situation, and families are usually appreciative of such support and outflowing of feeling. Although sacramental occasions may be important to some Protestants, more important is the quality of the relationships between the minister and the family and between the congregation and the family. The significance of these relationships often supersedes any past religious background, particular denominational affiliation, or specific set of theological beliefs.

Pastoral care offered by hospital chaplains is transdenominational and interfaith. The chaplain is available to all people, no matter what their religious affiliation or background. For a Jewish patient, the initial visit by the chaplain may be an occasion for curiosity and new learning. If the contact occurs at a time of crisis, the Jewish patient and family express surprise and much appreciation for the pastoral services given in the hospital context. To the Roman Catholic patient, the chaplain offers the possibility of a pastoral relationship that complements and supplements the sacramental work of the priest. If the experience of such a personal relationship with a religious authority figure is new, this may become a source of growth in the Catholic patient and his faith. For the Protestant, the visit of the hospital chaplain (who is most likely not of the same denomination) offers an opportunity to talk freely about religious matters with someone who is knowledgeable, caring, and able to be helpful in sorting out whatever issues, emotional or religious, may be aroused by the onset of illness. In all of these situations, the hospital chaplain is able to both respect religious differences and transcend them.

HEALTHY AND UNHEALTHY FAITH

The degree to which a person's faith is healthy or unhealthy depends on the extent to which it is a helpful and responsive resource, both in the midst of the ups and downs of daily life and in the midst of the turmoil of crisis. Although specific expressions of religious faith may vary considerably, ranging all the way from daily prayer and weekly worship to sporadic poetic expression and no formal religious affiliation at all, the extent to which such faith is a congruent and integrated part of the personality will determine its usefulness. If the person is made to feel judged and inadequate by a faith system outside himself and alien to his ego, then such a system becomes a negative rather than a positive influence in the healing process. In this sense it is unhealthy. On the other hand, if the faith system is experienced as accepting and nurturing and forgiving, and if it seems to grow out of inner conviction, decision, and desire, then this expression of faith can be a positive force in the healing process. Depending on the individual's personality structure, either of these systems or their several variations might be healthily employed. In this respect it is more important how a person uses his faith than what he actually believes.

To determine whether a person's faith is healthy or not, several questions can be kept in mind. First, to what extent does expression of faith allow for simultaneous and spontaneous ventilation of real feelings, especially anger (at God), fear, and self-doubt? On the other hand, to what extent is the person's faith a denial of feelings and therefore a defense? Second, if a person's faith is a defense, is it serving the person in positive ways (giving strength, hope, ability to endure), or is it shutting off the person from himself and other people? Third, to what degree is the faith system flexible and adaptable to changing circumstances and needs? And finally, can the person allow someone of a different faith (or none at all) to be close and caring during a crisis time? With these questions, hospital staff as well as chaplains can evaluate their patients and families and anticipate religious needs as well as potential problems in the course of the illness and the healing process.

WHERE IS GOD?

Theologians through the ages have struggled over the nature of evil, its entry into the world, and its relationship or lack thereof to a Supreme Being or Source of all life. The illness and death of a child, perhaps more than any other single event, raises urgent questions for all of us about evil and the nature and meaning of life and death and disease and suffering. For the Jew, the Messiah who will redeem this world and its evils is yet to come. For the Christian, that source of salvation has come in Jesus Christ, who chose to participate in life at the very heart of its pain on a cross. For the cynic, the quest for meaning is pointless. But for the healer or caregiver, whether doctor or nurse or social worker or minister or parent or friend, to be called to stay with a child in illness and then in death is fundamentally a privilege. Such an experience brushes close by the mysterious center of things where there are no longer questions or answers, good or evil, life or death, but only a special Presence that transcends the ordinary and marks the beginning of something new.

ADDITIONAL READINGS
Journals

The Journal of Pastoral Care
Pastoral Psychology

Books

Bruder, E.: Ministering to deeply troubled people, Englewood Cliffs, N.J., 1964, Prentice-Hall, Inc.

Clebsch, W., and Jaekle, C.: Pastoral care in historical perspective, Englewood Cliffs, N.J., 1964, Prentice-Hall, Inc.

Clinebell, H.: Basic types of pastoral counseling, New York, 1966, Abingdon Press.

Dicks, R.: Principles and practices of pastoral care, Englewood Cliffs, N.J., 1963, Prentice-Hall, Inc.

Jackson, E.: Understanding grief, New York, 1957, Abingdon Press.

Jackson, E.: Telling a child about death, New York, 1965. Hawthorn Books, Inc.

Mitchell, K.: Hospital chaplain, Philadelphia, 1972, The Westminster Press.

Nouwen, H.: The wounded healer, New York, 1972, Doubleday & Co., Inc.

Satir, V.: Peoplemaking, Palo Alto, 1972, Science & Behavior Books, Inc.

CHAPTER 21

On the right to information and freedom of choice for the dying: is it for minors?

LORETTA KOPELMAN

Persons must attain a certain degree of maturity before they achieve full civil rights. As a matter of administrative convenience, an arbitrary age (such as 18 or 21 years) is selected when, unless there are extenuating circumstances such as severe retardation, it is assumed that the person is then sufficiently mature to be granted full civil rights. This selection of an arbitrary chronological age for determining the age of maturity seems proper under most circumstances. However, in the case of the dying child or adolescent we ought to set aside the fiction that persons on the occasion of a particular birthday suddenly achieve sufficient maturity to judge what is in their own best interest and to direct their own affairs. In the following pages I shall defend the view that out of respect to persons who are dying, they, regardless of their age, should have the prima facie right to direct their own affairs as they wish. (That is, the right is not absolute and can be overridden in some situations.)

I shall argue that this view has support within our legal system for adults. However, while there has been some recognition of the rights of children and adolescents to self-determination in other matters, there is little attention currently being paid to them in the recent wave of Natural Death Acts and bills before state legislatures. This could be rectified by replacing the chronological age requirements that appear on most of these bills and acts for the execution of directives with statements about the competency of persons to direct their own affairs regardless of their age.

There is uniform agreement about the desirability of the goal of compassionate care and support for all terminally ill persons, although opinions differ about how this goal should be achieved, what should be communicated to whom, and what may be the treatment of choice for a particular patient. Even though a general range of professionally acceptable behavior is agreed on by physicians and other health professionals, there can be room for substantial disagreement among them about what course best suits (and here one does not mean only medically) a particular patient. For example, some persons who are terminally ill welcome comfort care, or aggressive medical or surgical management, or participation in a research protocol; others object. Evidence does indicate that most patients want to be informed.[8] In a better world than this one, patients would always have families and attending physicians whose beliefs, attitudes, and values are close to their own in these matters.

SOME LEGAL CONSIDERATIONS

In the United States the courts have supported the position that a person has the right of self-determination. This right to control one's destiny is not lost in a medical setting. In Natanson vs. Kline, Justice Schroeder writes:[11]

> Anglo-American law starts with the premise of thoroughgoing self determination. It follows that each man is considered to be master of his own body, and he may, if he be of sound mind, expressedly prohibit the performance of lifesaving surgery or other medical treatment.

This position is modified in his statement made shortly after that given above:[11]

> The duty of the physician to disclose, however, is limited to those disclosures which a reasonable medical practitioner would make under the same or similar circumstances. . . . So long as the disclosure is sufficient to assure an informed consent, the physician's choice of plausible courses should not be called into question if it appears, all circumstances considered, that the physician was motivated only by the patient's best therapeutic interest and he proceeded as a competent medical man would have done in a similar situation.

According to this decision, physicians must inform the patient in accordance with standard medical practice and to the extent any reasonable person would want or need to make a decision in a similar situation. Where there is a dispute on this issue, the court decides whether adequate information was provided for such a decision and whether it was in accordance with standard medical practice. Twelve years later in the decision Canterbury vs. Spence, delivered by S. W. Robinson III,[2] the court reaffirmed the position that a physician is obligated to provide enough information for the patient, in light of his needs, to make an intelligent treatment choice; the patient should be provided with the information a prudent and reasonable person would want in making his decision. Two exceptions are cited by the court: "The first comes into play where the patient is unconscious or otherwise incapable of consenting, and harm from a failure to treat is imminent and outweighs any harm threatened by the proposed treatment."[2] That is, when there is an emergency and the patient or family is unable to consent, the court recognizes an exception to the general rule of disclosure. The court writes, "The second exception obtains when risk-disclosure poses such a threat of detriment to the patient as to become unfeasible or contraindicated from a medical point of view."[2] The court further states[2]:

> The physician's privilege to withhold information for therapeutic reasons must be carefully circumscribed, however, for otherwise it might devour the disclosure rule itself. The privilege does not accept the paternalistic notion that the physician may remain silent simply because divulgence might prompt the patient to forego therapy the physician feels the patient really needs. That attitude presumes instability or perversity for even the normal patient and runs counter to the foundation principle that the patient should and ordinarily can make the choice for himself. Nor does the privilege contemplate operations save where the patient's reaction to risk information, as reasonably foreseen by the physician, is menacing. And even in a situation of that kind, disclosure to a close relative with a view to securing consent to the proposed treatment may be the only alternative open to the physician.

Thus the court tempers its libertarian judgement by acknowledging, first that physicians are not under the impossible obligation to give each patient a medical school course, and second that there are therapeutic privilege exceptions.

Adults as medical consumers have been able to speak for themselves and demand certain rights. Minors, however, are not generally able to organize themselves to demand that certain claims be fulfilled. It is only lately that they have been recognized as individuals in need of specifically recognized rights.[12,13,15-17,20] Society has acknowledged it has specific obligations to the children and not simply to the guardians of children.[12,13,15-17,20] The recognition of children's rights is a departure from the past, when it was assumed that parents and guardians had the right to control their children's destinies, because it was believed that (1) children were their property, or that (2) children, until they reached a particular birthday, were always incompetent to make rational decisions, or that (3) guardians and parents had the right to the labors of their children, or that (4) thoroughgoing direction was necessary to help children properly develop their potential.[20] However, in recent years it has been acknowledged that children should be granted certain rights independently of their parents or guardians.[12,13,15-17,20] In the area of medical care, many rights have recently been guaranteed to minors by the United States Supreme Court under the right of privacy.[15] These include the right to contraceptive information and contraceptive devices, treatment for veneral disease, and treatment for alcoholism and drug-related problems.[12,13,15] Minors may obtain such information or treatment without parental consent. Moreover, health professionals are, by law, immune from prosecution by parents or guardians who object to the provision of such services to minors.[15] In the Danforth case of 1976, minor girls are given the right to elect abortions without parental consent.[13,14] Children are slowly winning the right to have their own representation in court cases.[17] Child abuse laws are being carefully reworked with great concern as to (1) what constitutes abuse or neglect, (2) who should be required to report it and to whom, (3) the granting of immunity from prosecution for those reporting cases, (4) possible penalties for failure to report, (5) waiver of privileged communication so that reporting can be done, and (6) the conditions under which central registers can be appropriately kept and used.[17] Many of these problems are complicated because they involve not only the right of the child to due process but the right of the parent or guardian to due process as well.[13]

STATEMENT OF TWO TENETS

In the following pages I shall defend two tenets. First, people have the right to be informed about their medical condition and treatment and the right to participate in treatment decisions.[4,6] To withhold important information that would affect the way people might conduct their lives or to disallow their participation in treatment decisions, even for allegedly altruistic motives, is an unwarranted interference with their freedom of choice; it constitutes an illicit use of power or authority over them.

To say that anyone has a right to something, however, means that they have a justifiable claim to it *if they want it,* and that unless there are extenuating circumstances, we (society) owe it to them to fulfill that claim. This does not mean that persons are morally obligated, or even that they should be pressured, to exercise this right to know and to participate in treatment decisions if they choose not to do so.

The second tenet I shall defend is that although we can agree that under certain circumstances some people cannot or should not be informed, the burden of proof is on those who withhold information to show compelling reasons why the person should not be informed or participate in treatment decisions. An example of appropriate withholding of information would be a case where the person clearly indicates that he wants neither to have this information nor to make such decisions. Another justifiable exception would be where there is no opportunity to inform or counsel the person (such as in an emergency) or where the person is clearly incompetent to be informed or participate in the choices (for example, infants or profoundly retarded persons). My purpose is not to list all manner of exceptions nor to address difficult practical problems, such as when and how persons can and should be informed, or how physicians can be protected from those who, with the advantage of hindsight, take legal action charging that no real informed choice was made because they do not like the consequences of the choice made. Rather, my purpose is to defend certain principles that may be valuable to those sorting out these and other practical matters—namely, that we as social creatures have certain obligations to other persons in our society, obligations that do not cease or diminish because they are dying. These obligations stem from the considerations that, in general, persons have the right to conduct their lives as they wish as long as they do not interfere with others and that they have the right to the medical information about themselves that will influence these choices.

Neither of these two tenets makes a reference to age. Thus, a minor who is capable and who wants to be informed and participate in treatment decisions has the *right* to do so. His claim is justifiable and we (society) are morally obligated, if possible, to provide him with the opportunity to control his own destiny even when—or especially when—he is terminally ill. Because of the different developmental and intellectual abilities and attitudes of minors at a particular chronological age, it would be inappropriate to specify at what chronological age a minor is capable of being informed or of participating in treatment choices. However, any person's expression that he wants such knowledge or participation is certainly evidence of a claim upon us that he deserves candor.

ARGUMENTS TO SUPPORT THESE TWO TENETS

Two kinds of arguments will be offered to support this defense; one type concerns the fair treatment of such dying persons, and the other type concerns the benefits to society in not denying this to them. First, by refusing them this control, we unjustifiably deny them their last opportunity for asserting their own individuality, personal growth, and self-development.[4,6] The right of self-determination for adults can be lost, but not because one is dying. It can be lost if one's actions interfere with the welfare of others.[10] The dying person's desire to be informed, to participate in treatment decisions, and to maintain control over his own destiny does not interfere with the rights of others. It is sometimes supposed to be sufficient for restricting the liberty of another that the person's action represents a substantial threat to his future well-being. However, this consideration lacks credibility when the person is dying. Thus the dying person's desire to maintain control represents a just claim. The adult should not lose the right of self-determination simply because he is dying.

Dying minors have never attained full civil rights, but a similar argument for their prima facie right to control their own destiny can be supported. First, just as with dying adults, it is their last opportunity for the expression of their own individuality. Second, in such circumstances, the protective function of third party consent for minors becomes less important; there is little left to protect them from, and no long-term benefits are justified by the intervention. Thus, if the minors sincerely desire such control, the burden of proof should fall to those who judge that they should be denied it.

In addition to considerations of the above arguments regarding the just or fair treatment of the individual in society, there are other arguments involving benefits to society in allowing the dying to control their lives. One benefit is that we can profit by learning from the successes or failures of the different choices made by others. If their choices are imprudent, we may be able to reason out why such choices fail. This may help us with our own decisions about ourselves or how to counsel others. If their choices succeed, they can serve as examples to us of the variety of alternatives open to ourselves and others. And, if the choices are partially successful, we can perhaps clarify our thoughts about the components contributing to success or failure.[10]

A second benefit to us all is that we profit from disallowing such a restriction on personal liberty. We would not want to adopt as a general rule that a person can interfere with someone's liberty because he (albeit a well-meaning family member or physician) happens to believe it is "for someone's own good." But if we disallow that others can decide when to restrict someone's freedom, even though they sincerely judge it is for his own good, then we should not adopt it for a particular group of persons, namely, dying persons. Not only is such a rule dangerous but, benevolent intentions aside, it is arrogant for us to adopt such a rule. It presupposes that we know the course of action that will suit another better than he knows it himself. In view of the diversity of opinion and rapidly changing views about the care of the terminally ill, unless the person is shown to be incompetent or does not want the information or responsibility, such judgments are unwarranted. The general problem being addressed here with reference to the dying is: What are the legitimate bounds of paternalism?[3] A society that permits its citizens, children as well as adults, to engage in life-threatening activities for sport (for example, hang gliding) should not restrict the freedom of persons simply because they are dying on the grounds that it is "for their own good."

I anticipate an important objection to this second consideration (that allowing the dying person control over his life results in a greater advantage to society than when others control his choice): advancement of scientific knowledge is an extremely important value, and if the dying person participates in a research protocol, there may be a significant contibution to society in the form of improved care for others. Present successful treatments are directly related to past studies, which systematically examined alternative methods of treatment. Therefore, there is an advantage, this argument might continue, to having some of the choices made by others. I am not opposed to the continuation of this important research if there is consent from the subject or patient. The person who stays in a study for the good of others or to advance scientific knowledge performs a morally commendable action beyond what is required of him or her. Still, it is unjustifiable to manipulate consent or require the participation of someone in a study for the good of others. To place scientific advancement as a higher value than freedom of choice would have the unacceptable consequences of allowing medical personnel and researchers to override our decisions for the sake of what they might learn. (Few would condone such behavior.) Thus, freedom of choice is the higher value; and even if the advance of science is slowed, this is a consequence that must be accepted in the defense of a higher value. However, it does seem to me that such an argument is narrow in its conception of what can be learned from the dying. It may be that we will learn at least as much from the variety of choices people make for themselves as we can from scientific investigation of the somatic response of the disease process to alternative therapies.

LEGISLATION REGARDING DYING PERSONS

It has been argued that the two tenets that have been defended are justifiable in themselves and that there is support for them within our legal system. Following is a brief discussion of some current legislation regarding the dying. These laws or bills attempt to clarify the rights of competent persons to accept or refuse treatment and decide who should make medical decisions in cases where the person is incompetent.[18,19] I question whether such laws should adopt a specific age limit as a necessary condition for determining competency.

As of September 1977, 40 states had introduced bills, and eight states had passed legislation attempting to set public policy. The first state to do so, in September 1976, was California.[1,5] In 1977, seven other states enacted Natural Death Acts: Idaho (S1164) and Arkansas (H826) in March, New Mexico (S16) in April, Nevada (AB8) in May, and Oregon (S438), Texas (S148), and North Carolina (S504) in June.

The California law permits patients to sign directives (revocable by them at any time) to their physicians that express the patient's desire to refuse medical treatment should he or she be unable to give instructions. The law states that it is a misdemeanor to conceal or destroy a directive and that it should be considered unprofessional conduct to ignore it in appropriate circumstances. It provides for the withdrawal of mechanical or artificial means of sustaining life at the patient's request. The law also contains (1) means for protecting the patient, such as requiring a consultation, (2) conditions concerning witnessing, and (3) the requirement that a waiting period elapse before the directive goes into effect.

This law was the first to state that the written directive of a person can be binding upon the attending physician(s) even when the person is no longer competent to direct his treatment. The other states have, in general, followed this.[18,19] They also usually specify that the request to have treatment withheld or withdrawn under certain circumstances should not be viewed as a suicide. (Life insurance policies typically contain a clause stating that they are voided in the event of suicide.) Most of the other bills and laws also affirm the right of medical personnel to withdraw from a case where they disagree with the course selected by the patient, next of kin, or the person designated by the patient.[18,19]

It has been argued that some minors are competent to make these choices. But, of course, many of them are unable to make them. Where persons are incompetent, do we need a public policy stating who should make medical decisions for them? The physician might be a good choice, but in a society with as much difference of opinion as ours regarding these matters, it is entirely possible that the physician will not know or be comfortable with the choices that the family knows the patient would want to make. Veatch argues that "the most reasonable first line of authority would be someone the patient himself might have designated while competent"[18]; otherwise the authority would be given to "the next of kin until such time as the next of kin's decision is judged so unreasonable that society must intervene and appoint a new guardian."[7,18] One wants to protect the patient from the enthusiasm of a maleficent, illinformed, or irrational family, and giving the authority to the physician might do this; on the other hand, most families do know the choices the patient would want to make, and they have the best interest of the family member as their goal.[9] Giving the authority to a physician, who could have entirely different attitudes, beliefs, and values from those of the family or who could be preoccupied with other concerns, can cause another dimension of grief and sorrow for them. In practical terms, the family can always have some control by the selection or dismissal of the attending physician, and the physician can appeal to the courts where the choice of the family or guardian is unacceptable or inappropriate. This provides a system of checks and balances.

Veatch argues that a model bill should state an age requirement. Presumably persons below that age should be regarded as incompetent to sign such a directive. "A minimum age for execution of a treatment acceptance or refusal document should be stated, probably the age of majority in the state for purposes of legally accepting or refusing medical treatments in general. . . ."[18] Most of the current acts or bills now before state legislatures specify age 18 or 19 as the age at which a person may be considered competent to sign a directive.[19] Should a model bill have an age requirement?

CONCLUSION

Natural Death Acts and model bills protecting freedom of choice for dying persons should not have an age requirement. Many minors, particularly adolescents, want to have the information and the option to make choices and are as capable as, or no less incapable than, many adults to deal with these matters. The critical question is whether a particular minor has the competency and desire to participate in these choices. The age requirement could direct our attention away from this central consideration. Moreover, the setting of an arbitrary age limit runs counter to current legal trends, some of which have been mentioned, regarding the rights of minors to self-determination.

At least, physicians could make it clear from the outset that they will not lie to the minor. If the minor specifically asks the attending physician, or a member of the health care team, such as a nurse or a resident physician, about his prognosis or treatment program, then the attending physician could and should feel at liberty to answer these questions forthrightly.

To summarize, I have defended two tenets: first, that people have the right to be informed about their medical condition and treatment and to participate in treatment decisions, and second, that the burden of proof is on those who would deny such information or choice to show compelling reasons why the person should not be informed or participate in treatment decisions. Neither of these two tenets makes any reference to age. Both have legal support for competent adults, and neither requires anyone to exercise these rights.

The object of this chapter has not been to minimize the difficulties of the practical situations. Disagreements arise about whether or not the person can be or wants to be informed or participate in decisions. Rather, the goal has been to suggest and defend certain principles that may be helpful in deciding what should be done. What John Stuart Mill wrote about living applies to dying.[10]

> Mankind are greater gainers by suffering each other to live as seems good to themselves than by compelling each to live as seems good to the rest.

REFERENCES

1. A. B. 3060 California Legislature (1976).
2. Canterbury vs. Spence 464, F.2d 772 (1972).
3. Engelhardt, H. T.: A demand to die, Hastings Center Rep. pp. 10 and 47, June, 1975.
4. Fletcher, J.: Medical diagnosis; our right to know the truth. In Morals and medicine, Boston, 1972, Beacon Press, pp. 34-64.
5. Garland, M.: Politics, legislation and natural death, Hastings Center Rep. **6:**5, 1976.
6. Kant, I.: On the supposed right to lie from altruistic motives. In Beck, L. W., editor and translator: Critique of practical reason, Chicago, 1949, University of Chicago Press.
7. Kaplan, R. P.: Euthanasia legislation; a survey and a model act, Am. J. Law Med. **2:**41, 1976.
8. Kelly, W. D., and Friesen, S. R.: Do cancer patients want to be told? Surgery **27:**822, 1950.
9. Maguire, D. C.: Death by choice, Garden City, N.Y., 1974, Doubleday & Co., Inc.
10. Mill, J. S.: On liberty, New York, 1974, Penguin Books.
11. Natanson vs. Kline 350, P. 2d 1093 (1960).
12. Paul, E. W.: Legal rights of minors to sex-related medical care, Columbia Human Rights Law Rev. **6:**357, 1974.
13. Paul, E. W., Pilpel, H. F., and Wechsler, N.: Pregnancy, teenagers and the law, 1976, Fam. Plann. Perspec. **8:**16, 1976.
14. Planned Parenthood of Central Missouri vs. Danforth, United States Supreme Court, 1976.
15. Raitt, G. E., Jr.: The minor's right to consent to medical treatment; a corollary of the constitutional right of privacy, South. Calif. Law Rev. **48:**1417, 1974-1975.
16. Rodham, H.: Children under the law. In The rights of children. Harvard Educ. Rev. Reprint Series No. 9, pp. 1-28, 1974.
17. Sussman, A.: Reporting child abuse; a review of the literature, Fam. Law Q. **8:**245, 1974.
18. Veatch, R. M.: Death and dying; the legislative options, Hastings Center Rep. **7:**5, 1977.
19. Veatch, R. M.: Analysis of legislative proposals on euthanasia and treatment refusals; bills that would clarify rights of competent patients, Research Group on Death and Dying, The Hastings Center, 1977.
20. Worsfold, V. L.:. A philosophical justification of children's rights. In The rights of children, Harvard Educ. Rev. Reprint Series No. 9, pp. 29-52, 1974.

CHAPTER 22

A teaching program for death education

JEFFREY D. REYNOLDS

Our high school, with an enrollment of about 1,300 students, is situated in a city with a metropolitan population of 300,000. About 13% of the students are handicapped in some way (orthopaedic, hearing impaired, visually impaired, slow learner, mentally retarded, and so on).

We have developed a program that helps prepare these exceptional students for the "real world." The program is designed to teach basic survival skills related to both personal safety and mental health, because in special education, social awareness is as important as academic excellence.

Three years ago, while I was teaching first aid (a basic survival skill for our students), one student asked, "What do you say to a dying person?" At first, I did not respond, and frankly, I did not answer the question. But this issue surfaced again and again. While I was teaching sex education, students wanted to know why a fetus might die. Curiosity about death mounted, topic after topic. Sometimes the students asked questions of a more personal nature, for example, "Why would a person take an overdose of drugs to kill himself?" The questions did not stop, and to me the students seemed "possessed" with questions concerning death.

I began to feel troubled. I thought, why are these students asking these questions? Have they no idea what death is all about? Have they never seen a corpse? After all, they live in the inner city and are exposed to violent crimes all the time—or at least this is the consensus of opinion. I was wrong. I found that my students were not exposed in a "natural way" to dead people. Exposure was limited, usually with no explanation of the events leading up to the death, the death itself, and the events after death.

John witnessed the shooting of his aunt. Because of the ambulance personnel, police, and subsequent investigation at the scene, John's exposure was short and "violent." When it was over, no one offered him any explanation. Later, the funeral was arranged and John attended, but for him there still was no satisfactory explanation of the death. He had witnessed the killing but not the actual death. Later he asked me, "Do you think she was in pain? What does death look like?" Was John asking me to describe a state that he could relate to in order to fill his need for reassurance? Did he have some fundamental concepts about death already in mind? I realized that the exposure, basically unexplained, had been left to the boy to work out by himself.

A different case again emphasized a basic need of our students.

> Cynthia, after a trip to a funeral home remarked, "You know, my Dad died a couple of weeks ago." "Why didn't you tell me?" I asked. She replied, "I was afraid you wouldn't let me come on the field trip. You know, I wish someone had told me all these things before, because now I feel better." The "things" Cynthia was referring to were explanations of what happens to a dead body. Some of her anxiety about her father's death had been relieved.

Discussion about death as a separate topic began 3 years ago as a 2-week miniunit and included a visit to a funeral home. During the first year, the emphasis of the program was on protecting the students from "being taken advantage of," an approach used in teaching other survival skill topics (sex education, drivers' education, drugs, first aid, and so on).

The result was a disaster. First of all, I found out that I was faced with a group of students who became depressed easily. Furthermore, they had little knowledge of basic terms and concepts. Last, only half the class attended the visit to the funeral home. Of those who did attend, most were not prepared emotionally for the visit. I decided that this topic was not teachable.

But this failure bothered me. I realized I was not listening to what the students were actually saying. They wanted to learn, but this desire was not in tune with my methods.

The course was redesigned to extend over a 10-week period, although the actual work was done only twice a week, usually Tuesdays and Thursdays. This learning module that replaced the earlier miniunit was a marked success from various standpoints. First, students did not become depressed during class discussions. They had time to think things out. In turn, the questions became more thoughtful and increasingly difficult to answer and were often in areas that I had not anticipated. Most important, I found that I had to come to grips with my own eventual death as a prerequisite to being an effective teacher.

Most of the students progressed with certain amounts of individualized instruction from one objective to the next without anxiety. They made value judgments for themselves and began to be interested in concrete things that they could do with regard to their own deaths, such as writing their own wills. Finally, on the days of off-site instruction, the students were ready to go. During the last 2 years, class attendance has been perfect for the funeral home visit.

THE EDUCATOR'S ROLE IN DEATH EDUCATION

The student seeks an explanation for everything, but certain subjects have greater emotional meaning for both the educator and the student. Death, an inescapable part of our lives, is not usually included as an acceptable classroom topic. Death education has been relegated to a position formerly reserved for sex education in the curricula of public schools—taboo. Because death is a tragic circumstance of life, faculty and students must see the need to learn about it. Thus the basic job of educators becomes guiding students toward greater understanding, even if it is painful for both those who teach and those who are taught.

Educators have long suppressed a frank discussion of death and dying with their students. This is a stand that is becoming more difficult to defend in an environment of increasing violence, drug abuse, potential nuclear holocaust, automobile accidents, natural catastrophies, and various other types of accidental death.

Besides, what is more essential to our students' success and happiness than good mental as well as physical health? Educators themselves must understand the emotional needs of their students and teach those survival skills that allow a student to satisfy his own needs openly for optimal psychological development. In other words, students are constantly seeking the "whole story" about life and death. As educators, we can help make sense out of what is going on around them while filling this need.

Educators should prevent unnecessary anxieties and fears. Sometimes it is difficult for a teacher to do this because he has not come adequately to grips with his own death. However, unless one can deal with whole truths, the students see the learning exercise as artificial and become disinterested.

TEACHING ABOUT DEATH
Who studied about death and dying and why?

At our high school, we have designed a program specifically to help our achievement students learn about death and dying. Achievement students are slow learners who are functioning in the low-normal IQ range (76-89). These students are between 14 and 18 years old with mental ages 3 to 4 years below chronological age. They are mainstreamed partially during grades 8, 9, and 10 and fully integrated into the regular program after successfully completing 10A (the achievement grade that is the equivalent of regular tenth grade).

The fact that achievement students were the original participants in this program has far-ranging implications. They represent the student population between educable mentally retarded students (EMR) and "normal-regular" students. Thus, the basic format can probably be used with minor modification for teaching EMR as well as regular students. Only the teaching procedures and software need to be changed.

Instructions for presentation of death education material

The quantity, quality, depth, and breadth of the learning that occurs with this topic are direct functions of material preparation and presentation. Two important facts must be remembered. First, it is essential to evaluate the maturational or developmental levels of the students. Second, abstractions, theories, or logical relationships should not be presented without having adequate background definitions and facts that can be manipulated easily by the student at his own level.

When questions are raised, answers depend on understanding what the student is really asking. The following is an example of a situation in which the student's question needed to be answered at a basic, concrete level, but was initially misunderstood by a resource person. Dan is one of the students. Mr. Hall is a funeral director.

> **Dan:** "What happens to the body of a dead person?"
> **Mr. Hall:** "It is embalmed."
> **Dan:** "Then what happens?"
> **Mr. Hall:** "Then it is placed in a coffin and buried."
> **Dan:** "But what happens to the body?"

Dan was persistent, seeking the answer that finally met his own need.

When subjects are introduced, the approach has to be gentle and indirect, but always genuine. At first the student should be allowed to initiate the discussion. This can be done by seeking topics that act as springboards. First aid is an excellent topic, because its emphasis is the prevention of death. When performing artificial respiration, one always says that death can occur after 6 minutes without oxygen. Then the instructor (or the student) might ask what death is or if anyone has seen a dead body.

One crucial point to remember is that death cannot be talked about all the time. One should avoid a general sense of depression in the class by purposely allowing time between discussions, as we learned by expanding the time frame for covering the topic without increasing the actual number of hours designated for death education.

Above all, parents and school administrators should be informed of the exact nature of the curriculum design. Inviting them to the classroom to observe and/or participate in instruction often reduces their own anxiety about what is being taught.

Student participation in off-site instruction trips should not be forced. Announcement about a visit to a funeral home at least 2 weeks in advance allows students to prepare themselves emotionally. A "happy" occasion might be planned for the same day. One tool I find useful is treating the students to breakfast. (Plan for full attendance the day of your trip.)

The learning module for death education

Objectives. The first phase in the development of an educational tool is the identification of behavioral objectives for the program. In the learning module for death education, objectives can be stated most easily in behavioral terms that describe what any learner should be able to comprehend on completing the module. For example, as a result of this program students should be able to (not in any order):

1. Describe the social, emotional, and practical aspects of death.
2. Describe the biological aspects of death.
3. Discuss the various ways different age groups view death.
4. Describe how American society views death.
5. Describe various ways to deal with grief.
6. Describe various funeral rituals.
7. Discuss the roles of the various helping professionals who can assist when death is near or has occurred (for instance, doctors, nurses, funeral directors).
8. Discuss various emotions as they relate to death, such as anger, despair, envy, grief, jealousy, resentment, love, hope.
9. Discuss the purposes of wills, lawyers, insurance, and so on.
10. Discuss planning for the event of one's own death.

Both teacher and students should be allowed some choice about specific course objectives and the order in which they would prefer to accomplish them.

Pretest. The second phase in developing the learning module for death education is to administer a pretest to help the teacher decide at what level to begin the discussion. Such objective evaluation of the students' "needs realm" (strengths and weaknesses) also defines areas that will need particular emphasis or extensive discussion. Here is an example of the pretest for part of this module:

A. State the purpose of a will.
B. From the following list, select the words that best describe the major areas associated with a will:

_____ Lawyer   _____ Insurance
_____ Car   _____ Taxes
_____ Court   _____ Executor
_____ Professions   _____ Relatives
_____ Money   _____ Bills

Content development. Content development is the third phase in developing the learning module. A basic vocabulary should be introduced and certain terms defined if necessary (such as fatal, deathbed, euthanasia, suicide, and bereavement).

This often leads to discussion of the student's own immediate associations with death. Has he ever seen someone die? Has a relative or friend recently died? Movies and filmstrips about death can be particularly helpful in initiating discussion during the first few sessions when there may be some hesitancy about sharing personal experiences or feelings. Some that are available commercially are listed at the end of the chapter.

Students should be introduced to the helping professionals who deal with death on a daily basis, such as doctors, nurses, coroners, lawyers, policemen, and funeral directors. It is also important to provide an opportunity for discussion of the ways various religions deal with death. Here the teacher may want to describe his own beliefs about an afterlife and reincarnation. In general, however, any detailed explanations should be left to various clergypeople invited to the classroom or visited in the community. (Parents sometimes express a genuine concern in this area.)

A discussion of facilities designed for the terminally ill patient is important. Along with this, the general concept of euthanasia (with specific reference to current topics, such as the Karen Ann Quinlan case), the ethics of abortion, capital punishment, or suicide might be addressed.

An explanation of current funeral home practices is extremely important, because they are very often misunderstood or not understood at all by the students.

Finally, a discussion of the process of dealing with one's own eventual death is crucial. The psychological resistance to probing into this last developmental milestone is painful and universal, so it is natural for the educator to feel this way, and he should not hesitate to admit his own fears to the students.

There is a need with this topic to establish stages for the accomplishment of chosen objectives. These stages should present a sequence of challenges and experiences that provide students with the necessary expertise for meeting successive objectives. Underlying all of this, however, must be a framework that helps the learners understand how completion of the learning module on death education is important to them.

Activities. The fourth phase, off-site instruction, is designed to help students bridge the gap between the classroom and the community. The teacher is invaluable in the process, for it is the teacher who suggests particular activities to the learners and acts as a resource person.

In a unit on death education, off-site instruction is important. On many occasions, our high school special education classes have visited funeral homes. It would be easier to invite a funeral director to the classroom, but taking the students directly to the home helps familiarize them with the setting and alleviate fear of the unknown. Once they have visited as part of the class and met the personnel, they will be less fearful or anxious when they have to go there on their own. Other people and places to visit to discuss death include a doctor's office, a hospital, a coroner's office, and a police station.

Posttest. The fifth phase of the learning module is measuring the students' objective achievement. Students may take the posttest whenever they feel confident that they have achieved the objectives of the module, and they should be encouraged to question the teacher about incorrect answers.

Evaluation of the learning module. The program as designed has been continuously monitored in the following areas by the instructors:

1. What are students' past experiences with death, and what are their major questions?
2. What information needs to be presented, and how will it be done? Options include off-site visits, films, speakers, and so on.
3. What are the participants' and educators' major areas of responsibility in this program? Who does what, when, how, where?
4. What resources are needed?
5. How is performance, that is, the quantity and quality of feedback, to be measured?
6. How do students' expectations compare with those of the faculty?

Observations

Following are some observations about the learning module for death education that must be emphasized. First, students often misunderstand some part of the course, sometimes immediately, sometimes in retrospect weeks or months later. Thus, channels of communication must be kept open to clarify information and minimize misconceptions. In addition, the student feels more comfortable if he perceives that the educator is receptive to and answers all questions as honestly as possible. Some of the questions most frequently asked by students are:

Why is death scary?
Why is black associated with death?
Is death painful?
Is death ever a good thing?
What is suicide?
Do funeral directors make a lot of money?
How do you embalm someone?
Why are funeral homes so cold, dark, and weird?
What do you say to a dying person?

Any emotional reaction a student has can be considerably lessened if the student feels that he knows what is going on and what is specifically expected of him. For this reason, it is helpful to schedule a continuous awareness of the method of approach. For example, before starting class, the teacher should outline what is to be covered. This relieves anxiety and allows the student time to plan questions. Finally, when the program ends, it is vital to log what actually happened. This provides a valuable tool for future planning.

After experiencing the learning module on death education, most students have some self-realization about death. At the end of each module, I have presented an oral attitude information survey. Some of the questions and most frequent answers follow.

Q: To what extent do you believe in life after death?
A: They strongly believe in it, or they are convinced it does not occur.

Q: To what extent do you believe in reincarnation?
A: Convinced it cannot occur.

Q: How often do you think about your own death?
A: Occasionally.

Q: What does death mean to you?
A: The end. The final process of life.

Q: What aspect of your own death is most distasteful to you?
A: All my plans and projects would come to an end.

Q: When you think of your own death, how do you feel?
A: Discouraged, fearful.

Q: If you had a choice, what kind of death would you prefer?
A: Quiet, dignified, sudden, but not violent.

Q: What are your thoughts about leaving a will?
A: I have not made a will but plan to someday.

Q: To what extent do you believe in life insurance to benefit your survivors?

A: I believe in it and plan to get it someday.

Q: What are your thoughts about funerals?

A: Inclined to feel they are valuable.

The students' concerns seem closely related to their home and community environments. Their abilities to understand concepts depend on
their intellectual maturity. Political, social, and religious attitudes also
contribute to their concept of death. With this in mind, the teacher must
remember that although what is said is important, how it is said sometimes has an even greater bearing on whether the student develops anxiety and fear or acceptance of the facts about death that are being presented.

We have found with achievement students that it is wise to avoid
abstract philosophical interpretations. Also, difficult terms will slip by the
student. He will take only those words he is familiar with and include
them in his concept of death. When teachers supply answers to their students, they are frequently only partially heard and often misunderstood.
Thus, if a student does not fully comprehend an explanation, he should
be encouraged to ask further questions. In such an atmosphere of openness, students do not stop questioning until they are completely satisfied
that nothing is being hidden from them.

The student may begin to ask questions to test the teacher. It is important to understand the train of thought leading to each question. What
is the student really asking? As an example: "Do you have a will? If so,
show it to us." You must ask yourself, "Is the student searching to further
his horizon by understanding the will, or is he testing me for some other
reason? Does he want real, tangible evidence that I do what I espouse
verbally?"

Religious concepts regarding death should be developed in conjunction with the clergy. This helps to alleviate most parental concern. It is
best either to present the death concepts from a variety of faiths or to plan
on excluding the topic altogether; the second alternative seems less advisable.

Above all, before the unit is introduced, a letter should be distributed
to parents that *precisely* explains the course objectives. It has been my
good fortune not to have had any parents deny permission for their
children to study death (in contrast to sex education). Furthermore,
formal permission for every off-site instruction should be obtained. The
purpose of a given trip should be clearly stated on the forms for
parental signature.

Summary of learning module for death education

Education is concerned with the individual's ability to perform at a given level, not only academically but also psychosocially. The learning module for death education goes beyond behavior and performance objectives, for it allows learners to progress at their own rate and identify their needs realm while it provides opportunities for community-based activities.

CONCLUSION

This chapter represents approximately 3 years of work in developing a learning module for death education. The strategies are derived from a working program, and are neither prescriptive nor predictive. They have been suggested because of our success in correlating methods and materials with our own specific goals. However, goals will (and should) vary from program to program; modifications will be necessary to meet individual class needs. The learning module for death education, at least at our high school, is expanding. For example, there are plans to have students work with terminally ill patients on a volunteer basis.

During the production of this chapter, I had the opportunity to present this module to Project Upward Bound students. These are regular-grade students who are taking courses at the University of Rochester for high school credit. Although the results have not yet been tabulated and evaluated, it is enough to say that the needs realm of these students is roughly equivalent to those of achievement students, which lends credibility to the potential applicability of the module to the regular classroom.

ADDITIONAL READINGS
Books

Alsop, S.: Stay of execution, Philadelphia, 1973, J. B. Lippincott Co.

Becker, E.: The denial of death, New York, 1973, The Free Press.

Davidson, G.: Living with dying, Minneapolis, 1975, Augsburg Publishing House.

Gunther, J.: Death be not proud, New York, 1965, Harper & Row, Publishers.

Kübler-Ross, E.: On death and dying, New York, 1969, Macmillan, Inc.

Kübler-Ross, E.: Questions and answers on death and dying, New York, 1974, Macmillan, Inc.

Lund, D.: Eric, Philadelphia, 1974, J. B. Lippincott Co.

Mitford, J.: The American way of death, New York, 1963, Simon & Schuster, Inc.

Rosenthal, T.: How could I not be among you? New York, 1973, George Braziller, Inc.

Vogel, L.: Helping a child understand death, Philadelphia, 1975, Fortress Press.

Audiovisual materials

Death and Dying—Closing the Circle: Guidance Associates, producer and distributor, 757 Third Avenue, New York 10017. A series of five full-color filmstrips and five records discussing the meaning of death.

Mechanized Death: Highway Safety Foundation, producer, 890 Hollywood Lane, P.O. Box 3563, Mansfield, Ohio 44904.

The Poetry of Death: Spectrum Educational Media, 105 Beverly St., Morton, Ill. 61550. Two color filmstrips, two cassettes plus reading script.

Peace Bird: by Deanna Edwards, Teleketics, 1220 South Santee Street, Los Angeles, Calif. 90015. Long-playing record album.

Perspectives on Death: by David Berg and George Dougherty, P.O. Box 213, DeKalb, Ill. 60015. Thematic teaching unit: two filmstrips and two audio cassettes.

Signal 30: Safety Enterprises, producer; EdCom, distributor, 26991 Tungston Rd., Cleveland, Ohio 44132.

You See, I've Had a Life: by Ben Levin, Educational Film Library Association, 17 West 60th Street, New York, N.Y. 10023. Film: 16 mm. sound, b/w, 32 minutes.

CHAPTER 23

Books about death for children, young adults, and parents

SISTER MARY FRANCES LORETTA BERGER

Recently, while watching a baseball game on television, an Illinois boy found out that he had had bone cancer for 3 years. While visiting the boy's home, one of the players had said that he would try to hit a home run for him. In the next game he hit not only one but two. The announcer, not knowing all the circumstances of the boy's illness, said that the runs were for a boy who lay dying of bone cancer. This was the first time the lad knew of the cause of his illness. He immediately became angry and distrustful of his parents for not having faced up to and discussed his diagnosis with him. About 1 week later the boy was dead.

Statistics show that there are 300,000 new cases of terminal illness diagnosed in the United States each year. Suicide is the second highest cause of death among adolescents. Violent and accidental deaths of children are in the papers daily. Until very recently, society has tried to avoid frank discussions of death. Although today we find a resurgence of literature on death and persons wanting to discuss the topic intelligently and sympathetically, this vacuum has already caused serious psychologic problems among many young people and adults.

I have witnessed a variety of confrontations with death during the past several years. Two nephews, the oldest children of a large family, had fatal accidents within a 2-year period. Several students of the school in which I taught met with personal tragedies that affected the entire student population: shortly after graduation an eighth-grade boy committed suicide; leukemia, cancer, and a brain tumor caused the deaths of three other children. The sudden death of a young basketball coach and teacher resulted in some pronounced changes in the life-styles and attitudes of his students. Parents of some members of the student body died as a result of cancer, automobile accidents, and fire.

I have had considerable success in using literature as a vehicle for teaching moral and social values. With a desire to use such materials in a similar way to teach about death, I decided to search for texts that would be appropriate. As a result, a bibliography of books that treat the topic, either directly or indirectly, was developed for use by children, young adults, and parents.

A varied selection of books was chosen for inclusion in this chapter, because each reader's cognitive and psychologic limitations are different. Sometimes an adult may select a book for a child reader; at other times it would be more profitable for the reader to make his own selection. Regardless of the selection method, however, what transpires is that the reader works out his particular frustrations, anxieties, or other feelings in concert with the characters in the story. This process of interaction is called *bibliotherapy*.

Not all of the books listed are necessarily "good" literature. Some treat the topic beautifully and delicately; others use violence. Parents will not always approve of the choices made by their children, but forcing a child to read, or depriving a child of, a particular book may be harmful. Parents should, instead, strive to be open and receptive if their children want to discuss a book with them or their peers. Usually, this is the time of most fruitful reflection.

Because individual responses to death are so variable, it seemed helpful to categorize as many titles as possible under one or more of the five stages of dying outlined by Kübler-Ross: denial and isolation, anger, bargaining, depression, and acceptance. In addition, I have added the categories of fear and grief, and a final category, hope.

The bibliography is not all-inclusive. Nearly all of the books have been published since 1970. Titles recommended for the young child are preceded by an asterisk (*). Some books will appeal to all age groups.

Death is a problem that each person faces individually, and each reader will respond according to his needs and convictions. However, I hope that some of these titles will provoke many fears, false concepts, and other misunderstandings to be changed to freedoms that transcend death.

ANNOTATED BIBLIOGRAPHY
Fiction

Armstrong, William H. Sourland. New York: Harper & Row, 1971.
Moses Waters helps the Stone children come to an understanding of death, injustice, and dignity. Some in the community, blinded by prejudice, cannot tolerate the black teacher's goodness and so are ultimately responsible for his death.   *(Acceptance)*

Bartoli, Jennifer. Nonna. New York: Harvey House, 1975.
A family's response to the death of Nonna is touchingly told. The narrative, with its delicate illustrations, provides a sympathetic mood toward death for both the child and the adult.   *(Acceptance)*

Beckman, Gunnel. Admission to the Feast. New York: Holt, Rinehart and Winston, 1971.

With no sensitivity, a doctor bluntly informs his patient that she has leukemia. Frightened by the knowledge, the young girl flees from those she loves until she is calm. In her solitude she reminisces about the plateaus in her life and is strengthened by her reflections.

(Depression/Acceptance)

Beckman, Gunnel. That Early Spring. New York: Viking, 1977.

After the divorce of her parents, Mia suggests that her father invite Gran to live with them. The remaining time with Gran is short, but it is a tonic and comfort to Mia. The healthy association allows Mia to grow and accept her grandmother's death with maturity. *(Acceptance)*

Benchley, Nathaniel. A Necessary End. New York: Harper & Row, 1976.

Ralph Coffin keeps a diary after he becomes Seaman First Class during World War II. Accounts are not extraordinary, but the reader gets a flavor of life in the Pacific Fleet. His teacher is entrusted with his memoirs until he returns home. The diary becomes a memorial, for the ship hits a mine, and all are lost except one. *(Denial/Acceptance)*

Bond, Nancy. A String in the Harp. New York: Atheneum, 1977.

A mother's untimely death builds tensions in a loving family. The author, by weaving sixth century lore with twentieth century realism, resolves some of the problems. The family responds to the needs of one another. *(Denial/Anger/Acceptance)*

Bradbury, Bianca. I'm Vinny, I'm Me. Boston: Houghton Mifflin, 1977.

Vinny and her brother vow to stay together after the death of their mother. With the support of the community and their own resourcefulness, they prove that they can provide for and take care of themselves. Reflections on the death of each parent are thought-provoking.

(Acceptance)

Bridges, Sue Ellen. Home Before Dark. New York: Knopf, 1976.

Having never had roots, the mother of a migrant family fears a permanent home. Lightning takes her life, yet the reader feels that she is happier. Accustomed to tragedy, the family accepts the death without incident. *(Acceptance)*

Brown, Roy. Find Debbie. New York: Seabury, 1976.

The twin brother of a psychotic child realizes that some members of the family are very near the breaking point because of the child's tantrums. Secretly, he takes the girl out to the country where she had been cared for on previous occasions. Unfortunately, this time the caregiver puts the child to rest. *(Despair/Acceptance)*

Bulla, Clyde. The Beast of Lor. New York: Crowell, 1977.

This story takes place during the first Roman invasion of England. Lor lives in the forest with a woman he thinks is his grandmother until the neighbors declare her a witch. One night as they close in on her, Lor has to flee for his life. As he wanders he meets a wounded traveler who tells him about other lands and gives him a stone to wear that changes Lor's life. The dying message of the friend gives the boy new courage to live.   *(Hope)*

*Carrick, Carol. Accident. New York: Seabury, 1976.

Christopher's dog is accidently killed by a passing truck. After witnessing the incident, he pretends it was a dream. A perceptive father helps to ease the blow by accompanying the boy as he searches for a suitable marker.   *(Denial/Anger/Acceptance)*

Cleaver, Vera and Bill. Grover. Philadelphia: Lippincott, 1970.

Grover realizes that his mother is ill, but he is confused because no one will discuss her condition with him. When his mother commits suicide, the boy responds more maturely to the tragedy than his preoccupied father does. (This story emphasizes the need for communication.)

(Denial/Acceptance)

*Coerr, Eleanor. Sadako and a Thousand Paper Cranes. New York: Putnam, 1977.

Sadako was 2 when the atom bomb was dropped on Hiroshima. She had been a happy, active child who loved to run. Now, after one sprint, she is exhausted. She has leukemia. Eleanor Coerr tenderly unfolds how the child bargains with the gods for life and quietly accepts death. (Both children and adults benefit from reading this warm narrative.)

(Bargaining/Acceptance)

*Cohen, Barbara. Thank you, Jackie Robinson. New York: Lothrop, Lee & Shepard, 1974.

This is a compassionate story of 12-year-old fatherless Davy, whose life centers on baseball, especially the Brooklyn Dodgers and Jackie Robinson, even though he has never attended a game. Fortunately, his mother's new cook shares his enthusiasm and takes Davy to his first game. When a heart attack fells his friend, Davy manages to get an autographed ball from Jackie and the team before the old man dies.

(Acceptance)

Collier, James and Christopher. The Bloody Country. New York: Four Winds, 1976.

The treachery of war and land greed result in the loss of many lives during the Revolutionary War. The Buck family lose their mother and brother-in-law, yet they do not despair.   *(Fear/Acceptance)*

Cormier, Robert. I Am the Cheese. New York: Pantheon, 1977.

Adam Farmer stands alone, having lost both of his parents in a premeditated automobile accident. Events leading up to the "accident" are stark and frightening, because his father had given valuable information that led to the conviction of many in prominent places. Three years later the boy is trying to fill in the blanks as he is interrogated by a government agent.   (*Fear*)

*Coutant, Helen. The First Snow. New York: Knopf, 1974.

A young Vietnamese child does not understand the term "death" when she overhears her parents using it in conversation. When she asks what it is all about, her grandmother uses the first snow as the image to teach her a memorable lesson of life and death.   (*Acceptance*)

Craven, Margaret. I Heard the Owl Call My Name. New York: Doubleday, 1973.

Faith, compassion, and understanding of his people prepare a young minister to grasp the true meaning of life and death. Realizing that life will be short for him, he is prepared when the owl calls his name.

(*Acceptance*)

Crawford, Charles. Three-Legged Race. New York: Harper & Row, 1974.

The misery of being in the hospital is dispelled for three young people as their friendship grows. The time of separation is difficult for Kirk, because Brent is released and Amy dies.   (*Bargaining/Acceptance*)

Degens, T. Transport 7-41R. New York: Harper & Row, 1974.

Selfishness and greed are characteristic of most of the passengers on Transport 7-41R. Befriended by a young girl, an elderly gentleman manages to get his dying wife safely through to Cologne to fulfill her last wish: burial in her native land.   (*Acceptance*)

Dixon, Paige. May I Cross Your Golden River? New York: Atheneum, 1975.

Jordan is a vigorous young man who suddenly discovers that he has Lou Gehrig's disease. Courageously he battles the disease. Family members are concerned and caring yet resigned at the time of his death.   (*Acceptance*)

Donavan, John. Wild in the World. New York: Harper & Row, 1971.

This is an unusual tale in which every member of the family dies in a short period of time. The peace and serenity that prevail in the account help the reader accept this procession of deaths.   (*Acceptance*)

*Duncombe, Frances. Summer of the Burning. New York: Putnam, 1976.

Through a young girl's ingenuity, a family is kept together after the mother's death until the father is exchanged as a prisoner during the Revolutionary War.   (*Acceptance*)

Estes, Winston. Homefront. Philadelphia: Lippincott, 1976.

Here is a World War II story about the folks at home, specifically the

Holly family. Paul survives the battles in Europe, but his deaf-mute brother dies in a freak accident. *(Acceptance)*

*Farley, Carol. The Garden Is Doing Fine. New York: Atheneum, 1975. Denying that her father is terminally ill, Carrie fights a difficult battle. As she hears others speak glowingly of her father's loving kindness, Carrie concludes that she must allow his hopes and dreams to develop through her. *(Denial/Acceptance)*

Fassler, Joan. My Grandpa Died Today. New York: Human Sciences Press, 1971.

Grandpa knows that his days are drawing to a close. He counsels his grandson, David, that he is "not afraid to die because I know how to live." When death takes the old man a short time later, David is well prepared. *(Acceptance)*

Feagles, Anita MacRae. The Year the Dreams Came Back. New York: Atheneum, 1976.

After her mother's death, Nell hopes for closer ties with her father. Absorbed in his own sorrow, he ignores her needs until he finds someone who can bring joy to his life again. *(Isolation/Hope)*

Garden, Nancy. Loners. New York: Viking, 1972.

Paul is challenged to be his own person. Gramps seems to be the only one who can communicate with and support him until Jenny comes along. Then he is stripped of everything: Gramps dies, and Jenny wants another world. Finally Paul looks into himself. *(Hope)*

Greene, Constance. Beat the Turtle Drum. New York: Viking, 1977.

This book has a unique theme. Many books emphasize sibling rivalry; this one emphasizes affection. Unfortunately, the younger, most loved, meets with an accident resulting in instant death. Anger, depression, and consolation are emoted as various members of the family rebel at the untimely death. *(Anger/Depression/Hope)*

Guest, Judith. Ordinary People. New York: Viking, 1976.

Wrought with guilt over his brother's death, Conrad Jarrett attempts suicide. The mother, unable to accept the death of her older son, freezes emotionally toward the younger boy, further adding to his problem. Once Conrad understands that he cannot live in the shadow of his deceased brother, he is able to make a new start.

(Denial/Depression/Acceptance)

Guy, Rosa. The Friends. New York: Holt, Rinehart and Winston, 1973. Beginning life anew in a strange country is perplexing for Rosa. Her invalid mother dies, and the young girl is irreconcilable. Her older sister's patience and her father's determination enable Rosa to adjust, and eventually a more united family evolves. *(Depression)*

Hall, Lynn. Flowers of Anger. Chicago: Follett, 1976.

Grief and revenge are the major themes throughout this book. Ann refuses any consolation and so resorts to extreme actions after her horse is killed for trespassing on a neighbor's property.   *(Anger/Depression)*

Hall, Lynn. Sticks and Stones. Chicago: Follett, 1972.

Tom Naylor does not realize that he is the victim of vicious gossip until he is informed by the school principal that he cannot participate in the state music festival. Accusations that the boy is a homosexual cause the boy to react with anger, disbelief, and determination to prove the rumor false. Unfortunately, there is an accident in which Tom is injured and the instigator of the rumor is killed.   *(Hope)*

*Henry, Marguerite. A Pictorial Life Story of Misty. Chicago: Rand McNally, 1976.

Horse lovers will delight in this pictorial of Misty's life. The author completes the life cycle of the horse, yet her life will continue through her children, grandchildren, and great-grandchildren.   *(Acceptance)*

Hinton, S. E. That Was Then, This Is Now. New York: Viking, 1971.

This is a perceptive book dealing with the pressures of today's society. Two young friends are brought up as brothers after the death of Mark's parents. Together they share many of the trials and mistakes of adolescence. They witness an older friend's life being taken to protect them. Each seems to go his own way. Byron has a girl friend, and Mark gets involved with drugs. Byron is forced to make a decision. Should he inform authorities about Mark and his drug problem?

(Anger/Acceptance)

Holland, Isabelle. Alan and the Animal Kingdom. Philadelphia: Lippincott, 1977.

Preservation of his animals is uppermost in Alan's mind when he learns of his great-aunt's death. For the fifth time he is being uprooted from a home and losing his treasured animals to accommodate others.

(Isolation/Hope)

Holland, Isabelle. Of Love and Death and Other Journeys. Philadelphia: Lippincott, 1975.

Meg Grant's mother cannot fit into her husband's culture, so she leaves him before her daughter is born. Mother and daughter lead a casual life in Europe until the mother discovers that she has not long to live. Meg is introduced to her father for the first time. Shocked by the loss of her mother, the girl tries to isolate herself from others. However, she gains a new outlook on life as she helps the poor patients in her stepmother's clinic.   *(Isolation/Depression)*

Holland, Isabelle. The Man Without a Face. Philadelphia: Lippincott, 1972.

Home becomes intolerable for Chuck, even though he finds friendship for the first time with McLeod, his tutor. While Chuck is away at school, McLeod dies of a heart attack. All of his personal treasures are left to Chuck. (There is a hint of homosexuality in the novel, which the author handles discreetly.)   *(Hope)*

*Hunt, Irene. William. New York: Scribner's 1977.

Here is a memorable story of a courageous mother's resistance to the inroads of cancer as she prepares her three children to carry on after her death. For 4 years the young woman whom she befriends when in need keeps the family together.   *(Acceptance)*

Hunter, Mollie. Sound of Chariots. New York: Harper & Row, 1972.

Bridie McShane is close to her father. When word comes from the hospital that he is dead, she isolates herself in her grief. Reconciliation to his death is difficult until she perceives that death is not an end in itself, but a beginning. Her challenge is to live for him.

(Depression/Hope)

Hunter, Mollie. The Stronghold. New York: Harper & Row, 1974.

Coll is left crippled and orphaned following one of the many raids on his island home. He spends long hours formulating plans to barricade the island from further attack. Leadership rivalry develops, and the chief is ordered to sacrifice his daughter to the gods for the protection of the people. The special one, Coll's younger brother, sacrifices himself in her stead. (Characterizations are powerful.)   *(Hope)*

Jansson, Tove. The Summer Book. New York: Pantheon, 1974.

Seventy years separate Sophia and her grandmother, yet together they explore their Nordic archipelago. They reflect about the sea, weather, birds, plants, boats, death, and life. Sophia is educated for life and death by this companionship.   *(Acceptance)*

*Kantrowitz, Mildred. When Violet Died. New York: Parents, 1973.

When Violet dies, the children are not surprised, because she gave them warning. The children prepare for a simple burial service. They discuss the finality of death and one of them, Eva, discovers how to preserve life a bit longer.   *(Hope)*

*Kennedy, Richard. Come Again in the Spring. New York: Harper & Row, 1976.

An elderly man bargains with death as he proceeds to carry out the task of feeding the birds through the winter.   *(Bargaining)*

Kingman, Lee. Break a Leg, Betsy Maybe. Boston: Houghton Mifflin, 1976.

Betsy's parents are killed in an automobile accident. She must pick up life anew as she goes to live with an aunt and uncle. In her new surroundings she blossoms into a much-loved young lady.   *(Acceptance)*

*Klein, Norma. Confessions of an Only Child. New York: Pantheon, 1974.

A family of three console one another when the new baby dies. Each individual is sensitive to the moods of the others.   *(Acceptance)*

Klein, Norma. Sunshine. New York: Avon, 1971.

Jacquelyn Hilton fights for 18 months to keep alive. The young mother wants to leave something so that her infant daughter will have some idea of her mother's identity. Norma Klein weaves the recorded taped diary into a novel that bespeaks determination, resoluteness, and valor.

(Acceptance)

Lawrence, Louise. Sing and Scatter Daisies. New York: Harper & Row, 1977.

Nickey Hennessy is not a lovable young man at 17. He uses others, he is selfish, and he has many problems of his own making. Because of the influence of the spirit of John Hollis, Nickey begins to develop a mature attitude toward life. *(Acceptance)*

Lee, Mildred. Fog. New York: Dell, 1974.

This is a perceptive portrayal of a young man as he advances into adulthood. Ordinary events are described with clarity and precision. The pivotal point in the story is the tender and loving responses by the members of the family to one another after the sudden death of their father. *(Acceptance/Hope)*

***Lee, Virginia. The Magic Moth.** New York: Seabury, 1972.

This is an exceptional story depicting care, concern, and preparedness for the death of 10-year-old Marianne. The narrative tingles with love and devotion without sentimentality. *(Acceptance)*

Lorenzo, Carol Lee. Heart-of-Snowbird. New York: Harper & Row, 1975.

Laurel Ivy does not remember her real mother. When she is 14, her stepmother dies, shattering, at least for a time, her desire to become a dental hygienist. *(Acceptance)*

Lowry, Lois. A Summer to Die. Boston: Houghton Mifflin, 1977.

Compassion and love conquer jealousy when Meg is made aware of the illness of her older sister. Lowry writes with dexterity. Her characterizations are realistic, forceful, and lovable. The problems of life and death are skillfully developed. *(Acceptance)*

Lutters, Valerie A. The Haunting of Julie Unger. New York: Atheneum, 1977.

Hidden guilt prevents Julie Unger's acceptance of her father's death. Life becomes lonely and she is unlovable until she rids herself of her father's ghost. *(Anger/Denial)*

Mann, Peggy. There Are Two Kinds of Terrible. New York: Doubleday, 1977.

Robbie finds it difficult to accept the fact that his mother is going to die. Yet even more terrible is his father's withdrawal into his own world, leaving Robbie in utter isolation until the boy begins to understand his father's grief. *(Grief/Hope)*

Mathis, Sharon. Listen for the Fig Tree. New York: Viking, 1974.
Overcome by despair, the result of the brutal slaying of her husband on
Christmas Eve, Leola Johnson drowns out her sorrow with alcohol.
Though blind, her 16-year-old daughter struggles to manage the
apartment and tries to help her mother cope with her many problems.
(Despair/Acceptance)

Mathis, Sharon. Teacup Full of Roses. New York: Viking, 1972.
Pride in the eldest son obscures Mattie Brooks's recognition of the
achievements of the two younger boys and the weakness of the oldest
son. However, realizing the talent of his younger brother, Joe tries to
make provision for him. Some money is stolen, Davy is killed in trying
to retrieve it, and Joe decides that perhaps Davy is better off without the
problems of the world.   *(Hope)*

Mazer, Norma Fox. A Figure of Speech. New York: Delacorte, 1973.
Jenny is the only one who cares for her grandfather. When the young
girl discovers that her parents plan to place him in a nursing home, she
steals away with him to his boyhood home. Exhausted by the trip, the
old man dies. Jenny is upset by the callousness of her family and
friends as they refer to the old gentleman.   *(Denial)*

McCaffrey, Anne. Dragonsong. New York: Atheneum, 1976.
This is a stimulating narrative based on a young girl's love of and competence in music, which were instilled in her by the old Harper. No girl
ever had this privilege before, and when the old Harper dies, the girl
labors under great difficulty and suspicion while trying to maintain the
musical traditions of her people.   *(Hope)*

*Miles, Miska. Annie and the Old One. Boston: Little, Brown, 1971.
A Navajo grandmother forewarns her family that her life is ending.
Annie tries to hamper the approach of death, but the Old One counsels
her that this cannot be done.   *(Denial/Acceptance)*

Mohr, Nicholasa. El Bronz Remembered. New York: Harper & Row,
1975.
This is a collection of twelve stories about Puerto Rican Americans living in the Bronx. Some depict the harsh realities that these people are
forced to face throughout life.   *(Acceptance)*

Mohr, Nicholasa. Nilda. New York: Harper & Row, 1973.
Life in the Puerto Rican barrio of New York City is a painful experience
for Nilda Ramirez. Her mother is determined to raise her family with
dignity but burns herself out in the attempt. Her final admonition to
Nilda is "hold on to your creative gift." As life goes on, the girl begins to
understand her mother's advice.   *(Acceptance)*

Moody, Anne. Mr. Death: Four Stories. New York: Harper & Row,
1975.

These four stories are grim yet meaningful for the special reader accustomed to some of the legends among blacks in the South. As grim as the stories are, however, death is intertwined with love.

(Fear/Acceptance)

Morgan, Alison. Ruth Crane. New York: Harper & Row, 1974.
Responsibilities are suddenly forced upon Ruth Crane when her father is killed and her mother and sister are seriously injured in an automobile accident. Because the father was cold and austere, his death does not seem to move the children. With fear and trepidation, Ruth plunges into the household duties until her mother is released from the hospital. *(Acceptance)*

O'Dell, Scott. Child of Fire. Boston: Houghton Mifflin, 1974.
A probation officer shows that he has a personal interest in his charges. Among them is Manuel Castillo, whom the officer tries to rehabilitate. Manuel, however, is an activist, and when he realizes what is happening to the farm laborers in the valley, he protests the use of a new machine. It is this machine that takes the young boy's life.

(Bargaining)

O'Dell, Scott. Zia. Boston: Houghton Mifflin, 1976.
In the Island of the Blue Dolphins, Karana is accidentally left behind as the members of her tribe seek safety on a ship. For 25 years she lives alone except for her dog until she is rescued by a small craft and brought to a mission. While in the company of others, she is lonely, because she is not accustomed to living in such surroundings. Karana contracts a bad cold and dies, but this experience gives her niece new hope, new courage, new life. *(Hope)*

Orgel, Doris. The Mulberry Music. New York: Harper & Row, 1971.
Doris Orgel writes sympathetically about a young child coming to grips with her devoted grandmother's illness and possible death. The child's parents are aware of the child's need to talk about her grandmother. Wisely, they allow the child to have a decisive role in preparing a suitable funeral service for the unusual Grandma Liza. *(Acceptance)*

Paterson, Katherine. Bridge to Terabithia. New York: Crowell, 1977.
Jess Aarons has an intense desire to prove himself among his peers by being the fastest runner in the group. Unfortunately, he and all the other boys are defeated by Leslie Burke, an unusual girl, who has just moved to the area. A wholesome friendship develops between Jess and Leslie, enabling both to enjoy and become enriched by their surroundings until tragedy strikes. *(Acceptance)*

Peck, Richard. A Day No Pigs Would Die. New York: Knopf, 1972.
A Shaker father is aware that he will soon die. He instructs his young son about his responsibilities as head of the family. After he finds his

father dead on his round of chores, the boy stoically announces to the family that on this day "no pigs will die."   *(Acceptance)*

Peck, Richard. Dreamland Lake. New York: Avon, 1974.
Death haunts Brian Bishop. After he and Flip find a dead man in the weeds at Dreamland Lake, his days and nights are filled with horror. Life becomes more complicated when he faces death again. Each new experience is more than he is able to handle successfully.   *(Fear)*

Platt, Kin. Hey, Dummy. Philadelphia: Chilton, 1971.
This is a sensitive yet harsh story of Neil Comstock's endeavors to befriend brain-damaged Alan. Suspected of beating a little girl, Alan is sought by a frenzied mob, and Neil tries to hide him. They are mistaken for prowlers behind a supermarket. Alan is killed, and Neil rejects the normal world.   *(Denial/Isolation)*

Rabe, Bernice. Naomi. New York: Nelson, 1975.
Naomi needs reassurance that she is going to live. Daringly, she visits a fortune teller, who reluctantly reveals that the child will die within 2 years. Fear of death permeates the story until Naomi safely reaches her fourteenth birthday.   *(Fear)*

Rabin, Gil. Changes. New York: Harper & Row, 1973.
Chris's father dies, and the family is forced to move from Aberdeen, South Dakota to New York. Shortly after their arrival, Chris's grandfather becomes blind, and Chris's mother is forced to place her father in a rest home. The old man's deterioration is swift, and Chris is not able to watch the living death. Conflicting feelings and his grandfather's death are difficult for the young boy.   *(Denial)*

Rinaldo, C. L. Dark Dreams. New York: Harper & Row, 1974.
A young boy continues to dream about his dead mother until he is befriended by a sympathetic man. He learns to ease these fears when he has to deal with the fact that his friend also is going to die.   *(Fear/Hope)*

*Rock, Gail. The Thanksgiving Treasure. New York: Knopf, 1974.
Determined to make a friend out of her father's enemy, Addie Mills offers to take care of the old man's horse. Her concern mellows the gentleman to a degree and brings peace to him in death.   *(Isolation/Hope)*

Rushing, Jane Gilmore. Mary Dove. New York: Avon, 1975.
A young girl loses her father in a spring storm. He is the only human being whom she remembers. Resourceful, she saves her food, finds shelter for the remaining animals, and plans for a new season. Unexpectedly, a cattle man discovers her, the only man she has seen other than her father. She experiences love, joy, pain, hatred, and contempt as she comes in contact with other human beings.   *(Acceptance)*

Samuels, Gertrude. Run, Shelley, Run. New York: Crowell, 1974.
Labeled a person in need of supervision, Shelley is confined to a deten-

tion home. In her third attempt to run away, she is accompanied by Deedee. Shelley is discovered; Deedee finds the pressures too great and takes her own life. Shelley, grief-stricken, reacts violently and is placed in confinement. A judge visits the institution. Appalled by the conditions she finds there, she endeavors to remedy the situation immediately. Shelley is given a new lease on life.   (*Despair/Anger*)

Scoppettone, Sandra. Trying Hard to Hear You. New York: Harper & Row, 1974.

Camilla Crawford has a summer of learning. Her best friend, Jeff, and the boy she thought she loved become involved with one another. Friends in their group have great difficulty in coping with the relationship between the boys. Confusion, anger, disappointment, harassment, and death are a part of the summer experience. (A sensitive treatment of homosexuality is depicted here.)   (*Anger/Acceptance*)

*Slote, Alfred. Hang Tough, Paul Mather. Philadelphia: Lippincott, 1973.

Paul Mather loves baseball and excels at the game. But he has a greater game to play—a battle with leukemia. In this first person narrative are revealed the courage of a boy and the pangs of a family watching his life being snuffed out.   (*Acceptance*)

Smith, Doris Buchanan. A Taste of Blackberries. New York: Crowell, 1973.

A touching story of the emotional trauma that a young boy experiences when he realizes that his best friend is dead. Even more important is the concern he has for his friend's family as they mourn their loss. (Excellent for adults as well as children.)   (*Hope*)

Stolz, Mary. By the Highway Home. New York: Harper & Row, 1971.

Catty is the only one in her family who is willing to talk about her brother's death. She is aware of her family's tension and feels that if only they would discuss the event openly, the hurt would ease. Other unfortunate circumstances eventually bring the family closer together. They are finally able to talk about the fun-loving son and brother who is gone.   (*Denial/Acceptance*)

Stolz, Mary. The Edge of Next Year. New York: Harper & Row, 1974.

An automobile accident takes the life of the mother of two young boys. Guilt causes the father to resort to drinking. He ignores his responsibility toward the sons until one day he is completely inept. The older boy, who has assumed responsibility, leaves a condemning note for the father, which brings him to an awareness of the need for change.

          (*Isolation/Despair*)

Taylor, Mildred. Roll of Thunder Hear My Cry. New York: Dial, 1976.

A highly motivated black family is forced to make many adjustments during the depression of the thirties. Although they are subject to bitter prejudice, they are determined to remain independent as they witness unscrupulous killing and destruction of property because of greed and ambition.   *(Hope)*

Taylor, Theodore. Teetoncey. New York: Doubleday, 1974.
The banks of North Carolina are considered the Atlantic graveyard. Ships are crushed by storms off the shores. Sometimes there are survivors; other times not. Members of families are lost in trying to save others. In the O'Neal family, the father and son are lost, leaving Mrs. O'Neal with an utter contempt for the sea. New life brightens the home when Ben finds a young girl washed up on the shore and brings her home for his mother to care for.   *(Fear)*

Thiele, Colin. Fire in the Stone. New York: Harper & Row, 1974.
Ernie Ryan works hard trying to provide for himself in the open fields of Australia. He finds a precious opal and then is robbed of his claim. In trying to retrieve his property, he loses his best friend in an explosion. He then decides to leave the frontier with the knowledge that man must struggle against nature, but even more difficult is the struggle against himself.   *(Despair)*

*Viorst, Judith. The Tenth Good Thing About Barney. New York: Atheneum, 1971.
To help soften the heartaches caused by the loss of a cat, a young boy's mother suggests that he think of ten good things about Barney. The boy is stumped after number nine until he helps his father plant some seeds. Then, realizing that death can bring new life, he has the tenth good thing about Barney.   *(Hope)*

Walsh, Jill Paton. Unleaving. New York: Farrar, Straus & Giroux, 1976.
Here is a complex book about many deaths; one is peaceful and two others are tragic. The atmosphere is eerie, and characterizations are strong as death affects different personalities.   *(Acceptance/Fear)*

Wersba, Barbara. Run Softly, Go Fast. New York: Atheneum, 1970.
Searching for his real self, Davy recalls, step by step, his relationship with his father. As a young boy it was love and admiration; as he grew older it was revulsion. The father's death forces him to face the fact that "each wanted the other to live in the image of their making."   *(Anger)*

*Whitehead, Ruth. The Mother Tree. New York: Seabury, 1971.
Pneumonia takes the mother of the Foster family when Tempe is 11 years old. This places many burdens on the young girl, the heaviest being the effects of the mother's death on 4-year-old Laurie, who is still waiting for her mother's return. Although the family finds this disturbing, they patiently allow nature to heal the wounds.   *(Denial)*

Wilkinson, Brenda. Ludell and Willie. New York: Harper & Row, 1977.

Ludell lives with her grandmother, whom she calls "Mama," from infancy until her senior year in high school when Mama dies from exhaustion and overwork. Without any thought of Ludell's feelings or desires, Dessa, her flighty, unstable mother, demands that Ludell begin life anew in New York.   *(Acceptance/Hope)*

Windsor, Patricia. The Summer Before. New York: Harper & Row, 1974.

Alexandria meets with social disapproval because her constant companion is a boy. When he is killed, she loses the only person she ever loved. Psychologic adjustments are difficult until she is able to help herself.   *(Fear)*

Wojcieshowska, Maia. Don't Play Dead Before You Have to. New York: Harper & Row, 1970.

Five-year-old Charlie has been living an overly protected life. Byron wants to help him. While the younger boy is away at school, the older boy writes about his experiences with the patients in the hospital. Byron matures during this process as he gains an understanding of death, and more important, of what it means to live.   *(Acceptance)*

Woodford, Peggy. Please Don't Go. New York: Dutton, 1973.

Mary Meredith gains confidence and introspection as she shares two summers with a family in France. After the sudden death of a young friend, she is aware that "the essential factor that makes life beautiful and significant is death."   *(Acceptance)*

Woods, George. Catch a Killer. New York: Harper & Row, 1972.

This book probes the theme of man's inhumanity to man—in this case, the cruelty of the group toward one individual. The victim is forced to run constantly because of the indignities he undergoes. This results in his taking the life of another and falling to his own death. (This book might awaken the sensitivities of some young people to the dangers of the pressures that they place on their peers.)   *(Fear)*

Zindel, Paul. Pardon Me, You're Stepping on My Eyeballs. New York: Harper & Row, 1976.

Marsh has not been able to admit to himself that his father is dead. Edna, his friend from the therapy group at school, helps him to face up to his problem. (Some of the bizarre activities that take place could have been omitted without affecting the message of the story.)   *(Denial)*

Zolotow, Charlotte. My Grandson Lew. New York: Harper & Row, 1974.

Lew misses his grandpa and often has pleasant dreams about him. One day he confides all of this to his mother. She is amazed, because grandpa has been dead for 4 years. Lew had not been told of the grand-father's death, and had been waiting for his return. Now mother and child are able to share the loss and thus lessen their loneliness.

(Acceptance)

Nonfiction

Anonymous. Go Ask Alice. Engelwood Cliffs, N. J.: Prentice-Hall, 1971.

A 15-year-old girl records in her diary her experience with drugs. Peer pressure is the most disturbing element of this book. Alice seems to realize what is happening to her, and tries to pull away, only to be mysteriously dragged down again. What is it that caused her to take her life? Was it fear of the group? Did she really take her life?

(Despair)

Bernstein, E. Joanne. Loss and How to Cope With It. New York: Sea-bury, 1977.

This book is written especially for the young reader. Reflections are current and meaningful. The book also contains a current bibliography of both fiction and nonfiction titles plus a listing of nonprint materials that are available commercially. This is currently one of the most valu-able books published on the topic of death because of its simplicity and practicality.

Carr, Austin C., and others. Grief: Selected Readings. New York: Health Sciences, 1973.

Among the readings included in this text is "Grief in Childhood." The article is technical and uses psychologic jargon, but it might be of in-terest to a limited audience.

Cook, Sarah Sheets. Children and Dying. New York: Health Sci-ences, 1973.

Here is an explanation and selected bibliography of a child's perception of death. The essays are compatible with current thinking; however, the bibliography is dated.

Friedman, Marcia. Story of Josh. New York: Praeger, 1974.

"Josh had a great sense of self-value, a great desire to live." Yet in his twenty-first year, he began his struggle with a brain tumor. The young man's mother narrates his story from the discovery of the disease until his death, using the tapes that Josh made as he bravely fought the rav-ages of the illness. *(Fear/Acceptance)*

Grollman, Earl. Explaining Death to Children. New York: Beacon, 1967.

The author provides a series of thought-provoking readings by au-thorities well versed in their field. Included in the readings are theological approaches to death by a number of religious groups and ways to handle death in a school environment. A bibliography on death is also included; however, more current lists are available on this subject.

Grollman, Earl. Talking about Death: A Dialogue between Parent and Child. New York: Beacon, 1976.

Here the author uses a sensitively illustrated discussion about death for parent and child. Vivid examples are cited to highlight various attitudes toward death. Also included is a working bibliography of organizations, books, tapes, and films that can be used as further sources of information.

Hendin, David. Death as a Fact of Life. New York: Norton, 1973.

The author's experience as a medical journalist adds to the clearness of his presentation. The chapter "Children and Death" is practical and provides concrete examples of how parents can deal with the topic of death with their children.

Irish, Jerry A. A Boy Thirteen. Philadelphia: Westminister, 1975.

Here is a reflective response to the death of a vibrant young boy by his father, mother, and younger brother. Two deaths within 4 years cause a father to cry out with anger and loneliness. The father movingly explains how he found "Death to be utterly unacceptable, in anger; how he knew complete abandonment, in aloneness; and how he discovered an occasion to love, in freedom."   (*Anger/Acceptance/Hope*)

Klagsburn, Francine. Too Young to Die: Youth and Suicide. New York: Houghton Mifflin, 1976.

Suicide rates in the United States continue to rise each year. Klagsburn provides a survey of why teenagers commit suicide and what can be done about it. Young people who have attempted suicide are interviewed, furnishing the reader with a picture of the mental attitude of the survivors as well as of those who influence their lives. Information about crisis centers and professional treatment is also included, making this a valuable resource.

*Klein, Stanley. The Final Mystery. New York: Doubleday, 1974.

Stanley Klein discusses many facets of death in simple language that can be readily used with a mature child or young adult.

Kollar, Nathan R. Death and Other Living Things. Dayton: Pflaum/Standard, 1973.

The theologic emphasis here is Roman Catholic; however, the message is acceptable to any Christian denomination. The chapter "Preparing the Children" is worthwhile.

Krant, Melvin J. Dying and Dignity. Springfield, Ill.: Charles C Thomas, 1974.

Scholarly but not technical, this book includes two chapters that are especially pertinent in dealing with the child and death: "Families of the Dying" and "Some Proposals for Education."

Kübler-Ross, Elisabeth. Death: The Final Stage of Growth. New York: Prentice-Hall, 1975.

The examples and case studies presented provide the reader with many thought-provoking and consoling reflections by persons whose lives grew as death approached.

Landau, Elaine. Death's Everyone's Heritage. New York: Messner, 1976.

Landau begins her book with a basic message on death. The book's strength lies in the author's sensitive awareness of the reactions of those who know that death is imminent and the responses of their families.

Langone, John. Death Is a Noun. Boston: Little, Brown, 1972.

Langone helps the reader form an intelligent approach to death. Topics such as euthanasia, abortion, murder, suicide, and immortality are discussed, leaving the reader to form his own conclusions about morality and ethics. The chapter, "Facing Death," brings to the forefront a critical issue.

Langone, John. Vital Signs. Boston: Little, Brown, 1974.

The author states in his introduction that he believes that terminally ill patients should serve as teachers. Talking and listening to and taking an interest in these patients provide fruitful experiences for many.

L'Engle, Madeleine. The Summer of the Great-Grandmother. New York: Farrar-Straus, 1974.

This is a beautiful family response to the final days of mother and grandmother. The family ties grow firmer as they observe the gentle slipping away of the old woman. When death does come, they all share in the satisfaction that their caring has strengthened their bond of love.

(Hope)

LeShan, Eda. Learning to Say Good-By—When a Parent Dies. New York: Macmillan, 1976.

The accounts presented in the book deal with children's experiences with death that will benefit the reader. The adult reader learns how to work intelligently with a child who has suffered the loss of a loved one. Adults who have been emotionally damaged by death when young are given insights into ways of dealing with their problem.   *(Hope)*

Lifton, Robert J., and Olson, Eric. Living and Dying. New York: Praeger, 1974.

The authors point out that the acceptability of death depends on the psychologic context in which it occurs. The reader is made aware of the shifts in historical and cultural attitudes that have had a profound effect on how man perceives the future. The book is for mature readers and is extremely helpful for those who instruct young adults.

(Hope)

Lund, Doris. Eric. Philadelphia: Lippincott, 1974.

A mother relates how her 17-year-old son battled with leukemia for 4 years. With courage and tenacity the boy does not give in to the disease but enrolls in college, plays on the soccer team, has many trips to the hospital between remissions, consoles and brings joy to other patients, falls in love, and fights for his life to the end. *(Acceptance)*

Mannes, Marya. Last Rights. New York: Morrow, 1974.

Marya Mannes' message is that every human being should be able to choose his manner of dying with dignity. She talks with many who are facing death, relatives of the dying, and those who care for them, challenging society's approach to age and death.

Miller, Randolph Crump. Live Until You Die. Philadelphia: United Church Press, 1973.

A renowned religious educator, Miller stresses the concept of death education by providing timely reflection on various aspects of death.

Morris, Jeanne. Brian Piccolo: A Short Season. Chicago: Rand McNally, 1971.

Courage, determination, and trust are evidenced throughout Brian Piccolo's bout with cancer. Suffering does not dampen the spirits of this resolute young football player; he is a source of inspiration.

(Acceptance)

Pringle, Laurence. Death Is Natural. New York: Four Winds, 1977.

Here is an informative description about the death of many living things. An underlying theme is the fact that death is necessary for new life.

Read, Piers Paul. Alive. Philadelphia: Lippincott, 1974.

Read lets the story of the survivors of a plane crash in the Andes unfold as simply as he can. He tells the story as it was, without emotionalism or heroics. The message is inspiring.

Schoenberg, Bernard, and others, editors. Anticipatory Grief. New York: Columbia University, 1974.

High-quality readings on anticipatory grief make up this unique book. Chapters of particular interest to those dealing with the child and death are those on introductory concepts and childhood illness.

Snow, Lois Wheeler. A Death with Dignity. New York: Random House, 1974.

When the Chinese come, they bring a new concept of life and death to the Snow family. Their philosophy of "total care" puts the Western world to shame. Death is no longer feared by the family but instead becomes a reminder to change the "loneliness, the selfishness that distort the potential worth of all men's lives."   *(Acceptance/Hope)*

Vogel, Linda Jane. Helping a Child Understand Death. Philadelphia: Fortress, 1975.

Linda Vogel offers practical help for the parent who is looking for ways to handle the problem of death with children. Her theory for good mental stability includes understanding the child and permitting him or her to work through particular emotions. A short but useful bibliography is included in the text.

Wolfenstein, Martha. Children and the Death of a President. Glouster: Peter Smith, 1969.

The research done after the assassination of President Kennedy offers many excellent suggestions on how to deal with the subject of death with children. Case studies, statistics, and conclusions of the team of researchers point out the great need for a change of attitude toward death.

EPILOGUE TO THE LOSS OF A CHILD

STANFORD B. FRIEDMAN

There is no end.

In this book, the "professionals" discuss such issues as the "acute grief reaction," "mourning," "normal versus abnormal grief," "adjustment to loss," "psychological sequelae to the death of a child," "grief counseling and grief counselors," "mental health intervention," and "support systems." Have we professionals developed such categories to promote the development of a scientific approach to death? Or a systematic clinical way of looking at the death of the child? Or to psychologically protect ourselves for our own death? Or to further our own careers?

To be psychologically naked among the clothed is frightening. Yet that is the essence of the next two sections. Two individuals, Lori and Carolyn Szybist, share their thoughts and feelings. This is the Epilogue of this book. The loss of a child—in this case an infant dying of sudden infant death syndrome—cannot be compartmentalized or divided into convenient time periods. The Epilogue is a plea to listen, to realize there is no "period of grief." Rather the loss of a child may cross generations.

In the Szybist family there is a husband (Tony) and a wife (Carolyn), a 14-year-old daughter (Lori) and an 8-year-old son (Gerald Patrick). *And* Larry, who died at 3 months of age—12 years ago.

We do not know the long-term effects to a family experiencing the loss of a child. Because of the absence of data, there has been, therefore, much opportunity to speculate. Psychological and emotional problems, alcoholism, divorce, physical illness, and other "detrimental" effects on parents have been attributed to the death of a child. However, others have suggested that such a tragedy strengthens a family. Still others believe the grief process, when "complete," allows the family to resume their "normal lives."

Lori and Carolyn Szybist, as a surviving sibling and a mother, give us enough of a glimpse into their lives to indicate clearly that the death of a child becomes an integral part of them—forever.

279

THOUGHTS OF A SISTER

LORRAINE ANNE SZYBIST

In 1965, during the spring before my second birthday, my brother, Lawrence Anthony, was born. My mother tells me that I was fascinated by him and called him my sister. She tells me lots of funny stories about my floating cookies in his bathtub, wanting him to play with me and my toys, and trying to take care of him for her. My mother also tells me that this was a happy time for our family, even when my brother and I both decided to cry at the same time. The pictures in our family album are those of a pretty, dark-haired baby that looked like my dad.

I don't remember my brother Larry very well. On a cool summer morning, just before he was 3 months old, we woke up to find that he had died during the night in his sleep. He died with no warning, no sounds, no signs of being sick. We hadn't expected him to die. Our doctor had seen him 6 days before and thought he was a beautiful baby.

I was too young then to remember much about the morning that my brother was found dead. My mother tells me that it was unreal, even in her memories. She told me about the neighbors who took me to their house while my parents were with my brother when he was pronounced dead at the same hospital where he was born. She told me that an autopsy was done and they couldn't find anything that caused him to die. She told me about the funeral and the tiny grave in the cemetery. I don't remember the sadness exactly, but my mother tells me that after that day, I never again would play with dolls the size of a baby.

My brother was a victim of crib death. Since 1969, it has been called sudden infant death syndrome (SIDS). Finally, in 1973, it was accepted as a disease process by the International Classification of Diseases. No one knows why it happens. Even today it is a disease that is called "unpredictable" and "unpreventable"; no cause or cure is known. It is the leading cause of death in infants after the first week of life. Most of all, sudden infant death syndrome is a disease that takes the lives of 8,000 brothers and sisters of kids like me every year in the United States alone.

I am 14 years old now, and it's been a long time since my brother died. But in lots of ways I still think about him a lot. The problem is that, except for my mom, no one wants to talk about it. When I ask questions,

280

it makes them feel bad, which makes me feel bad that I asked. He was *my* brother, and I want to know what happened and how people felt. I get curious about it sometimes.

I have read a lot of information about SIDS, but what bothers me is that no one knows for sure what causes it. You'd think someone would have come up with an answer by now. My grandmother says that "God" took him away. Did He? Why would He just take anyone away? I can't accept that. It seems so easy to tell people that there was nothing they could have done, but what if there was? And what if it had been me taking care of a baby? That's one of the things I think about. I have a dream that I will someday be the one who finds the cure for SIDS, and then it will all be over.

Most of my friends babysit. I usually don't, especially if the people have a small baby. One of the first things I think about is what would happen if the baby died while I was watching it? It could happen. I know that lots of other things could happen, but they don't bother me. I don't think about the other things. My aunt has two little girls. When they were babies I used to think about them dying of SIDS. I like it better now that they are older.

When you think about it, crib death is scary.

Death is scary, too. Sometimes when I think about my brother who died, I think about other people dying. It's easier to think about someone else dying. I don't like to think of me dying; it makes me feel trembly. It's sort of like crib death. No one knows for sure, so that's why it's scary. I read some of the newspaper stories about death. There don't seem to be any experts or anybody who really knows. I get interested in the stories about the people who died and were brought back to life. One day in religion class at school we talked about death. It wasn't so scary when we all talked about how we felt, and we all felt uneasy. It was an interesting class. It's funny, though, how I can talk about death except when it concerns me. I wonder what really happens.

I have tried to talk about my brother's death with other people. My grandmother gets upset and sounds as if she's going to cry, even now. What she remembers is his smile, and then she wonders why God took him away. My dad doesn't talk about it at all. I've tried to ask him questions, but I can tell he doesn't want to think about it. My dad was with me and my brother when my brother died, and I think that still bothers him. My mom is the only one I can talk to about my brother. She listens and tells me how she feels, too. I'm glad that someone will talk to me about it and feel that what I have to say is important. I think that's good, because I also need someone to talk to sometimes. When we talk about how I reacted, it seems as if we are talking about another person entirely. It's strange to imagine that it really all happened. My mom told me that she didn't take me to the funeral. I don't remember that, but it makes me mad now to think that they left me home with someone else. It sometimes amazes me how freely my mom can talk to me about my brother when I ask. I'm glad that she can. But I've also noticed something else. Every year around the time of my brother's birthday, my mom gets weird. I don't know how else to explain it, but I know she must think about him a lot then. And it was so long ago! She doesn't cry, it's just something that I feel must be happening to her. That bothers me a lot.

I have a brother who was born after Larry died. He's 8 years old, and if someone mentions Larry to him, he gets upset. That puzzles me because he wasn't even alive when Larry died. I wonder if he acts upset because he really is or if he feels he should be upset. When we get mad at each other and fight, sometimes I tell him that I wish that he had died instead of Larry. That makes him even madder. Sometimes he tells me that he wishes I were dead. Neither one of us means it, and maybe if we hadn't lost a brother, we would say those kinds of things to each other and they wouldn't mean anything. I don't know.

Someone asked me if the fact that I had a brother who died had changed my life or the life of my family. I'm sure that in some ways it did. My mother spends a lot of time with SIDS, and I know a lot about it. I have met a lot of people who have lost babies to SIDS, and most of them are really nice people. I sometimes get angry that people can't talk to each other and that there is no cure for SIDS. Maybe if my brother hadn't died, I wouldn't be afraid to babysit. And maybe if my brother hadn't died, we wouldn't have the brother I have now, and I wouldn't like that. I think that maybe there were some good things, though. We all care about each other a lot. Maybe we would have done that anyway. Mostly when I think about my brother, what I really feel is that something is missing.

THOUGHTS OF A MOTHER

CAROLYN SZYBIST

I am the parent of a child who has died. The real significance of that fact is that it took me so long to come to terms with the ultimate reality of it, to accept that which is true. You don't get over the loss of a child. You don't replace him. Grief will surface unexpectedly, softer at the edges with the passage of time, but grief nonetheless. Like many of the components of each of our lives, the death of a child is something that finally you incorporate into yourself. Instead of waking up one morning being healed from your grief, you learn to live with it.

There is no easy way to lose a child. There is no disease or event that is preferable, and no age or point in time that makes a difference. Although parents who lose children may frequently empathize with others and say things like, "I'm glad that didn't happen to me," we usually mean, "I'm glad that didn't happen to me in addition to what did." As time passes, we feel an almost universal kinship with anyone who has lost a child and have a strong sense that of all our grief experiences, the death of a child is the most difficult. We all have the conception that in the scheme of things, parents are *not* supposed to outlive their children.

I am a different person from the young woman I was just before my child died. I don't feel changed in a radical sense, but I am changed. It's sometimes difficult to relate to that person: to the youth, invincibility, and near simplicity. Sometimes I have difficulty remembering that young woman who was the mother of two children, a daughter nearly 2 and a son aged 3 months, a person who could resent the moments when everybody was cranky and hungry at once and sleep seemed a remote experience, and a person who also reveled in the joys and experiences of motherhood. Tucked into those days were the joys and strains of a young marriage as my husband and I adapted and attempted to grow: the children and the two of us, completing educational goals and beginning professional careers. It was a good time, laced with all the happiness and minor dissensions that are part of living.

And in one hellish moment, all of that changed. Changed as swiftly as if a bomb had been dropped into the core of our lives. Changed on a bright, sunny summer morning when I picked up the rigid, lifeless, distorted body of our young son. Changed as swiftly as he must have died. Part of the hell was the fact that his death was not expected. Part of the hell was the fact that the year was 1965 and his death from crib death was a phenomenon not well understood, especially by me, his mother, who as a nurse took pride in some knowledge of disease. Most of the hell came simply from the fact that he was dead and from all the events that followed because he was dead.

I'm grateful for the haziness that enveloped me from the beginning of that terrible moment. The attempts by my husband to resuscitate the tiny little body, and my own rejection of the deadness of him. After that first moment of discovery, my inability to touch him. The horrendous anger of my husband (that was shared with me later), that while he tried to revive our son, what he wanted to do was hurl his body across the room as if to deny that the cold body could have ever held the personality of his son. The silly decisions that come with what to do with the young daughter, confined to her own crib, who is baffled by the madness of her parents. The wild dash to the hospital emergency room, the irrevocable pronouncement of death, the shared disbelief of the physician who had brought this child into the world and cared for him in those early days. The convergence of relatives from across the country interspersed with autopsy reports and questions, asked and unasked. The image of the distorted face of my son's body from the mottled blueness of death, an image eased somewhat by the dressed and made-up body in the tiny white casket. And the pain that came from deep inside my chest and radiated relentlessly to every part of my body. The inability to eat or sleep, and the insane ability to talk to people about things I didn't care about. I know I smiled at the funeral, thanked people for coming, laughed about the population explosion that we would participate in, as if another baby would make things right. I also know that I wasn't really there. I performed as carefully as a well-rehearsed script, except that the performance was staged in unreality, done to ease the pain of others but done mostly because it really wasn't happening and tomorrow I could wake up to my two children and only think of the nightmare I must be dreaming.

The first twinges of reality came the evening of his funeral, came with the onset of a thunderstorm and the realness that my son was out in the rain, sleeping in a small grave among other children. I had never left a child in the rain before and the franticness of that reality was a reality in itself. The haziness was comfort; reality was sheer terror.

There is discomfort in looking back and remembering the endless days that followed the funeral. The discomfort comes from the human desire to acknowledge the fragility of others, but not of ourselves. They were days that passed for living. And days when other events were irrevocably locked into the kind of living that we did. The sudden death of my husband's 22-year-old male cousin from unclear causes came 3 weeks after my son's death. The fact that we shared the same last name brought with it my own thoughts that we were locked into a bizarre twist of fate where all the members of our family would die. I checked sleeping people in our household with the regularity of an intensive care facility and felt singularly responsible for their ability to breathe.

I became the perfect, overprotective, smothering, all-consuming parent to my young daughter. I was afraid to let her from my sight but also afraid to accept the responsibility for her care. It was a time of decisionless decisions. I was her constant companion and playmate. I needed others to help with her care, but resented their helpfulness. I marvel that either of us survived those early months when her life was changed from the patterns that she knew. And again the jolts of reality among the haze. The jolt that came with the Christmas that followed the foggy months of summer and fall and the present to my daughter, gaily wrapped and delivered with affection by a caring relative. A present torn from its wrappings with the toddler fingers to discover under the lid of the box a life-size baby doll. A present greeted with screams of pain and attempts to cover and rewrap it with the shreds of paper. And the attempts to hide from her sight what jolted us all: the return of the baby brother whose swift departure had never been acknowledged or shared with her. The sobs that finally resulted in sleep said much about our own denial that our child had died.

Denial comes in many ways. It sits beneath the surface of our statements of truth. I wanted another baby, and I was terrified of having one. It disrupted my relationship with my husband in many subtle ways. We talked, but we didn't talk. We shared, but we didn't share. He was alternately strong and compassionate and angry and unfeeling. And sometimes we hated each other and ourselves, but never openly. Our sex life was mostly bad. Tenderness and need can get lost in fear of pregnancy and fear of being incapable of good parenting. And just fear in general.

When I look back, one word describes it best of all. Lonely. No matter what the activity, or how many people were around, it was a lonely, vacant time. And disruptive to our total sense of living. I like to think that we did a good job of covering up our feelings, that on the surface we performed normally. It was the feelings just under the surface of that cover that were either astir or just an enormous void. It was hard to talk to anyone about that baby. A mention of even good times involving him could bring a conversation to an uncomfortable standstill.

There were moments when I began to search relentlessly through the medical literature and libraries for information about crib death. And days when I believed that he had died of the interstitial pneumonitis that appeared on the all-knowing death certificate. Those were the days that I knew I must be a terrible mother and obviously a lousy nurse. Pneumonia was curable. But not for my child and probably because of me. No one ever really accused me, but frequently I accused myself. And there were days when I couldn't bear to hear about him at all, much less any speculation of why he died. The very mention of the word dead or death in the lightest of conversation sent sensations of pain all the way to my toes.

The pregnancy in the following spring that resulted in a miscarriage was probably the lowest point of all. The pain was real, and this time there was really no one to share that with, or so it seemed. The death of that son was a closed book. And the months that followed were as sterile as my inability to become pregnant again.

When do you start to "get better"? The landmarks don't exist until you can get far enough away to start to look back at them. And landmarks are really events that you are finally ready for. For me, there was the article in a woman's magazine about crib death. An article I read exactly 3 years after the death of my son. I had read other articles, but this one sparked something inside of me. Perhaps I was ready for what it had to say. That article somehow led me to a list of names of other people, who in turn were given my name. In one overwhelming week, I found myself talking on the telephone to 14 other parents. For each of us it was the first time we had ever really talked to anyone "like" us. And the release inside of me of so many locked up feelings can only be described as nearly exhilarating. It was a strange blend of hearing other people say what I had been feeling, and feeling along with them what I was hearing them say. When we all finally met as a group, it can only be described as a warm reunion of very old friends; there were no strangers.

To "get involved" with other parents was landmark in itself. The majority of my relatives and friends, particularly my health professional friends, were concerned and fearful that this kind of activity could only be destructive—especially 3 years later. How could I go about the business of forgetting, which I should have already done, and at the same time associate with families who had lost children? That landmark took on new meaning that I was much slower to perceive. The quiet, strong support for what was happening to me came from an unexpected, and yet should have been expected, source: my husband. The sharing that wasn't his need was acknowledged by him as being mine, and the real encouragement to "be involved" came from him. It sometimes baffles his children to this day that he doesn't talk much about that young son, but I know he feels. We all work out our greatest pains in our own ways, and there is no right or wrong for each of us. Just different ways. Grief is staggeringly self-centered. I sometimes feel a sense of sadness for the too many lonely days that might not have all had to be if we had known that simple truth, if someone had pointed out that those differences don't have to isolate you from each other. I'm only grateful that somehow we learned it.

To "be involved" with other parents and crib death in the 1960s was an experience of its own. The groups became islands for others like us in a world that knew very little about us. I never made a conscious decision to get involved in crib death as a cause. As with so many others like me across the country, it is better explained by saying that it happened by simply happening—whatever our needs or reasons.

At the very beginnings of my involvement with other parents came the long-awaited pregnancy and the arrival of another son. The baby, like the group involvement, was blessing and disruption, joyful and fearful, good and bad. Sometimes we worried about the baby. Other times we accepted that if he died, too, it might be beyond our control. There were moments when the awareness of crib death loomed over our heads, and that awareness was resented. There were more times when that knowledge was a comfort. And there were days when it was important to hide from the fact that other children were dying. And days when we could face that fact without discomfort. We survived our son's infancy, as did he, in a period of time that was its own landmark.

In the years that followed, I am fascinated by remembering the new kind of denial that took place, a denial that I have learned to accept with some semblance of amusement at myself. There were periods of time when I wanted to believe, like so many other people, that grief has a beginning and an end. That anything less than that might require acknowledging some human instability. There were times when I questioned how anyone could be involved in a cause that had claimed the life of their child without being somewhat strange, if not actually bordering on the mentally unhealthy. Being identified as a SIDS parent meant being less than credible, and perhaps the only objective individuals were those who had never touched on the grief experiences of life. So although I could talk about my son, I often considered that he was a closed chapter of my life, that he had been loved and mourned but that was finished.

Just as I now know that the brief life of the son who died has taught me much about myself and living, I also know that it took my living son to show me a great deal about death and accepting grief. It was the most important landmark for me, and I learned it from a 6-year-old on a cold, snowy day just before Christmas 2 years ago. I hadn't planned to drive down the street I had chosen, nor had I planned on the snow or the two bickering children jailed with an intolerant mother in a car doing last-

minute holiday shopping. But that street and that day took us past the
cemetery where a small marker is a reminder of that child that was. The
announcement by my daughter that we were passing the cemetery was
almost one of retaliation to her brother, an attempt to even the score of
the backseat hostilities with some special knowledge. And the announcement brought silence, a silence that was broken by the sudden demand of
my son to stop, to turn into the cemetery and to see his brother. It was a
turn that I made with reluctance; we so rarely stopped there anymore. It
was not where I wanted to be, but I went along with his request. But it
wasn't enough to trudge through the snow and locate the tiny grave. He
had asked to see his brother, and he wanted to do just that. To see him, to
touch him. And I knew, just as suddenly as the demand had been made,
that there was some new realization present, some new significance to
this brother who had been mentioned but didn't live with us. When it was
finally clear that we couldn't see the body, a series of relentless questions
began that were almost beyond the youngness of his mind. "Why did he
die?" "What did you do?" "Why couldn't you save him?" "What is this
disease?" "Are you sure?" "Why couldn't anyone save him?" "Why my
brother?" "Why me?"

And there they were, so many years later. All my questions coming
back to haunt me. All the questions of any parent who has ever lost a
child. And the snow became mixed with tears, mine and his, as we stood
there. I cried for him, that young son caught in unexpected grief for a
brother he never knew and would never know. And I cried for the daughter who somehow survived our inadequacies. And I cried for that child
who would never grow up. And I cried for me. I cried with the clear
knowledge that it was okay to cry, that remembering is not abnormal or
strange, that there is a time and a place for remembering, that you don't
ever really forget, that you learn to live with it.

I am many things. And among those things is the acceptance of an inescapable truth. I am the parent of a child who has died.

INDEX